Dementia in Parkinson's Disease - Everything you Need to Know

Edited by Lin Zhang and John M. Olichney

Published in London, United Kingdom

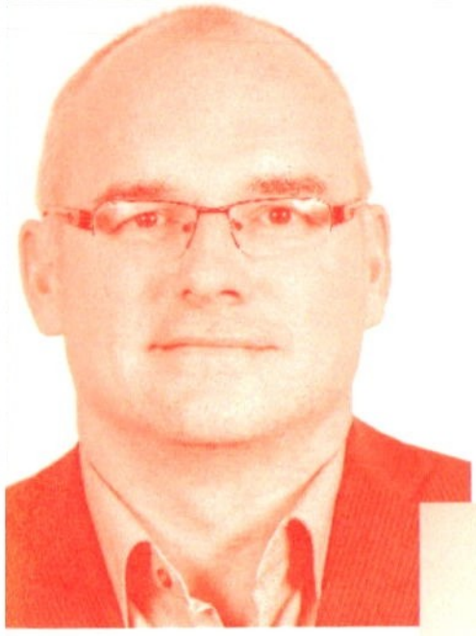
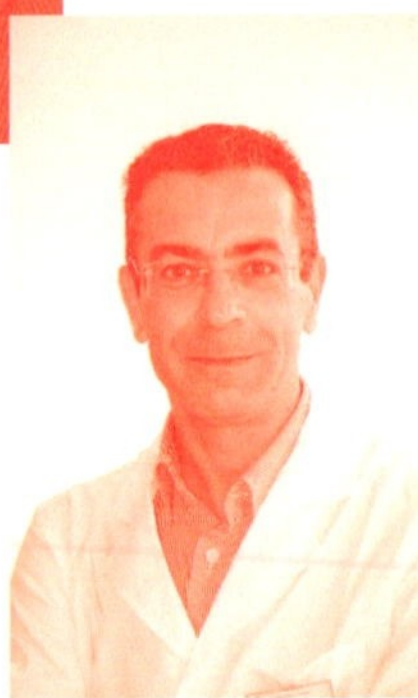
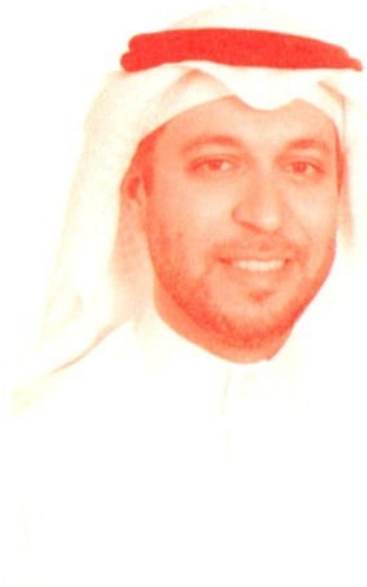
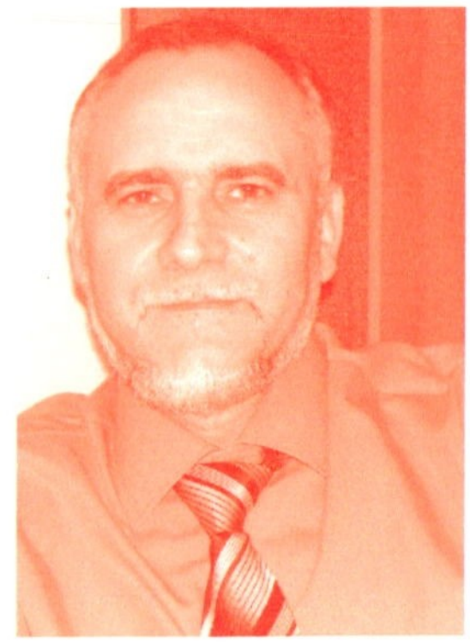
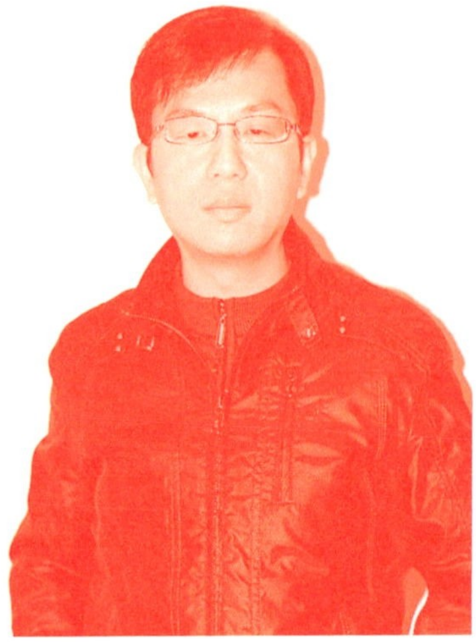
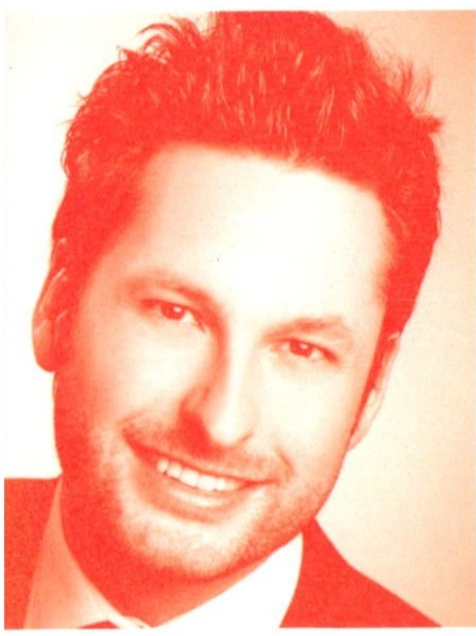
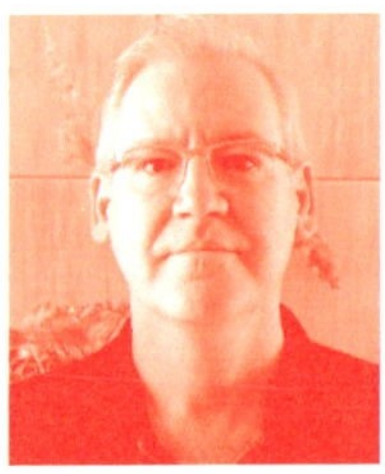

IntechOpen

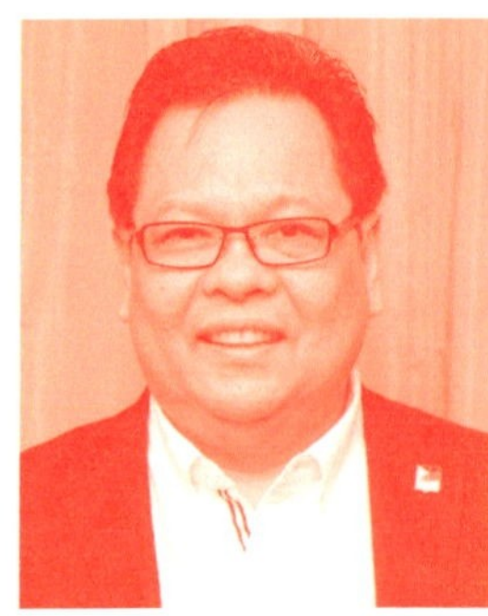
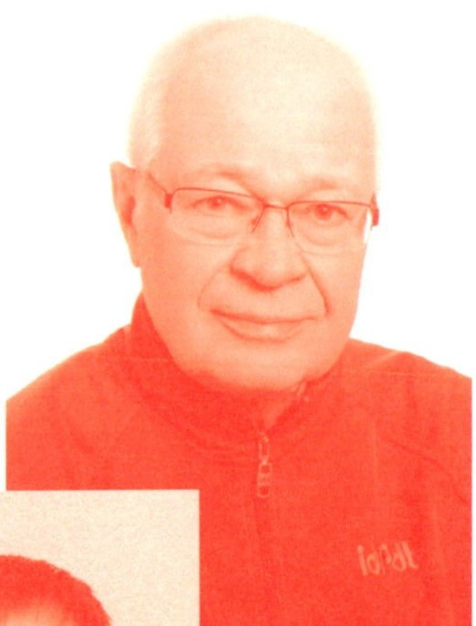
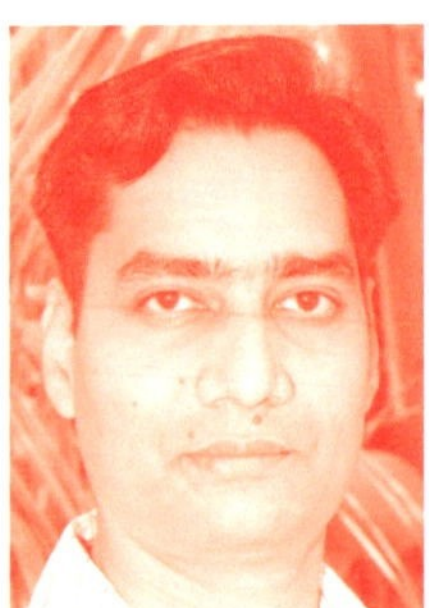
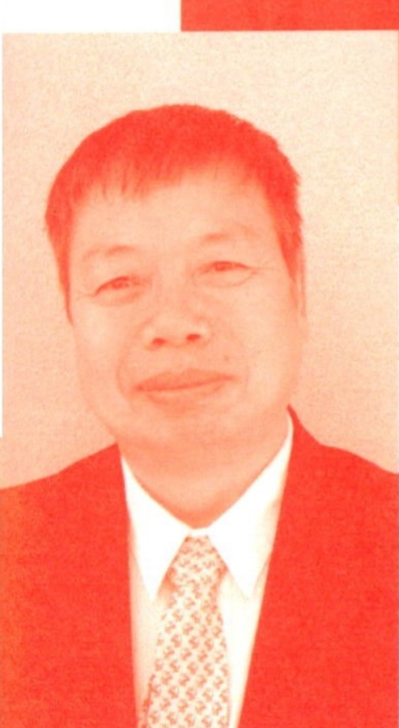
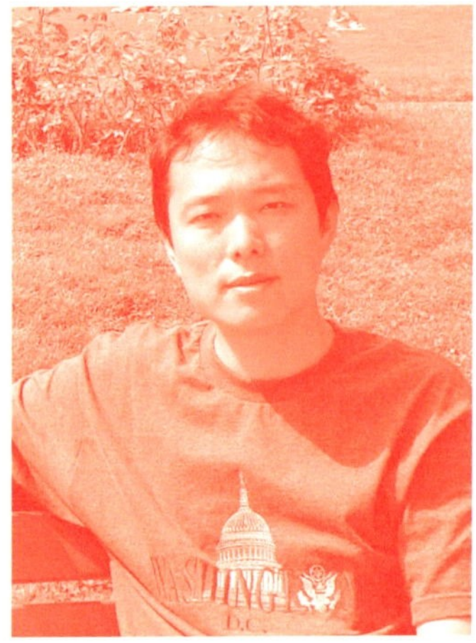
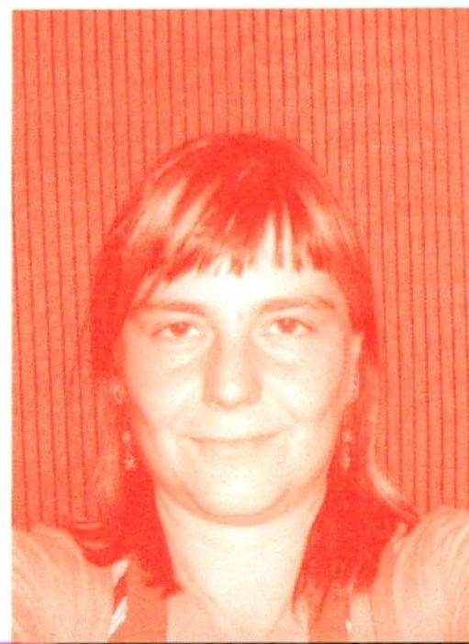

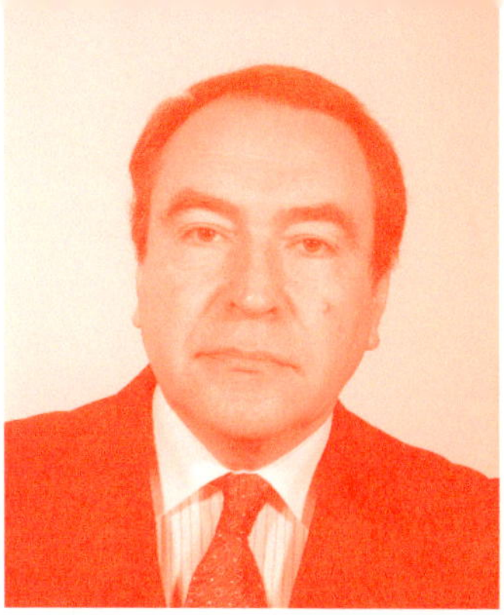
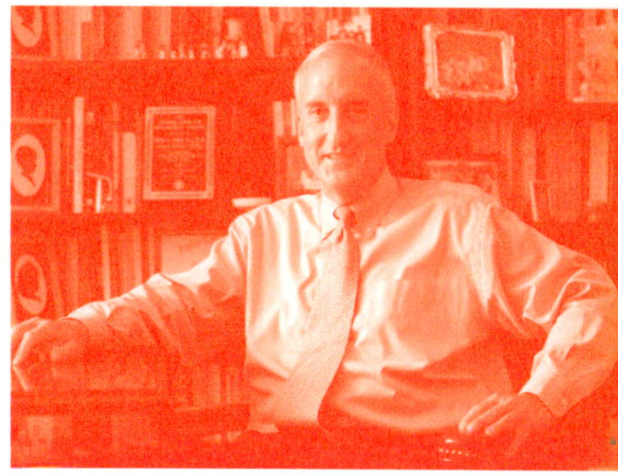
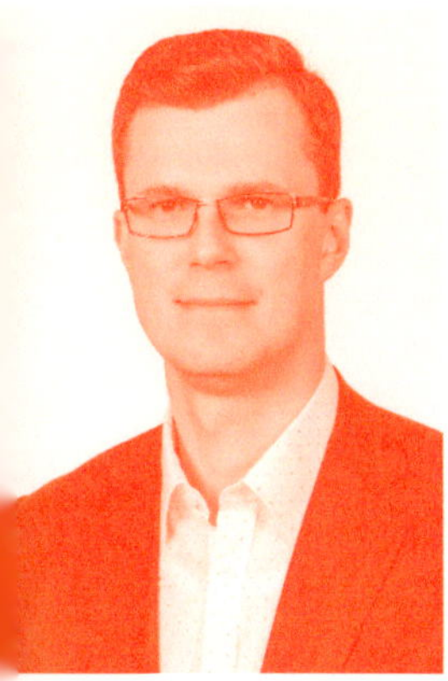
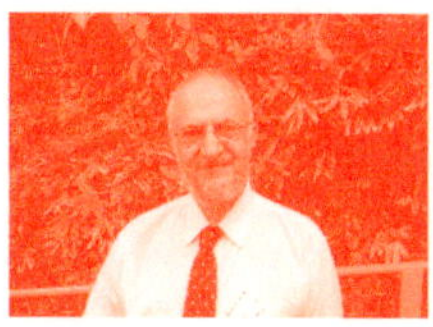
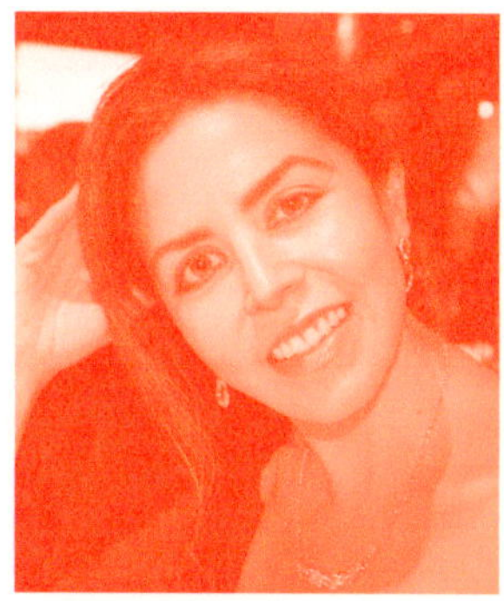

Supporting open minds since 2005

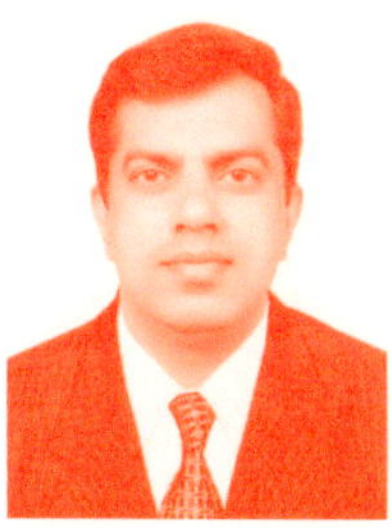
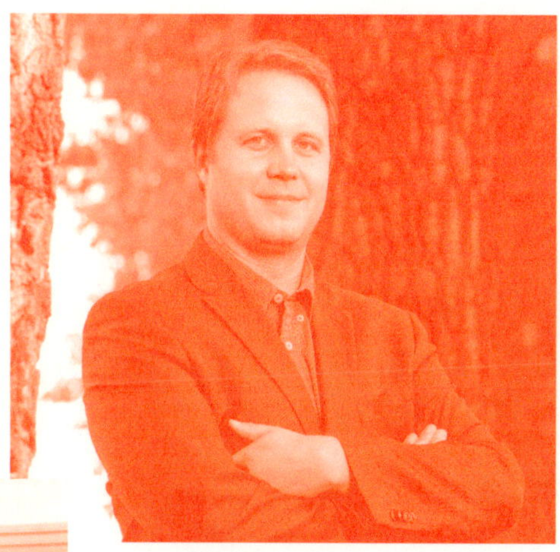
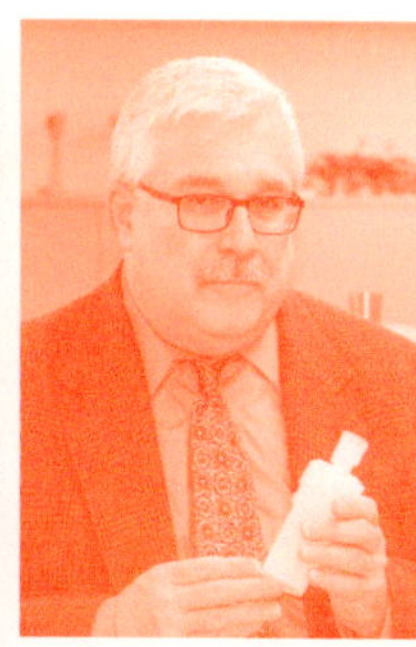
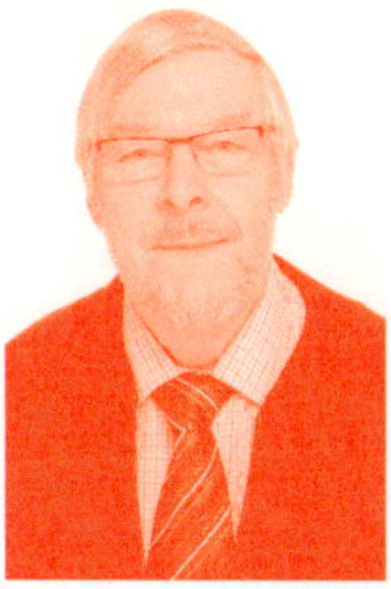
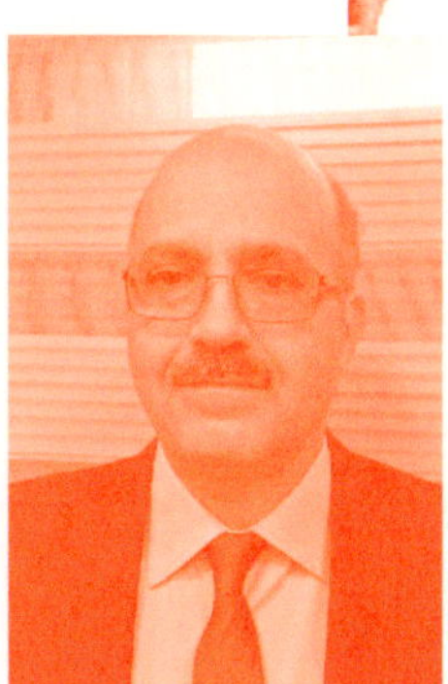
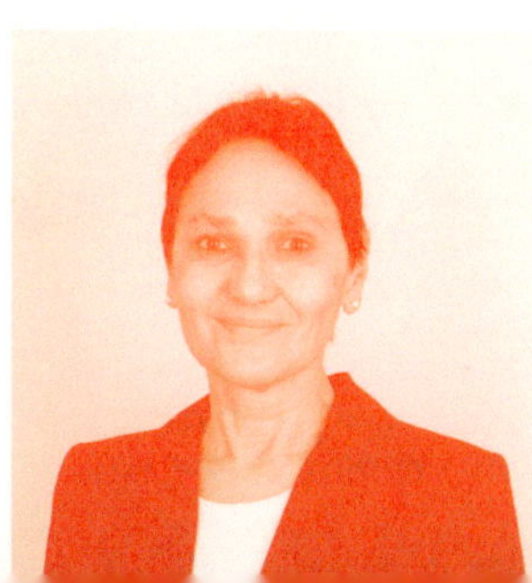
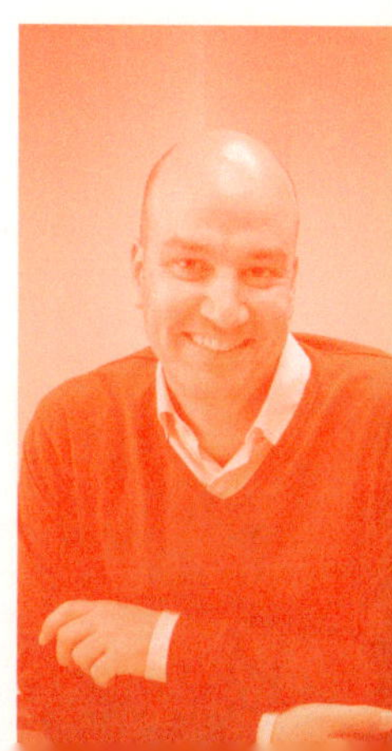

Dementia in Parkinson's Disease - Everything you Need to Know
http://dx.doi.org/10.5772/intechopen.91520
Edited by Lin Zhang and John M. Olichney

Contributors
Judit Ovádi, Judit Oláh, Attila Lehotzky, Tibor Szénási, Beatriz Munoz Ospina, Jorge L. Orozco, Yuri Takeuchi, Jaime A. Valderrama, Valentina Quintana-Peña, Daniela Alvarez, Constanza I. San Martín Valenzuela, Yuki Asahara, Taiji Mukai, Machiko Suda, Masahiko Suzuki, Justin Antony, J. Jeyaram Bharathi, Xin-Nong Li, Dawei Zheng, Laura McKae Sperry, Luhua Wei, Lin Zhang, Kiarash Shahlaie, Matthew Chow, Marc E. Lenaerts, Jin Jun Luo, Nae J. Dun, John M. Olichney, Wentao Li, Yasmine Gharbaoui, Alison P. Puiming Kwok, Jade E. Jenkins, Lisa Marie Mooney

First published in London, United Kingdom, 2022 by IntechOpen
IntechOpen is the global imprint of INTECHOPEN LIMITED, registered in England and Wales, registration number: 11086078, 5 Princes Gate Court, London, SW7 2QJ, United Kingdom
Printed in Croatia

British Library Cataloguing-in-Publication Data
A catalogue record for this book is available from the British Library

Additional hard and PDF copies can be obtained from orders@intechopen.com

Dementia in Parkinson's Disease - Everything you Need to Know
Edited by Lin Zhang and John M. Olichney
p. cm.
Print ISBN 978-1-83968-843-0
Online ISBN 978-1-83968-844-7
eBook (PDF) ISBN 978-1-83968-845-4

For EU product safety concerns:
IN TECH d.o.o., Prolaz Marije Krucifikse Kozulić 3, 51000 Rijeka, Croatia, info@intechopen.com or visit our website at intechopen.com.

Meet the editors

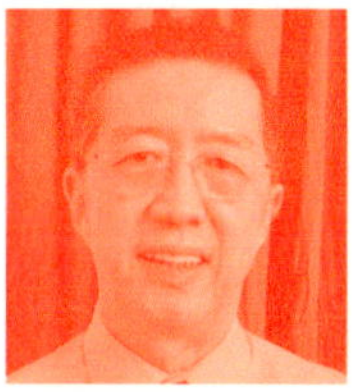

Lin Zhang MD, Ph.D., is a movement disorder neurologist and Professor of Neurology, University California, Davis (UCDavis). He serves as co-director of the UCDavis Deep Brain Stimulation Program and directs the Clinical Trial Unit for Parkinson's disease (PD) and dystonia. His research interests include the early diagnosis and pathophysiology of PD, neuromodulation, and neurotoxin therapeutics. He conducts clinical trials of movement disorders and studies the epidemiology of PD and its various phenotypes. He leads the international neuroscience program and has trained many international scholars and academic physicians. He was the recipient of the prestigious Movement Disorder Society international visiting scholarship and the Fulbright scholarship from the National Institutes of Health. He has co-authored more than sixty scientific articles and four book chapters.

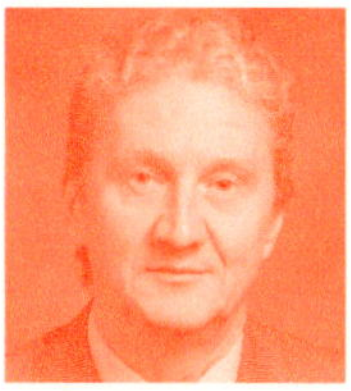

John Olichney, MD, is a behavioral neurologist, dementia specialist, and Professor of Neurology, with the University of California, Davis. He co-leads the UC Davis Alzheimer's Disease Research Center's (ADRC) Clinical Core, directs the Cognitive Electrophysiology and Neuroimaging (CEAN) laboratory in the Center for Mind and Brain (CMB), and directs a fellowship on "Behavioral Neurology and Neuropsychiatry in Neurodegeneration and Aging." His research interests include the early diagnosis and pathophysiology of neurodegenerative diseases, Alzheimer's disease (AD), Lewy body disease, and the interactions between AD and vascular pathology. He also conducts clinical trials, electrophysiological and neuroimaging studies of memory and language processes and their disruption in higher cognitive disorders. He has co-authored more than ninety scientific articles and seven book chapters.

Contents

Preface

An estimated 50% to 80% of individuals with Parkinson's disease experience Parkinson's disease dementia (PDD).

The goal, whatever the classification system, is to seek the most comprehensive and yet discriminating features that will produce the greatest clarity without losing the details diagnostically and therapeutically. Diagnosing and managing PDD is complex and difficult. This book presents a comprehensive overview of parkinsonology to aid health professionals in achieving diagnostic clarity.

Each chapter in this book is built on a structural framework that focuses on the diagnosis and management of all aspects of dementia associated with Parkinson's disease. Each chapter emphasizes tools for diagnosis, disease characteristics, and common problems, and includes tables and algorithms, references, and a bibliography.

This text is in no way a singular effort and reflects the expertise of all who contributed in so many ways.

We would like to acknowledge Ms. Heather Johnson, who was fundamental in gaining support from the university on funding all affiliated authors, and Mrs. Maja Bozicevic at IntechOpen, who proved a most efficient liaison between authors, editors, and publishers, and provided communication support and editorial assistance, and guidance. Most amazingly, she did not stop doing so during her pregnancy.

Lin Zhang, MD, Ph.D. and John M. Olichney, MD
University of California,
Davis, United States of America

Section 1

Etiology and Pathophysiology

Chapter 1

TrkA Signalling and Parkinson's Dementia

J. Jeyaram Bharathi and Justin Antony

Abstract

Cognitive impairment and dementia are the most frequently occurring non-motor symptoms in Parkinson's disease (PD), yet these symptoms are mostly overlooked and are not diagnosed and treated exceptionally like the cardinal motor symptoms in clinical practice. It is only in the late twentieth century that dementia has been recognized as a major clinical manifestation in PD. The possible mechanisms that cause dementia are complex with different patterns of cognitive behavior that disrupt the patient's quality of life. It is preeminently considered that the cholinergic denervation in the basal forebrain region mediates dementia in PD. So far, dopamine-based therapy is the key objective in the treatment of PD and the nonmotor symptoms are mostly neglected. Interestingly, the loss of Tyrosine kinase receptor-A (TrkA) signaling in basal forebrain results in neuronal atrophy, which precedes cholinergic denervation and cognitive impairment. Nerve Growth Factor (NGF) binds to TrkA receptors, inducing a cascade of events like PI-3Kinase/Akt and MAPK signaling pathways that render cholinergic degeneration and upregulate the choline acetyltransferase activity and neuronal differentiation. Hence, TrkA receptor activation by small molecules might attenuate the dementia symptoms associated with PD, and may be targeted as a novel treatment strategy along with regular clinical agents.

Keywords: dementia, Trk receptors, nonmotor symptoms, cholinergic neurotransmission, neuroprotective signaling pathways

1. Introduction

Parkinson's disease (PD) is a progressive neurodegenerative disorder with a wide range of clinical symptoms. Even though PD is traditionally considered a disorder of movement, mounting number of evidences emerged that concerned the connection of dementia and other nonmotor symptoms (NMS) that occurs from the early stages of PD and contradicted the statement of *James Parkinson's (1817) "the senses and intellects being uninjured"* [1, 2]. But more attention was paid to dementia and cognitive impairment associated with PD only from the levodopa era and most researchers agreed that dementia (particularly organic dementia) occurs more frequently in patients suffering from PD [1, 3].

Jeffery Cummings reported a mean dementia prevalence of 40% in his review of 27 studies that included 4336 patients with PD [4]. In spite of these studies being crucially considered, most studies represented patients with unselected PD population based on patients being referred to neurology clinics and some studies did not specify the exclusion of patients who were already diagnosed with

 IntechOpen

Dementia with Lewy Bodies (DLB) [4, 5]. Another systematic review of 13 studies employing strict methodological inclusion and exclusions screened 1767 patients, out of which 554 were diagnosed with dementia, reflecting a prevalence of 31.3%. This review also proclaimed the prevalence of dementia in general population that included PD patients, and revealed that 3–4% of dementia in patients was due to dementia associated with PD, which sums to a total of 0.3–0.5% among the overall general population aged 65 years and above [5, 6]. Most of the studies evaluating the incidence of dementia associated with PD are based on longitudinal study of community-based cohorts, from which the prevalence of PD has been estimated [5]. Some studies revealed incident rates of 95 [7] and 112 [8] in 1000 patient years, revealing that approximately 10% of the patients diagnosed with PD are at a higher risk category and develop dementia within 10 years [5, 7, 8]. In 2008, Hely and team reported the data from their 20-year follow-up multi-center longitudinal study, which demonstrated that up to 80% of patients with PD will develop dementia over a 20-year period and this finding implies that most patients with PD will eventually develop dementia if they live long enough [9].

Dementia currently is considered the most significant nonmotor symptom (NMS) in PD due to its crucial contribution towards the morbidity and mortality of the disease and has also evinced remarkable clinical consequences to the patients in terms of disability, increased risk of psychosis, and reduced Quality of Life (QoL) [5]. Recent advancements in treatment have increased patient survival, which has in turn increased the incidence and prevalence of dementia in PD population. Although a slight cognitive deficit is sometimes noticed in the initial stages of PD, overt dementia and cognitive impairment manifest more commonly in the later stages when the patient's age advances [2]. The prevalence of dementia and cognitive impairment remains controversial and eminently depends upon the study population and on the diagnostic tools and methods used. Various studies estimating the frequency of dementia and cognitive impairment in PD have used a variety of methods and study designs that may alter study outcomes [2, 5].

The cholinergic neurons are projected in three major areas in the brain: brainstem [10], striatum [11], and the basal forebrain (BF) region [12]. The cholinergic projection in the brainstem extends to the thalamus and it functions in risk aversion [11, 13, 14], while the cholinergic interneurons in the striatum play a key role in the regulation of dopamine secretion [11]. The basal forebrain cholinergic neurotransmission system principally originates in the medial septum, vertical limb of the diagonal band (MS/VDB), and the nucleus basalis, which extends to the olfactory bulb, neocortex hippocampus, and amygdala [12, 15]. Basal forebrain cholinergic neurons, especially the ones in the nucleus basalis, are reported to selectively degenerate in certain neurodegenerative disorders and have long been a key focus of research in the determination of the relation between acetylcholine (ACh) and memory [16].

It is widely accepted that the cholinergic neurotransmission system in the basal forebrain region is for normal cognitive function, especially memory and attention. Degeneration of the cholinergic neurotransmission is thought to be responsible for cognitive impairment and dementia associated with neurodegenerative disorders like PD and Alzheimer's disease (AD) [17–19]. Many studies have reported that deficits in cholinergic neurotransmission and signaling are often coupled with neurodegenerative and attentional disorders and impaired cognitive control [20]. While the possible mechanisms resulting in such manifestations are complex and heterogenous and lead to different patterns of cognition and behavior that majorly affects the patient's QoL. The preeminent mechanism through which cholinergic signaling influences cognition is predicted to be direct cholinergic stimulation of pre- and post-synaptic neuronal receptors. Neuroinflammation is considered to be the hallmark pathology in neurodegenerative disorders like Parkinson's and Alzheimer's and may also contribute to other neurodegenerative disorders [10, 21].

Neurotrophins are proteins that are identified as survival factors of sensory and sympathetic neurons and have been shown to have an imperative control of survival, development, and functioning of neurons in both the peripheral and central nervous system [22]. The neurotrophin family is comprised of nerve growth factor (NGF), brain-derived neurotrophic factor (BDNF), neurotrophin-3 (NT-3), and neurotrophin-4 (NT-4). Pro-neurotrophins bind to and signal via two principal receptor types: $p75^{NTR}$ and TRK receptors. There are three TRK receptors: TRKA, TRKB, and TRKC, and each receptor selectively binds to different neurotrophins: NGF binds to TRKA; BDNF and NT4 bind to TRKB; and NT3 binds to TRKC [23, 24]. TRKB and TRKC are widely found in neuronal populations throughout the central and peripheral nervous system in humans, while the distribution of TRKA is mostly restricted to the basal forebrain cholinergic region, the dorsal root ganglion, and sympathetic neurons [25]. Cholinergic neurons that do not transport NGF are severely shrunken and downregulate the expression of TRKA receptor [26]. Neurotrophins are thought to be a promising therapy for various neurodegenerative disorders including PD and AD. Because of their poor bioavailability and pharmacokinetic properties, make poor drug entities [27]. The major drawback in neurotrophin therapy is reduced passage of peptide hormones across the blood–brain barrier (BBB); peripheral administration of peptide hormones resulted in a slight increase in the intracranial neurotrophin concentration. Hence, considerable efforts are devoted towards the discovery of appropriate small molecule neurotrophin peptidomimetics that can mimic the binding of selective peptides and elicit neuronal regenerative responses like that of neurotrophins [28]. Hence, this chapter points out the risk factors, progression, and possible novel targets for Parkinson's dementia.

2. Risk factors of dementia in PD

Many demographic features, along with cardinal motor and NMS, have been identified as potential risk factors and predictors of dementia in PD [5, 29]. A study outlined that the patient's age was reported to be a common risk factor for dementia in a PD population [30] and some studies also suggested that advanced disease stage, specific subtypes of PD (e.g., akinetic-subtype), and certain NMS like olfactory dysfunction, mild cognitive impairment and mood disorders, rapid eye movement sleep behavior disorder (RBD), and hallucinations are reported to be strong predictors of dementia in PD [29].

2.1 Age

A number of studies have proposed that the patient's age and the age of onset of PD are both associated with a higher risk of dementia, and interestingly, patient's age along with increasing severity of the cardinal motor symptoms and duration of the disease are considered to be the key risk factors of dementia in PD [30, 31]. Based on such proposals, Levy concluded that aging may still play a substantive role in the pathogenesis and progression of the disease and the pathogenic cascades should further account not only for the relative selectivity of the disease process to the substantia nigra pars compacta but also for the widespread involvement of the cholinergic structures in late clinical stages of the disease [32].

2.2 Olfactory dysfunction

Olfactory dysfunction, or hyposmia, is frequently observed in the pre-motor (pre symptomatic stage) phase of the disease, even before dopaminergic denervation is evident and most of the evidence highlights the involvement of cholinergic dysfunction in hyposmia and several other aspects of olfaction [33]. The prevalence of hyposmia in PD patients is reported to be very high with up to 95% being affected [34]. A study conducted in 2012 including PD patients with hyposmia (prevalence ~55%) reported that in contrast to PD patients without hyposmia, PD patients with hyposmia exhibited mild impairment in general cognition, memory, and visuoperceptual functioning. After a follow-up period of 3 years, it was found that the cognitive impairment in the patients with hyposmia was more severe and their scores on Mini-Mental State Examination became significantly worse than compared with that of patients without hyposmia [35].

2.3 Cognition and mood disturbances

Cognitive impairment and dementia are frequent findings in PD patients. Approximately 75% of the PD patients who survive for more than 10 years are expected to develop dementia [36]. Neuropathological studies have shown that cognitive impairment in PD is associated with the cholinergic loss in BF. Reductions of acetylcholine esterase (AChE) activity in frontal cortex are found to be greater in Parkinson's disease dementia (PDD) compared to PD without dementia [37]. Major depression and apathy are commonly reported in PD; although alterations in the monoaminergic systems is thought to result in mood changes, there is evidence that the severity of cortical cholinergic degeneration is strongly associated with the presence of depression and apathy in PD [38]. Depression in PD appears to be associated with cognitive deficits, suggesting a common mechanism, and this hypothesis is justified by the observation that depression is one of the major risk factor for dementia in PD [39, 40].

2.4 Random eye movement sleep behavior disorder (RBD)

RBD is a commonly reported NMS in PD and is mostly reported to precede cognitive impairment and dementia associated with PD [41, 42]. RBD is mainly characterized by disturbed atonia during random eye movement sleep, which results in abnormal motor manifestations [42, 43]. The principal mechanism underlying RBD is considered to be cholinergic dysfunction, which is also assumed to play an imperative role between RBD and increased dementia in PD patients [42–44]. A brain imaging study exposed that cholinergic denervation was strongly associated with RBD, and 33.8% of 80 patients presented with RBD. The patients underwent acetylcholine esterase and dopaminergic dual-tracer PET scanning. The scan reports revealed that patients who presented with RBD and related symptoms exhibited decreased cortical, neocortical, and thalamic cholinergic innervations when compared to PD patients without RBD and related symptoms. This study also summarized that cholinergic denervation can occur in early stages of the disease [43–45].

2.5 Visual hallucinations

Visual hallucinations are generally considered as the main neuropsychiatric feature [46] and it is commonly observed in patients with PD [46, 47], particularly in patients with dementia [48]. A longitudinal study found that visual hallucinations are associated with higher risk of developing dementia [49]. The relationship between hallucinations and dementia is thought to be related to both Lewy body pathology [50] and cholinergic disturbance [51].

3. Pathophysiology of dementia in PD

The mechanism behind dementia in PD remains uncertain, and a number of neurochemical and neuropathological changes are assumed to be involved. Dementia in PD is thought to be a result of several cortical and subcortical changes, mainly involving the cortical cholinergic deficiency due to neurodegeneration in the nucleus basalis of Meynert (nbM) and the subcortical pathology, including dopaminergic deficiency in the caudate and in mesocortical areas [52]. It is also reported that additional AD-like pathology and the presence of Lewy bodies are likely to furthermore complicate cognitive impairment and dementia [53]. Cognitive impairment in non-demented PD patients is thought to be caused by the depletion of the dopaminergic system in the frontal cortex, which results from degeneration of the mesocortical dopaminergic system mainly projecting from the ventral tegmental area (VTA) [54].

It has also been reported that the loss of neurons in the locus coeruleus along with noradrenergic deficiency in the cortex region may result in dementia in PD. However, this neuropathology was not found or reported in other similar studies. The loss of serotonergic neurons in the dorsal raphe nucleus (DRN) is mainly reported to be associated with depression among PD patients and comparisons between demented and non-demented PD patients did not find differences in neuronal counts in the DRN [55].

In an attempt to establish a connection between dementia in PD and diminished monoaminergic activity in their study, instead identified the association between cholinergic deficiency and dementia and reported that cholinergic deficit is implicated in the neuropathology of dementia in PD and in DLB [52, 56]. It was also reported that more profound and definite cholinergic depletion was found in the nbM region in PD brains when compared to that of AD brains [57]. This hypothesis was further supported by the fact that anti-cholinergics elicited cognitive impairment in PD patients and by the therapeutic benefits of acetylcholine esterase inhibitors in the management of symptoms associated with dementia [58]. Adjacent to these neuropathological changes, important AD-like cortical changes have also been reported and implicated especially due to the abundant expression of AD-neurites in PD patients with dementia, which also correlates with the severity of dementia in PD [58, 59]. Basal forebrain (BF) cholinergic neurons within the nucleus basalis are the major source of cholinergic innervation to the cerebral cortex and play a key role in cognition and attention. In conditions like PD and AD, these cortical projection neurons undergo extensive degeneration, which correlates with clinical severity and disease duration. BF cholinergic neurons require Nerve Growth Factor (NGF) for their survival and biologic activity [60]. NGF mediates its actions on the BF cholinergic neurons via binding to the low-specificity, low-affinity p75NTR and the NGF-specific high-affinity TrkA receptor. Both the receptors are expressed and localized at cholinergic cell bodies and at nerve terminals [61]. The embryonic development of the BF cholinergic neurons is highly dependent on the expression of NGF and TrkA expression. Aging causes mammalian NGF expression and release to diminish to basal levels; however, the trophic dependence of cholinergic neurons on NGF remains critical even in the mature and fully differentiated CNS [61, 62].

4. TrkA receptor activation, a new target in Parkinson's dementia

Neurotrophins are proteins that were initially identified as survival factors of sensory and sympathetic neurons, and since have been shown to have an imperative control of survival, development, and functioning of neurons in both the peripheral and central nervous system [22]. The neurotrophin family comprises nerve growth factor (NGF), brain-derived neurotrophic factor (BDNF), neurotrophin-3 (NT-3), and neurotrophin-4 (NT-4). These neurotrophins are formerly synthesized in the endoplasmic reticulum as pre-proproteins, and cleavage of the signal peptide of pre-proproteins converts these into pro-neurotrophins. In the *trans*-Golgi network and in secretory vesicles, pro-neurotrophins dimerize and are proteolytically processed by proprotein convertase subtilisin kexin (PCSK) enzymes to their mature forms prior to their release from the cell. Pro-neurotrophins binds to and signals via two principal receptors: $p75^{NTR}$ and the TRK receptors. $p75^{NTR}$, a tumor necrosis factor (TNF) receptor family member that unselectively binds all of the neurotrophins and lacks known intrinsic enzymatic activity but recruits signaling adaptors and modulates molecular signaling via TRK receptors [25]. Depending on the expression of TRK receptors and other intercellular signaling adaptors, $p75^{NTR}$ induced effects vary a wide range including neuronal cell survival, regulation, proliferation, and inhibition of neurite growth and is also known to regulate various proteins and pathways like phosphoinositide 3-kinase (PI3K)–AKT pathway, nuclear factor-κB, (NF-κB), and mitogen-activated protein kinase (MAPK) [63–65].

There are three TRK receptors: TRKA, TRKB, and TRKC, and each neurotrophin selectively binds to different receptors: NGF binds to TRKA; BDNF and NT4 bind to TRKB; and NT3 binds to TRKC [23, 24]. In addition, there is heterologous binding, with NT3 and NT4 both provoking some activation of TRKA, and NT3 prompting some activation of TRKB [23, 25]. TRKB and TRKC are widely found in neuronal populations throughout the central and peripheral nervous system in humans, while the distribution of TRKA is mostly restricted to basal forebrain cholinergic region, the dorsal root ganglion, and in sympathetic neurons [25]. TRK signaling occurs

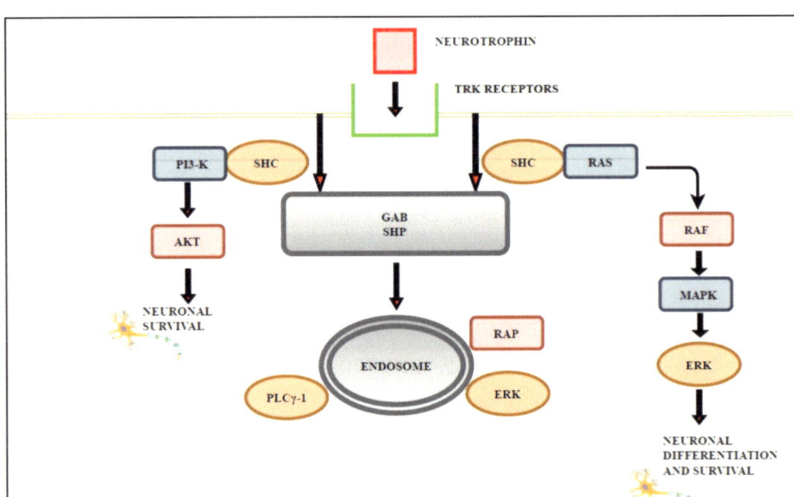

Figure 1.
Neurotrophin-TRK receptors signaling pathway. Neurotrophins binds and activates the TRK receptors, which phosphorylates the SCH domain that in turn triggers the RAS mediated MAPK signaling pathway and PI3-K/AKT pro-survival pathway that results in neuronal differentiation and survival.

Receptors	Preferred ligand	Non-preferred ligand	Non-ligand
TRKA	NGF	NT3, NT4	BDNF
TRKB	BDNF	NT3	NGF
TRKC	NT3	None	NGF, BDNF AND NT4
$P75^{NTR}$	NGF, BDNF, NT3, AND NT4	None	None

Table 1.
Binding specificity of neurotrophins.

principally through three tyrosine kinase–mediated pathways: MAPK–ERK (extracellular signal-regulated kinase) pathway, PI3K–AKT pathway, and phospholipase Cγ-1 (PLCγ-1)–PKC pathway (summarized in **Figure 1**). The effects elicited via these signaling pathways predominantly endorse cell survival and differentiation [24]. Even though these neurotrophin receptors possess overlapping expression patterns and functions, certain neural mechanisms, such as NGF-TRKA mediated basal forebrain cholinergic upregulation [66], BDNF–TRKB mediated improved synaptic plasticity, and NT3-TRKC mediated survival of peripheral proprioceptive neurons, are receptor specific. The receptor-ligand specificity is mentioned in **Table 1**.

4.1 TrkA neuroprotective signaling pathways

NGF was discovered as a molecule that promoted survival and differentiation of sensory and sympathetic neurons. Cellular responses to NGF are elicited through binding and activation of TRKA receptor [67]. Major pathways activated include Ras stimulated MAPK/ERK protein kinase pathway, PI3-K stimulation of AKT, and PLCγ1-dependent generation of IP3 and diacylglycerol (DAG) that results in mobilization of calcium stores and activation of Ca^{2+} and DAG-regulated protein kinases [22]. These signaling pathways prevent apoptotic cell death and promote cellular differentiation, axon regulation, and choline acetyl transferase (ChAT) upregulation [68]. NGF mediated neuroprotective signaling most likely depends on PI3K/Akt in PC12 cells, cerebellar cortex, sympathetic, sensory and motor neurons [69]. The neuroprotective pathways induced by TrkA receptor is summarized in **Figure 1**.

4.1.1 RAS signaling pathway

Reticular Activating System (RAS) regulates neuronal differentiation and also promotes neuronal survival, through either the PI3K or the mitogen-activated protein kinase (MAPK)/Extracellular-Signal-Regulated Kinase (ERK) pathways. In PC12 cells, different adaptors appear to facilitate transient versus prolonged activation of ERK signaling. In each case, phosphorylation of Y490 initiates the recruitment of an adaptor protein, initiating a cascade of signaling events [69]. Shc recruitment and phosphorylation in turn results in recruitment to the membrane complex of the adaptor Grb-2 and the Ras exchange factor son of Sevenless (SOS), thereby stimulating transient activation of Ras. Ras in turn activates PI3K, p38 MAPK/MAPK-activating protein kinase 2 pathway, and the c-Raf/ERK pathway [70].

4.1.2 PI3K signaling pathway

Trk receptors can activate PI3K at least via two distinct pathways, depending upon the neuronal subpopulations. In many neurons, Ras-dependent activation of PI3K is the most important pathway through which neurotrophins promote cell survival. In some cells, however, PI3K is also activated by three adaptor proteins, Shc, Grb-2, and Gab-1 [71]. Shc binding with phosphorylated Y490 results in recruitment of Grb-2. Phosphorylated Grb-2 provides a docking site for Gab-1, which is bound by PI3K [72]. In some neurons, the insulin receptor substrate (IRS)-1 is also phosphorylated by neurotrophins that recruit and activate the PI3K signaling pathway [73]. In addition to providing a linker for activation of PI3K, Gab-1 also nucleates formation of a complex including the protein phosphatase Shp-2, [74] which enhances activation of the Ras/ERK signaling pathway [72, 75].

4.1.3 PLC-γ1 signaling pathway

Phosphorylated Y785 on TrkA and similarly placed residues on other Trk receptors recruit the PLC-γ1 signaling pathway. The Trk kinase then phosphorylates and activates PLC-γ1, which acts to hydrolyze phosphatidylinositides to generate diacylglycerol (DAG) and inositol 1,4,5 triphosphate (IP3). IP3 induces the release of calcium ion (Ca^{2+}) stores, thereby increasing the levels of cytoplasmic Ca^{2+}, which in turn activates many pathways controlled by Ca^{2+}. It has been shown that NGF activates DAG-regulated protein kinase and protein kinase C (PKC)-δ, which is required for ERK cascade activation and neurite outgrowth [76]. PKC-δ appears to act between Raf and MAPK/ERK in this signaling cascade.

5. TrkA activation and cholinergic regeneration

TrkA gene expression is under positive feedback from NGF signaling, and this pathway may be disturbed by reduced retrograde transport of cortical NGF to nbM cholinergic consumer neurons [77]. In sustenance of this hypothesis, NGF levels are stable [78] or increased [79] in the cortex, whereas the levels of NGF are decreased in nbM [77]. Notably, defective retrograde transport of NGF within cholinergic projection neurons was reported in a transgenic mouse model of Down syndrome [80]. In aged rats, these neurons exhibited a pronounced reduction in NGF retrograde transport, TrkA protein expression, and severe atrophy. Defective NGF retrograde transport may therefore underlie the reductions in nbM TrkA gene and protein expression observed in single nbM neurons, leading to eventual reduction of TrkA protein in cortical projection sites [81] and further trepidations in NGF signaling within the nbM. This putative "off trk" cycle of deficient NGF signaling may contribute to the selective degeneration of cholinergic nbM neurons and deficits in cortical cholinergic tone [60, 82]. Several lines of evidence support the role of NGF in the survival of cholinergic neurons in the BF brain region. *In vitro* studies, using dissociated rat nbM cultures [83, 84] or organotypic nbM slices, [85] revealed that NGF treatment prevented the cholinergic neurodegeneration that was observed in untreated preparations. These results are similar to those demonstrating that infusion of NGF can prevent septal cholinergic neuron death following septo-hippocampal axotomy [86].

Finally, transgenic mice that express anti-NGF antibodies in adulthood display an age-dependent loss of CBF neurons [87]. These reciprocal correlations between reduced cortical TrkA and elevated pro-NGF levels with MMSE scores recommend that cholinotrophic aberrations play a significant role in cognitive impairment and may underlie the subsequent demise of nbM cholinergic neurons and extensive cholinergic deficits seen in the late stages of neurodegenerative disorders. Similar studies in nonhuman primates showed that recombinant human NGF reverses both age-related and lesion-induced cholinergic neuronal degeneration and promotes cholinergic neurite sprouting [88, 89]. In addition, exogenous NGF rescues age-related and cholinergic lesion-induced spatial memory deficits in rodents [90, 91]. Thus, restoration of NGF signaling may demonstrate efficacious for the prevention of cognitive deficits resulting from nbM dysfunction.

6. TrkA ligands

Initially, the approach for the development of ligands targeting the neuro trophin receptors was to create small synthetic peptides with amino acid residues corresponding to various domains of neurotrophins and to assess those small molecules for their ability to mimic or inhibit the neurotrophic functions of the neurotrophins. The discovery of synthetic peptic ligands that correspond to specific neurotrophic domains with agonist and antagonist activities enacted the vital proof that small molecules, including those that bind monomerically to the Trk receptors are able to modulate the receptor functions and also provide a useful basis for the discovery of new non-peptide small molecules [25].

6.1 Gambogic amide

Combinatorial compound library screening identified several TrkA activators, including asterriquinone (1H5) and mono-indolyl-quinone (E5E). These compounds activated the receptor possibly by binding to an intercellular site that promoted PC12 cell survival at micromolecular concentrations [92]. Another screening study identified Gambogic amide (MW 628), which prevented the death of TrkA expressing cell line [68]. It was also found that the gambogic amide binds to the intracellular juxta-membrane domain of the receptor instead of the extracellular ligand binding region, which suggests that gambogic amide results in allosteric activation of the receptor [93]. Gambogic amide was reported to activate TrkA and its downstream signaling pathways and promoted the survival of cells that were reported to express TrkA [68]. However, additional studies are required to establish the degree of specificity for the receptor.

6.2 Amitriptyline

The antidepressant amitriptyline was found to bind with the extracellular domains of the TrkA and TrkB receptors(?) and induce their activation, which promoted heterodimerization that does not occur with NGF or BDNF, which suggests that amitriptyline induces alternative signaling outcomes [94]. Amitriptyline was shown to prevent the apoptosis of cultured hippocampal cells and stimulate neurite outgrowth in PC12 cells. *In vivo* studies reported that amitriptyline abridged kainic acid–triggered neuronal cell death. Studies in inducible TrkA-null mice demonstrated the key role of TrkA in mediating the effects of amitriptyline. However, given the broad spectrum of mechanisms affected by amitriptyline, the issue of target specificity needs to be cautiously considered [94].

6.3 MT2

Several small peptidomimetics were also found to interact with the immunoglobulin-like domain of the TrkA receptor [95]. Interestingly, MT2 exhibits a dominant effect on the survival of PC12 cells, similar to neurotrophin NGF. It was

Compound	Structure	*In-vitro* activity
Gambogic amide	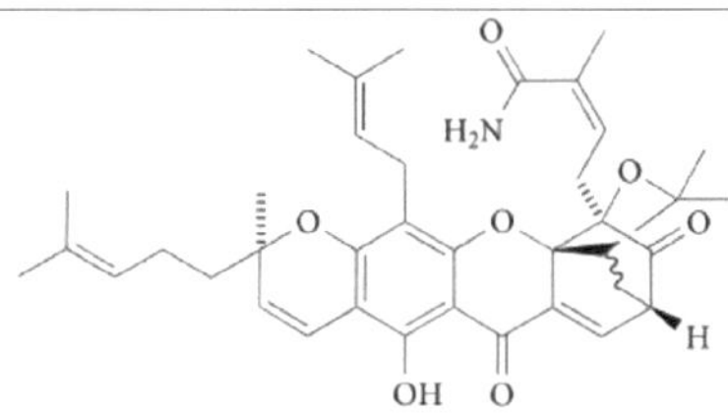	Inhibits the death of hippocampal neurons
MT2	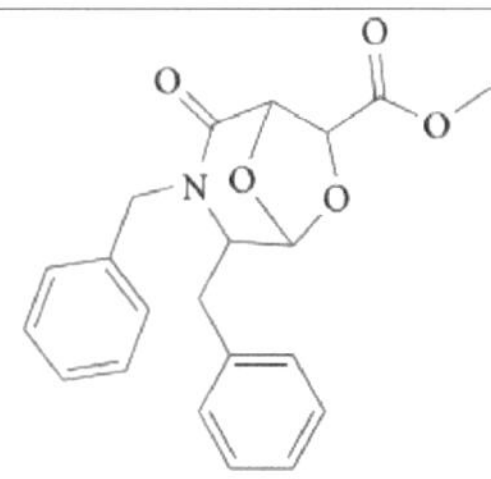	Inhibits the death of hippocampal neurons
Amitriptyline (binds to both TRKA and TRKB receptors)	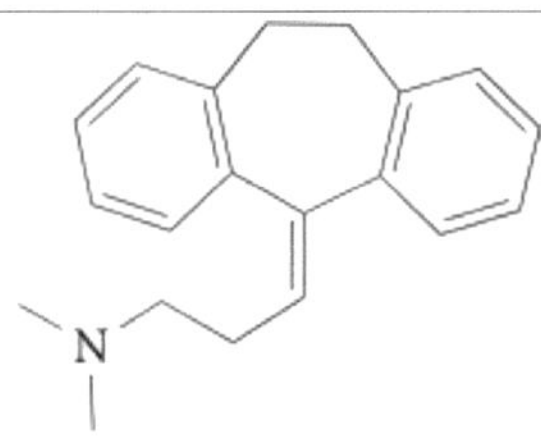	Inhibits the death of hippocampal neurons

Table 2.
Ligands targeting TrkA receptor.

also found that the compound was less capable of inducing TrkA phosphorylation. Additional analysis showed that MT2 and NGF stimulated TrkA-Tyr490 phosphorylation to a similar degree, where MT2 induced significantly less phosphorylation at Tyr674, Tyr675, and Tyr785, which insinuates that there is differential activation of signaling between the compound MT2 and NGF [95]. Whether this idiosyncratic signaling pattern provides any therapeutic compensations or disadvantages relative to NGF relics undetermined.

Taken together, these studies demonstrate that capable small molecules can be created or identified that activate TrkA receptors, in some cases through non-ligand receptor sites. A remaining challenge in most cases is demonstrating the degree of receptor specificity towards TrkA. TrkA receptor agonists and their *in vitro* activity are given below in **Table 2**.

6.4 Limitations of small molecule ligands

Although small molecule activators of the neurotrophin receptors have numerous advantages over native neurotrophins, there are potential limitations that should be considered during their development.

6.4.1 Inadequate receptor specificity

- These molecules bind only to a limited number of motifs present in the protein interaction regions, which leads to identical epitopes occurring in another protein interface, which could produce off-target effects.

- Protein interfaces largely cover several interaction hotspots comprising groups of amino acid residues. The structures and chemical constituencies of these hotspots are not unique, but their combination in a three-dimensional structure produces a larger interaction region with the potential for high degrees of specificity.

6.4.2 Continuous dosing requirement

- Unlike nucleic acids and other proteins, that are permanently transduced with viral vectors, small molecules cannot be readily produced endogenously and consequently, continued exogenous administration is likely required to maintain their therapeutic efficacy.

6.4.3 Neurotrophin receptor mediated side effects

- Even decidedly specific small molecules may produce abnormal signaling patterns through neurotrophin receptors via detouring the homeostatic mechanisms (for example, proteolysis and endocytosis), which would normally limit the extent of receptor activation.

- These considerations, along with the potential for broad tissue exposure, recommend that some small molecules may have the tendency to elicit on-target side effects like pain, epilepsy, promotion of neoplasia, or hypertension in neural and non-neuronal tissues.

7. Conclusion

The cholinergic system is widely affected in PD, with widespread denervation that contributes to a number of clinical features associated with PD, especially cognitive impairment, abnormal olfaction, and mood disturbances. Multisystem neurodegeneration may play an imperative role in the etiology of nonmotor as well as motor symptoms in PD. While nigrostriatal dopaminergic denervation occurs in all PD patients, there are PD patients with additional degeneration of non-dopaminergic systems (especially the cholinergic system), which significantly impacts the patient quality of life. NGF promotes survival and differentiation of sensory and sympathetic neurons and the cellular responses are elicited via binding and activation of TrkA receptors. BF cholinergic neurons are highly dependent on NGF, which mediates actions on the BF cholinergic neurons via NGF-specific high-affinity TrkA receptors. Cholinergic neurons that do not transport NGF are severely shrunken and downregulate the expression of TrkA receptors. Hence, restoration of NGF signaling may prove efficacious for the prevention of cognitive deficits resulting from nbM dysfunction in PD. The development of small-molecule neurotrophin receptor ligands has only recently begun and only a few ligands have been created and characterized. Nevertheless, observations in *in vitro* and *in vivo* studies using prototype compounds have indicated various vital mechanistic principles that could be used for the future expansion of such similar compounds. These include the discovery that small molecules might achieve patterns of signaling and biological end points that are distinct from those induced by the native neurotrophins. Additionally, 'monovalent' small molecules are capable of activating TRK receptors or modulating $P75^{NTR}$. These capabilities, along with the fundamental roles of neurotrophin receptors in several neurological disorders, will encourage the development and broad application of many more ligands. Moreover, several of the recently described compounds have favorable pharmacological features demonstrating that they could be advanced to clinical studies. However, the possible boundaries of small-molecule modulation of neurotrophin receptors should be taken into consideration, and it will be crucial to better characterize *in vivo* target binding and establish the pharmacodynamic properties of these compounds. Though, as neurotrophin receptor signaling mechanisms and pathways are better understood, it may be possible to design small molecules to achieve tailored signaling profiles, which could lead to the development of 'disease specific designer ligands'.

Author details

J. Jeyaram Bharathi and Justin Antony*
Department of Pharmacology, JSS College of Pharmacy, JSS Academy of Higher Education and Research, Nilgiris, Tamil Nadu, India

*Address all correspondence to: justin@jssuni.edu.in

References

[1] Marttila RJ, Rinne UK. Dementia in Parkinson's disease. Acta Neurologica Scandinavica. 1976;**54**(5):431-441

[2] Hanagasi HA, Tufekcioglu Z, Emre M. Dementia in Parkinson's disease. Journal of the Neurological Sciences. 2017;**374**(2016):26-31. Available from: http://dx.doi.org/10.1016/j.jns.2017.01.012

[3] Gaspar P, Gray F. Dementia in idiopathic Parkinson's disease—A neuropathological study of 32 cases. Acta Neuropathologica. 1984;**64**(1):43-52

[4] Cummings JL. Intellectual impairment in Parkinson's disease: Clinical, pathologic, and biochemical correlates. Journal of Geriatric Psychiatry and Neurology. 1988;**1**(1):24-36

[5] Aarsland D, Kurz MW. The epidemiology of dementia associated with Parkinson disease. Journal of the Neurological Sciences. 2010;**289**(1-2):18-22. Available from: http://dx.doi.org/10.1016/j.jns.2009.08.034

[6] Aarsland D, Zaccai J, Brayne C. A systematic review of prevalence studies of dementia in Parkinson's disease. Movement Disorders. 2005;**20**(10):1255-1263

[7] Aarsland D, Andersen K, Larsen JP, Lolk A, Nielsen H, Kragh-Sørensen P. Risk of dementia in Parkinson's disease: A community-based, prospective study. Neurology [Internet]. 2001;**56**(6):730-736. Available from: http://www.embase.com/search/results?subaction=viewrecord&from=export&id=L32240091%5Cnhttp://wt3cf4et2l.search.serialssolutions.com?sid=EMBASE&issn=00283878&id=doi:&atitle=Risk+of+dementia+in+Parkinson%27s+disease%3A+A+community-based%2C+prospective+study

[8] Goymer P. The frequency and associated risk factors for dementia in patients with Parkinson's disease karen. Nature Reviews. Cancer. 2006;**6**(6):695-701

[9] Hely MA, Reid WGJ, Adena MA, Halliday GM, Morris JGL. The sydney multicenter study of Parkinson's disease: The inevitability of dementia at 20 years. Movement Disorders. 2008;**23**(6):837-844

[10] Martinez-Gonzalez C, Bolam JP, Mena-Segovia J. Topographical organization of the pedunculopontine nucleus. Frontiers in Neuroanatomy. 2011;**5**(April):1-10

[11] Mesulam M-M, Mufson EJ, Levey AI, Wainer BH. Cholinergic innervation of cortex by the basal forebrain: Cytochemistry and cortical connections of the septal area, diagonal band nuclei, nucleus basalis (Substantia innominata), and hypothalamus in the rhesus monkey. The Journal of Comparative Neurology. 1983;**214**(2):170-197

[12] Perez-Lloret S, Barrantes FJ. Deficits in cholinergic neurotransmission and their clinical correlates in Parkinson's disease. npj Parkinson's Disease. 2016;**2**(1). Available from: http://dx.doi.org/10.1038/npjparkd.2016.1

[13] Ye M, Hayar A, Strotman B, Garcia-Rill E. Cholinergic modulation of fast inhibitory and excitatory transmission to pedunculopontine thalamic projecting neurons. Journal of Neurophysiology. 2010;**103**(5):2417-2432

[14] Goldberg JA, Reynolds JNJ. Spontaneous firing and evoked pauses in the tonically active cholinergic interneurons of the striatum.

Neuroscience [Internet]. 2011;**198**:27-43. Available from: http://dx.doi.org/10.1016/j.neuroscience.2011.08.067

[15] Woolf NJ. Cholinergic systems in mammalian brain and spinal cord nancy. Neurobiology. 1977;**37**:285-295

[16] Himmelheber AM, Sarter M, Bruno JP. Increases in cortical acetylcholine release during sustained attention performance in rats. Cognitive Brain Research. 2000;**9**(3):313-325

[17] Ballinger E, Ananth M, Talmage DA, Role L. Basal forebrain cholinergic circuits and signaling in cognition and cognitive decline. Physiology & Behavior. 2018;**176**(1):139-148

[18] Bartus RT, Dean RL 3rd, Beer B, Lippa AS. The cholinergic hypothesis of geriatric memory dysfunction. Science. 1982;**217**:408-417

[19] Zhagn L, Li Z. Alzheimer and the discovery of Alzheimer's disease. Zhonghua Yi Shi Za Zhi. 2014;**44**(5):288-290

[20] Ben Achour S, Pascual O. Glia: The many ways to modulate synaptic plasticity. Neurochemistry International. 2010;**57**(4):440-445. Available from: http://dx.doi.org/10.1016/j.neuint.2010.02.013

[21] Müller MLTM, Albin RL, Kotagal V, Koeppe RA, Scott PJH, Frey KA, et al. Thalamic cholinergic innervation and postural sensory integration function in Parkinson's disease. Brain. 2013;**136**(11):3282-3289

[22] Reichardt LF. Neurotrophin-regulated signalling pathways. Philosophical Transactions of the Royal Society B: Biological Sciences. 2006;**361**(1473):1545-1564

[23] Barbacid M. Structural and Functional properties of the TRK family of neurotrophin receptors. Annals of the New York Academy of Sciences. 1995;**766**(1):442-458

[24] Huang EJ, Reichardt LF. Trk receptors: Roles in neuronal signal transduction. Annual Review of Biochemistry. 2003;**72**:609-642

[25] Longo FM, Massa SM. Small-molecule modulation of neurotrophin receptors: A strategy for the treatment of neurological disease. Nature Reviews Drug Discovery. 2013;**12**(7):507-525. Available from: http://dx.doi.org/10.1038/nrd4024

[26] Mufson EJ. SEC and SDG. Cholinergic System. Pharmacology for Dental and Allied Health Sciences. 2017. 49-49 p.

[27] Fred JF. Risk in CNS drug discovery: Focus on treatment of Alzheimer's disease. BMC Neuroscience. 2008;**9**(SUPPL. 3):1-8

[28] Miller G. Drug targeting: Breaking down barriers. Science (80-). 2002;**297**(5584):1116-1118

[29] Xu Y, Yang J, Shang H. Meta-analysis of risk factors for Parkinson's disease dementia. Translational Neurodegeneration. 2016;**5**(1):1-8. Available from: http://dx.doi.org/10.1186/s40035-016-0058-0

[30] Levy G, Schupf N, Tang MX, Cote LJ, Louis ED, Mejia H, et al. Combined effect of age and severity on the risk of dementia in Parkinson's disease. Annals of Neurology. 2002;**51**(6):722-729

[31] Aarsland D, Kvaløy JT, Andersen K, Larsen JP, Tang MX, Lolk A, et al. The effect of age of onset of PD on risk of dementia. Journal of Neurology. 2007;**254**(1):38-45

[32] Levy G. The relationship of Parkinson disease with aging. Archives of Neurology. 2007;**64**(9):1242-1246

[33] Bohnen NI, Müller MLTM. In vivo neurochemical imaging of olfactory dysfunction in Parkinson's Disease. Journal of Neural Transmission [Internet]. 2014;**23**(1):571-576. Available from: https://www.ncbi.nlm.nih.gov/pmc/articles/PMC3624763/pdf/nihms412728.pdf

[34] Haehner A, Boesveldt S, Berendse HW, Mackay-Sim A, Fleischmann J, Silburn PA, et al. Prevalence of smell loss in Parkinson's disease—A multicenter study. Parkinsonism & Related Disorders. 2009;**15**(7):490-494. Available from: http://dx.doi.org/10.1016/j.parkreldis.2008.12.005

[35] Baba T, Kikuchi A, Hirayama K, Nishio Y, Hosokai Y, Kanno S, et al. Severe olfactory dysfunction is a prodromal symptom of dementia associated with Parkinson's disease: A 3 year longitudinal study. Brain. 2012;**135**(1):161-169

[36] Ruberg M, Ploska A, Javoy-agid F, Agid Y. Muscarinic binding and choline acetyltransferase activity in Parkinsonian subjects with reference to dementia. Brain Research. 1982;**232**:129-139

[37] Kulisevsky J, Pagonbarraga J, Pascual-Sedano B, García-Sánchez C, Gironell A. Prevalence and correlates of neuropsychiatric symptoms in Parkinson's disease without dementia. Movement Disorders. 2008;**23**(13):1889-1896

[38] Fields JA, Tr AI, Stalp LD, Koller WC, Paolo AM. Neuropsychological impairment in Parkinson's disease with and without depression. Archives of Neurology. 1995;**52**:1164-1169

[39] Cicerone KD. Depression, intellectual impairment, and parkinson disease: To the Editor. Neurology. 1982;**32**(4):455-458

[40] Grover S, Somaiya M, Kumar S, Avasthi A. Psychiatric aspects of Parkinson's disease. Journal of Neuroscience in Rural Practice. 2015;**6**(1):65-76

[41] Marion MH, Qurashi M, Marshall G, Foster O. Is REM sleep Behaviour Disorder (RBD) a risk factor of dementia in idiopathic Parkinson's disease? Journal of Neurology. 2008;**255**(2):192-196

[42] Vendette M, Gagnon JF, Décary A, Massicotte-Marquez J, Postuma RB, Doyon J, et al. REM sleep behavior disorder predicts cognitive impairment in Parkinson disease without dementia. Neurology. 2007;**69**(19):1843-1849

[43] Postuma RB, Gagnon JF, Montplaisir J. Cognition in REM sleep behavior disorder—A window into preclinical dementia? Sleep Medicine. 2008;**9**(4):341-342

[44] Kotagal V, Albin RL, Müller MLTM, Koeppe RA, Chervin RD, Frey KA, et al. Symptoms of rapid eye movement sleep behavior disorder are associated with cholinergic denervation in Parkinson disease. Annals of Neurology. 2012;**71**(4):560-568

[45] Postuma RB, Gagnon JF, Montplaisir JY. REM sleep behavior disorder: From dreams to neurodegeneration. Neurobiology of Disease. 2012;**46**(3):553-558. Available from: http://dx.doi.org/10.1016/j.nbd.2011.10.003

[46] Williams DR, Warren JD, Lees AJ. Using the presence of visual hallucinations to differentiate Parkinson's disease from atypical parkinsonism. Journal of Neurology, Neurosurgery, and Psychiatry. 2008;**79**(6):652-655

[47] Fénelon G, Mahieux F, Huon R, Ziégler M. Hallucinations in Parkinson's disease. Prevalence, phenomenology

and risk factors. Brain. 2000;**123**(4):733-745

[48] Aarsland D, Brønnick K, Ehrt U, De Deyn PP, Tekin S, Emre M, et al. Neuropsychiatric symptoms in patients with Parkinson's disease and dementia: Frequency, profile and associated care giver stress. Journal of Neurology, Neurosurgery, and Psychiatry. 2007;**78**(1):36-42

[49] Aarsland D, Andersen K, Larsen JP, Lolk A, Kragh-Sørensen P. Prevalence and characteristics of dementia in Parkinson disease: An 8-year prospective study. Archives of Neurology. 2003;**60**(3):387-392

[50] Harding AJ, Broe GA, Halliday GM. Visual hallucinations in Lewy body disease relate to Lewy bodies in the temporal lobe. Brain. 2002;**125**(2):391-403

[51] Perry EK, Kerwin J, Perry RH, Blessed G, Fairbairn AF. Visual hallucinations and the cholinergic system in dementia. Letters. 1989;**1**(1):88

[52] Bosboom JLW, Stoffers D, Wolters EC. Cognitive dysfunction and dementia in Parkinson's disease. Journal of Neural Transmission. 2004;**111**(10-11):1303-1315

[53] Wolters EC, Francot CMJE. Mental dysfunction in Parkinson ' s disease. Parkinsonism & Related Disorders. 1998;**4**:107-112

[54] Lange KW, Robbins TW, Marsden CD, James M, Owen AM, Paup GM. Psychopharmacology L-Dopa withdrawal in Parkinson ' s disease selectively impairs cognitive performance in tests sensitive to frontal lobe dysfunction. Psychopharmacology. 1992;**107**:394-404

[55] Scatton B, Javoy-Agid F, Rouquier L, Dubois B, Agid Y. Reduction of cortical dopamine, noradrenaline, serotonin and their metabolites in Parkinson's disease. Brain Research. 1983;**275**(2):321-328

[56] Perry EK, Mckeith I, Thompson P, Edwardson JA, Ince P, Blessed G. Topography, extent, and clinical relevance of neurochemical deficits in dementia of Lewy body type, Parkinson' s disease, and Alzheimer' s disease. Annals of the New York Academy of Sciences. 1990:197-202

[57] Perry EK, Curtis M, Dick DJ, Candy JM, Atack JR, Bloxham CA, et al. Cholinergic correlates of cognitive impairment in Parkinson's disease: Comparisons with Alzheimer' s disease. Journal of Neurology, Neurosurgery, and Psychiatry. 1985;**48**:413-421

[58] Pillon B, Dubois B, Duchesne N, Masson H. Acute and long-term administration of anticholinergics in Parkinson's disease: Specific effects on the subcortico-frontal syndrome. Brain and Cognition. 1999;**313**:289-313

[59] Harding AJ, Halliday GM. Cortical Lewy body pathology in the diagnosis of dementia. Acta Neuropathologica. 2001;**102**:355-363

[60] Counts SE, Mufson EJ. The role of nerve growth factor receptors in cholinergic basal forebrain degeneration in prodromal Alzheimer disease. Journal of Neuropathology and Experimental Neurology. 2005;**64**(4):263-272

[61] Gibbs RB, Pfaff DW. In situ hybridization detection of trka mRNA in brain: Distribution, colocalization with p75NGFR and up-regulation by nerve growth factor. The Journal of Comparative Neurology. 1994;**341**(3):324-339

[62] Holtzman DM, Li Y, Parada LF, Kinsman S, Chen CK, Valletta JS, et al. p140trk mRNA marks NGF-responsive forebrain neurons: Evidence that trk gene expression is induced by NGF. Neuron. 1992;**9**(3):465-478

[63] Roux PP, Bhakar AL, Kennedy TE, Barker PA. The p75 neurotrophin receptor activates Akt (protein kinase B) through a phosphatidylinositol 3-kinase-dependent Pathway. The Journal of Biological Chemistry. 2001;**276**(25):23097-23104

[64] Carter BD, Kaltschmidt C, Kaltschmidt B, Offenhäuser N, Böhm-Matthaei R, Baeuerle PA, et al. Selective activation of NF-κB by nerve growth factor through the neurotrophin receptor p75. Science (80-). 1996;**272**(5261):542-545

[65] Volonte C, Angelastro JM, Greene LA. Association of protein kinases ERK1 and ERK2 with p75 nerve growth factor receptors. The Journal of Biological Chemistry. 1993;**268**(28):21410-21415

[66] Sofroniew MV, Howe WC Mobley CL. Nerve growth factor signaling, neuroprotection, and neural repair. Annual Review of Neuroscience. 2001;**24**(5):1217-1281

[67] Bothwell M. Functional interactions of neurotrophins and neurotrophin receptors. Annual Review of Neuroscience. 1995;**18**:223-253

[68] Jang SW, Okada M, Sayeed I, Xiao G, Stein D, Jin P, et al. Gambogic amide, a selective agonist for TrkA receptor that possesses robust neurotrophic activity, prevents neuronal cell death. Proceedings of the National Academy of Sciences of the United States of America. 2007;**104**(41):16329-16334

[69] Nguyen N, Lee SB, Lee YS, Lee KH, Ahn JY. Neuroprotection by NGF and BDNF against neurotoxin-exerted apoptotic death in neural stem cells are mediated through TRK receptors, activating PI3-kinase and MAPK pathways. Neurochemical Research. 2009;**34**(5):942-951

[70] Xing J, David D, MEG G. Coupling of the RAS-MAPK pathway to gene activation by RSK2, a growth factor-regulated CREB kinase. Science (80-). 1996;**273**(August):959-963

[71] Vaillant AR, Mazzoni I, Tudan C, Boudreau M, Kaplan DR, Miller FD. 3-Kinase – Akt pathway to synergistically regulate neuronal survival. Cell. 1999;**146**(5):955-966

[72] Holgado-Madruga M, Moscatello DK, Emlet DR, Dieterich R, Wong AJ. Grb2-associated binder-1 mediates phosphatidylinositol 3-kinase activation and the promotion of cell survival by nerve growth factor. Proceedings of the National Academy of Sciences of the United States of America. 1997;**94**(23):12419-12424

[73] Yamada M, Ohnishi H, Sano SI, Nakatani A, Ikeuchi T, Hatanaka H. Insulin receptor substrate (IRS)-1 and IRS-2 are tyrosine-phosphorylated and associated with phosphatidylinositol 3-kinase in response to brain-derived neurotrophic factor in cultured cerebral cortical neurons. The Journal of Biological Chemistry. 1997;**272**(48):30334-30339

[74] Shi Z-Q, Yu D-H, Park M, Marshall M, Feng G-S. Molecular mechanism for the Shp-2 tyrosine phosphatase function in promoting growth factor stimulation of Erk activity. Molecular and Cellular Biology. 2000;**20**(5):1526-1536

[75] Yamada M, Ohnishi H, Sano SI, Araki T, Nakatani A, Ikeuchi T, et al. Brain-derived neurotrophic factor stimulates interactions of Shp2 with phosphatidylinositol 3-kinase and Grb2 in cultured cerebral cortical neurons. Journal of Neurochemistry. 1999;**73**(1):41-49

[76] Corbit KC, Soh J-W, Yoshida K, Eves EM, Weinstein IB, Rosner MR. Different protein kinase C isoforms

determine growth factor specificity in neuronal cells. Molecular and Cellular Biology. 2000;**20**(15):5392-5403

[77] Scott SA, Mufson EJ, Weingartner JA, Skau KA, Crutcher KA. Nerve growth factor in Alzheimer's disease: Increased levels throughout the brain coupled with declines in nucleus basalis. The Journal of Neuroscience. 1995;**15**(9):6213-6221

[78] Allen SJ, MacGowan SH, Treanor JJS, Feeney R, Wilcock GK, Dawbarn D. Normal β-NGF content in Alzheimer's disease cerebral cortex and hippocampus. Neuroscience Letters. 1991;**131**(1):135-139

[79] Crutcher KA, Scott SA, Liang S, Everson WV, Weingartner J. Detection of NGF-like activity in human brain tissue: Increased levels in Alzheimer's disease. The Journal of Neuroscience. 1993;**13**(6):2540-2550

[80] Cooper JD, Salehi A, Delcroix JD, Howe CL, Belichenko PV, Chua-Couzens J, et al. Failed retrograde transport of NGF in a mouse model of Down's syndrome: Reversal of cholinergic neurodegenerative phenotypes following NGF infusion. Proceedings of the National Academy of Sciences of the United States of America. 2001;**98**(18):10439-10444

[81] De Lacalle S, Cooper JD, Svendsen CN, Dunnett SB, Sofroniew MV. Reduced retrograde labelling with fluorescent tracer accompanies neuronal atrophy of basal forebrain cholinergic neurons in aged rats. Neuroscience. 1996;**75**(1):19-27

[82] Chu Y, Cochran EJ, Bennett DA, Mufson EJ, Kordower JH. Down-regulation of trkA mRNA within nucleus basalis neurons in individuals with mild cognitive impairment and Alzheimer's disease. The Journal of Comparative Neurology. 2001;**437**(3):296-307

[83] Hartikka J, Hefti F. Comparison of nerve growth factor's effects on development of septum, striatum, and nucleus basalis cholinergic neurons in vitro. Journal of Neuroscience Research. 1988;**21**(2-4):352-364

[84] Hatanaka H, Nihonmatsu I, Tsukui H. Nerve growth factor promotes survival of cultured magnocellular cholinergic neurons from nucleus basalis of Meynert in postnatal rats. Neuroscience Letters. 1988;**90**(1-2):63-68

[85] Humpel C, Weis C. Nerve growth factor and cholinergic CNS neurons studied in organotypic brain slices. 1990

[86] Williams LR, Varon S, Peterson GM, Wictorin K, Fischer W, Bjorklund A, et al. Continuous infusion of nerve growth factor prevents basal forebrain neuronal death after fimbria fornix transection. Proceedings of the National Academy of Sciences of the United States of America. 1986;**83**(23):9231-9235

[87] Capsoni S, Ugolini G, Comparini A, Ruberti F, Berardi N, Cattaneo A. Alzheimer-like neurodegeneration in aged antinerve growth factor transgenic mice. Proceedings of the National Academy of Sciences of the United States of America. 2000;**97**(12):6826-6831

[88] Burgos I, Claudio Cuello A, Liberini P, Pioro E, Masliah E. NGF-mediated synaptic sprouting in the cerebral cortex of lesioned primate brain. Brain Research. 1995;**692**(1-2):154-160

[89] Kordower JH, Winn SR, Liu YT, Mufson EJ, Sladek JR, Hammang JP, et al. The aged monkey basal forebrain: Rescue and sprouting of axotomized basal forebrain neurons after grafts of encapsulated cells secreting human nerve growth factor. Proceedings of the National Academy of Sciences of the

United States of America. 1994;**91**(23):10898-10902

[90] Fischer W, Wictorin K, Björklund A, Williams LR, Varon S, Gage FH. Amelioration of cholinergic neuron atrophy and spatial memory impairment in aged rats by nerve growth factor. Nature. 1987;**329**(6134):65-68

[91] Bäckman C, Rose GM, Hoffer BJ, Henry MA, Bartus RT, Friden P, et al. Systemic administration of a nerve growth factor conjugate reverses age-related cognitive dysfunction and prevents cholinergic neuron atrophy. The Journal of Neuroscience. 1996;**16**(17):5437-5442

[92] Lin B, Pirrung MC, Deng L, Li Z, Liu Y, Webster NJG. Neuroprotection by small molecule activators of the nerve growth factor receptor. The Journal of Pharmacology and Experimental Therapeutics. 2007;**322**(1):59-69

[93] Zhang B, Salituro G, Szalkowski D, Li Z, Zhang Y, Royo I, et al. Discovery of a small molecule insulin mimetic with antidiabetic activity in mice. Science (80-). 1999;**284**(5416):974-977

[94] Tang X, Jang S, Okada M, Chan C, Feng Y, Liu Y, et al. The antidepressant amitriptyline is a TrkA and TrkB receptor agonist that promotes TrkA/TrkB heterodimerization and has potent neurotrophic activity. Chemistry & Biology. 2010;**16**(6):644-656

[95] Scarpi D, Cirelli D, Matrone C, Castronovo G, Rosini P, Occhiato EG, et al. Low molecular weight, non-peptidic agonists of TrkA receptor with NGF-mimetic activity. Cell Death and Disease. 2012;**3**(7):e339-e313. Available from: http://dx.doi.org/10.1038/cddis.2012.80

Chapter 2

Etiology and Treatment Approach for Visual Hallucinations in PD Dementia

Yuki Asahara, Taiji Mukai, Machiko Suda and Masahiko Suzuki

Abstract

Visual hallucinations are a common symptom of Parkinson's disease dementia. These can cause delusions and violent behaviors that can be significant burdens on patients and caregivers. The cause of visual hallucinations is considered to be the dysregulation of the default mode network due to the presence of Lewy bodies in the cortex and the degeneration of dopaminergic and cholinergic neurons. Dopaminergic agents, especially non-ergoline dopamine agonists, can exacerbate visual hallucinations. Reducing the dosage can ameliorate symptoms in many cases; however, this frequently worsens parkinsonism. In contrast, the administration of cholinesterase inhibitors is effective and rarely worsens motor symptoms. In advanced cases, antipsychotic drugs are required; clinical studies have shown that some drugs are beneficial while the adverse events are acceptable. An optimal treatment protocol should be selected depending on the patient's condition.

Keywords: Parkinson's disease, dementia, hallucinations, dopaminergic agents, cholinesterase inhibitors, antipsychotic agents

1. Introduction

Advanced Parkinson's disease (PD) patients often have dementia due to widespread Lewy bodies in the cerebrum [1]. Lewy bodies are inclusion bodies consisting of a protein, named alpha-synuclein [2]. In Parkinson's disease dementia (PDD), visual hallucinations (VH), defined as hallucinations accompanied by delusions, which are abnormal beliefs that are endorsed by patients as real, that persist in spite of evidence to the contrary, and that are not part of a patient's culture or subculture, are a common symptom as in dementia with Lewy bodies (DLB) [3]. VH can cause delusions and violent behavior that can be a considerable burden on patients and their caregivers [4–6]; therefore, optimal treatments are indispensable.

In the early stages of PD, VH are usually a simple presentation like blurred moving images [3]. Complex VH, which are consisting of well-organized unreal visual perception, appear as the disease progresses. In a study of early-stage patients within 7 years from onset, VH were found in 17% during 4-year follow-up [7]. On the other hand, the lifetime incidence was reported as 50% [8].

The main form of treatment is the adjustment of medication dosage. In many cases, a reduction of the dose of dopaminergic agents ameliorates symptoms [2]. In contrast, the administration of antidementia medications, especially cholinesterase inhibitors, is an effective alternative that can relieve VH without worsening motor symptoms [2]. However, antipsychotic agents are required for some patients [2]. In this chapter, we review previous studies on drug management to propose a clinical approach for treating VH in PDD patients.

2. Etiology of visual hallucinations

Visual identification of objects processes from the occipital lobes to the temporal lobes [9]. The object is recognized when this visual information is linked to memories. It is considered that this linking occurs partly in a network called the default mode network (DMN) [3, 10]. The DMN is activated when a person does not focus on any task in particular [3, 11]. The DMN comprises multiple parts of the brain such as the medial prefrontal cortex, precuneus, posterior cingulate cortex, inferior parietal cortex, and lateral temporal cortex (**Figure 1**) [12]. In contrast, the network activated by attention-demanding tasks is called the task-positive network (TPN) [3, 11], which includes the lateral frontal cortex, superior parietal cortex, insula cortex, and frontal operculum cortex [12]. The TPN modulates the DMN, and it is hypothesized that overactivity of the DMN causes VH (**Figure 2**) [3].

Findings from a pathological study are consistent with this hypothesis. One study compared Lewy body deposits in patients with and without VH [13]. Patients with VH had more accumulation of Lewy bodies at many sites, and the most statistically significant difference was seen in the frontal cortex. Most of this area is part of the TPN, and the damage incurred by Lewy bodies can lead to the dysregulation of the DMN.

Furthermore, dopaminergic and cholinergic agents can affect VH [14]. Dopaminergic neurons and cholinergic neurons are associated with visual recognition. The prefrontal cortex and striatum receive dopaminergic stimulation and control attention and working memory [15–19]. The nucleus basalis of Meynert projects acetylcholine across the entire cerebral cortex [20]. These are related to the TPN; therefore, dopaminergic or cholinergic dysfunction can cause dysregulation of the DMN.

Although the pathophysiology of VH is not fully understood, it is reasonable to adjust dopaminergic agents and administer antidementia drugs to treat VH of PDD patients.

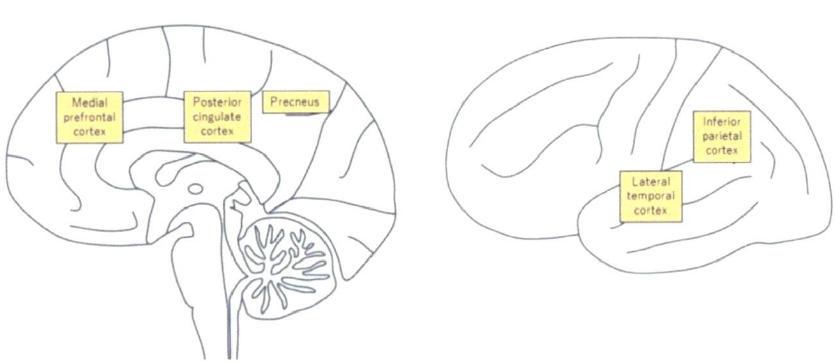

Figure 1.
DMN components. DMN is mainly composed of the medial prefrontal cortex, precuneus, posterior cingulate cortex, inferior parietal cortex, and lateral temporal cortex.

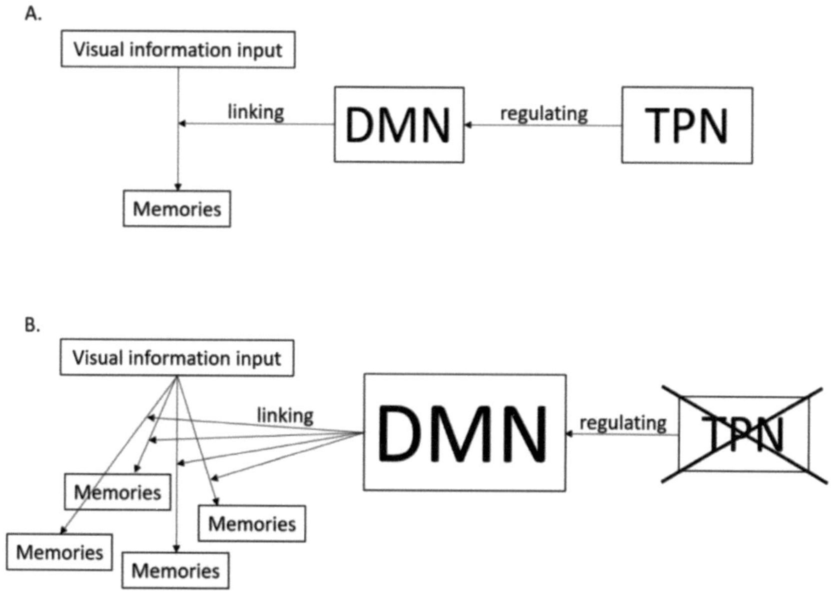

Figure 2.
Brain network process of linking visual input to memories. DMN properly links visual information input to memories under regulation by TPN (A). DMN links visual information input to inappropriate memories without adequate regulation by TPN (B).

3. Management of dopaminergic agents

Most PDD patients with VH use dopaminergic agents (e.g., levodopa, dopamine agonists, monoamine oxidase inhibitors, catechol-O-methyltransferase inhibitors, or amantadine) to ameliorate motor symptoms. However, these drugs may exacerbate VH in patients with PDD [14]. This exacerbation is considered to be due to the overactivity of the mesolimbic system caused by an unnatural dopaminergic stimulation. Of course, other drugs, such as anticholinergics, antidepressants, and N-methyl-D-aspartate (NMDA) antagonists, can cause VH; however, these are less frequently used, and most of them have a low risk [3, 14]. Thus, reducing the dose of dopaminergic agents ameliorates the symptoms of VH.

Not all patients require VH treatment since, in some mild cases, patients can understand that VH are unreal. In such cases, motor symptom treatment is prioritized; therefore, dopaminergic agents can be continued. Goetz et al. evaluated the prognosis of PD patients who have VH with insight [21]. Eighty-one percent of the patients progressed to VH without insight during 3-year follow-up (**Figure 3**). If VH cause delusions or violent behavior, doses of dopaminergic agents should be reduced. However, abruptly discontinuing them can cause severe rigidity and rhabdomyolysis, possibly leading to neuroleptic malignant syndrome [22, 23]; thus, gradual tapering is recommended.

Among dopaminergic agents, non-ergoline dopamine agonists pose a greater risk of VH than do others [24], which have different dopamine receptor binding profiles compared with dopamine [25]. It is considered that this profile difference causes VH. Four non-ergoline dopamine agonists, pramipexole, ropinirole, rotigotine, and apomorphine, received U.S. Food and Drug Administration (FDA) approval as PD treatment agents and are globally used. In PDD patients with VH using these drugs, a reduction in the dose is recommended. In particular, slow tapering is strongly recommended to avoid dopamine agonist withdrawal syndrome [26]. This syndrome can cause miscellaneous symptoms, such as anxiety,

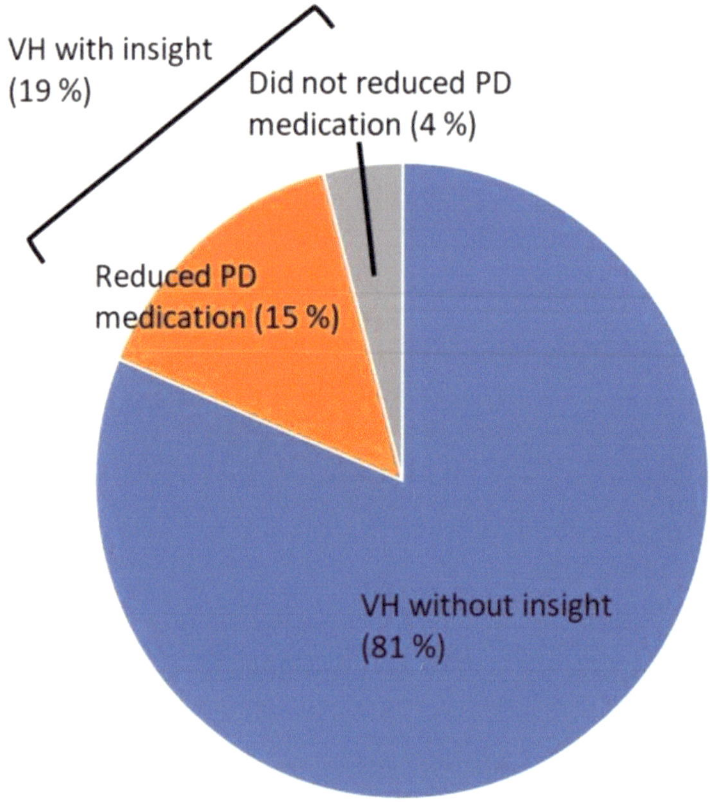

Figure 3.
Three-year follow-up result of PD patients who had VH with insight [21]. Eighty-one percent of the patients progressed to VH without insight. Fifteen percent reduced PD medication and retained insight.

depression, irritability, fatigue, nausea, pain, and suicidal ideation [27, 28]. Careful monitoring is required after reducing drug dosage, since patients can show symptoms even during slow tapering [27, 29].

Reducing dopaminergic agents worsens motor symptoms in most cases. Since most PDD patients are in the advanced disease stage, worsening bradykinesia due to the drug reduction can lead to fatal complications such as pneumonia [30]. Therefore, it may be necessary to change from a high-risk drug to a relatively safe drug rather than merely reduce it (e.g., non-ergoline dopamine agonist replacement by levodopa). However, all dopaminergic agents can cause VH [3, 14], and deterioration of motor functions may be unavoidable in some cases. This is a trade-off situation, and it is necessary to comprehensively consider the balance of all symptoms and adjust the optimal prescription for each patient [31].

4. Therapeutic drugs

4.1 Overview of therapeutic drugs

Several studies have reported the therapeutic effects of antidementia and antipsychotic drugs on VH. There are two types of globally used antidementia drugs, cholinesterase inhibitors and NMDA receptor antagonists. We reviewed key previous studies on these drugs.

Cholinesterase inhibitors reduce VH and mostly do not worsen parkinsonism [32–43]. They can be used as first-line drugs. Although there is no study showing that memantine ameliorates VH sufficiently, it may improve cognitive function [44]. It can be used as an additional drug. Antipsychotic drugs should be used in a minimal dose due to high risks of mortality and adverse events [45]. However, some of them reduce VH without causing intolerable adverse events [46, 47]. They should be used for cases that are difficult to control.

Hereafter, we will explain the studies on and detailed characteristics of these drugs and propose a treatment strategy.

4.2 Cholinesterase inhibitors

Previous studies have revealed that PDD patients have cholinergic deficits [48]. Alpha-synuclein pathology usually occurs in the nucleus basalis of Meynert, which projects acetylcholine throughout the cerebral cortex [20]. This can cause TPN dysfunction leading to VH [49]. Cholinesterase inhibitors ameliorate cognitive functions and reduce VH in PDD and DLB patients [32–43]. They rarely worsen parkinsonism. Research has been conducted on three agents: rivastigmine, donepezil, and galantamine. These drugs are clinically used in North America, Latin America, Europe, the Middle East, Asia, and Oceania.

Rivastigmine was the first cholinesterase inhibitor that showed a reduction in VH in DLB patients in a randomized controlled trial (RCT) [36]. It not only inhibits acetylcholinesterase but also suppresses butyrylcholinesterase [50]. It was suggested that this dual inhibition may be beneficial for the long-term treatment of Alzheimer's disease (AD) [51, 52]. As half of the PDD patients have AD pathology [53], this pharmacological characteristic may also be preferable for PDD treatment. A large double-blind RCT suggested that rivastigmine ameliorates VH as well as cognitive function in PDD patients [39]. In this study, significant improvements in both neuropsychiatric inventory (NPI) and mini-mental state examination (MMSE) scores were observed. Although it caused a significantly high frequency of gastrointestinal adverse events, a transdermal patch is available [54], which is less likely to cause gastrointestinal events [55]. Another study compared rivastigmine effect on PDD patients with and without VH [42]. The cognitive function improvement was greater in patients with VH. These previous studies suggest rivastigmine is beneficial for PDD patients with VH.

Donepezil is a selective acetylcholinesterase inhibitor and delays the hydrolysis of acetylcholine in the brain neuronal synapses [56]. Stinton et al. performed a systematic review and meta-analysis of donepezil studies for PDD patients [32]. They compared MMSE scores between donepezil and placebo groups in four double-blind RCTs [34, 38, 41, 43]. Donepezil group showed better scores, but without significant difference. They found significantly better scores of NPI [38, 41], which suggests a possibly beneficial effect of donepezil on VH. The most frequent adverse event was gastrointestinal symptoms [34, 38, 41, 43]. In the largest study, 21% of the donepezil group patients experienced nausea, and the frequency was significantly higher than in the placebo group [41]. However, no discontinuation rate difference was found. Mori et al. performed a double-blind RCT of donepezil for DLB patients [35]. In this study, the experimental group had fewer VH and significant improvement of NPI. Furthermore, a positron emission tomography study showed a significant change of glucose metabolism in occipital lobes after administration of donepezil [33]. Although we need to be aware of the side effects, donepezil is a reasonable choice for VH treatment. We have summarized the RCTs of donepezil in **Table 1**.

Authors	Year	Patients	Protocol	Improved primary outcome
Aarsland et al. [43]	2002	PD patients with cognitive impairment	Randomized double-blind placebo-controlled crossover study	Mini-mental state examination and clinician's interview-based impression of change plus caregiver input scale
Ravina et al. [34]	2005	PDD patients	Randomized double-blind placebo-controlled crossover study	None (not significant trend for better Alzheimer's disease assessment scale-cognitive subscale scores)
Leroi et al. [38]	2004	PD patients with cognitive impairment	Randomized double-blind placebo-controlled study	The memory subscale of the dementia rating scale
Dubois et al. [41]	2012	PDD patients	Randomized double-blind placebo-controlled study	Clinician's interview-based impression of change plus caregiver input scale

Each study did not show the beneficial effect of donepezil on VH. However, Stinton's systematic review showed significantly better NPI scores, which suggested that donepezil possibly ameliorates VH [32].

Table 1.
RCTs of donepezil on PDD or PD patients with cognitive impairment.

Galantamine is another acetylcholinesterase inhibitor commonly used. It is also an allosteric potentiating ligand for nicotinic acetylcholine receptors [56, 57]. (The pharmacological characteristics of each cholinesterase inhibitor are described in **Figure 4**.) We did not find a double-blind RCT for galantamine. However, a small open-label controlled trial showed significant amelioration of VH, as well as MMSE and NPI scores [37]. The drug-related adverse events were seen in 30% of the experimental group, and the most frequent one was drooling. Edwards et al. performed a 24-week open-label study on DLB patients [40]. This study suggested that galantamine ameliorates VH similar to rivastigmine and donepezil in DLB patients. Galantamine is a possible option in PDD patients with VH, based on these studies.

Cholinesterase inhibitors generally ameliorate VH without worsening motor symptoms. Each of them has a different advantage, and they should as such be selected depending on the patient's condition. Donepezil is the most clinically studied drug, and its efficacy is reliable [34, 38, 41, 43]. Besides, the administration burden is small since it requires oral intake only once a day due to its long elimination half-life [58]. In contrast, galantamine requires oral administration twice daily [59]. However, it can ameliorate agitation and disinhibition due to its nicotinic effect [60]. The most remarkable benefit of rivastigmine is the availability of the transdermal patch [54]. It can be administered to patients who refuse oral intake.

4.3 Memantine

Memantine is an antidementia drug that blocks NMDA receptors [61]. It is approved for clinical use in North America, Latin America, Europe, the Middle East, Asia, and Oceania. Many RCTs and meta-analytic studies have demonstrated the beneficial effect of memantine in AD patients [62–66]. In contrast, according to a meta-analysis of three RCTs of PDD and DLB patients, no significant amelioration of cognitive function or VH was found [32, 67–69]. However, another meta-analysis reported a small but significant improvement in the score of clinicians'

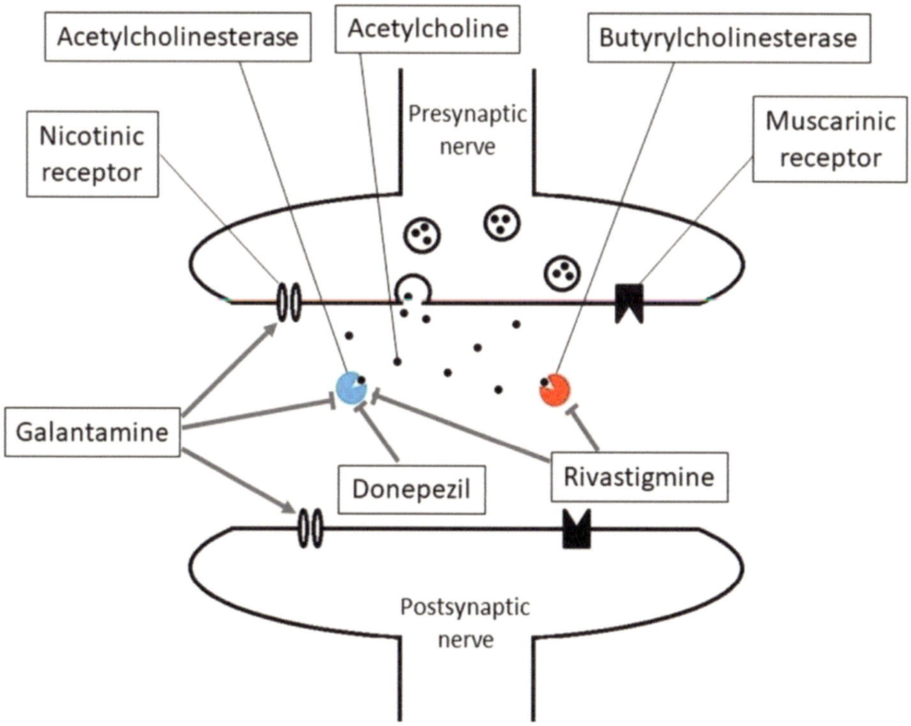

Figure 4.
The pharmacological characteristics of each cholinesterase inhibitor. Rivastigmine, donepezil, and galantamine inhibit acetylcholinesterase. Rivastigmine also suppresses butyrylcholinesterase. Galantamine binds to the nicotinic receptors and allosterically enhances their response to acetylcholine.

global impression of change [44]. Memantine has very few drug-related adverse events [67–69], and it can be used as an additional treatment for cognitive function improvement. However, findings from a case series suggested that memantine may exacerbate VH [70]. As other NMDA antagonists, such as ketamine, can cause hallucinations, memantine may have a similar effect [3]. Although the evidence suggesting exacerbation of VH is limited with most RCTs reporting no significant deterioration [67–69], memantine should be used with caution.

4.4 Antipsychotic agents

Antipsychotic agents compromise dopaminergic function and ameliorate psychiatric symptoms including VH. They should be used in a minimal dose owing to high risks of mortality and adverse events in these patients [45]. However, several studies have reported the beneficial effect of atypical antipsychotic agents.

A systematic review suggested that clozapine is efficacious in the treatment of psychosis in PD patients [46]. Two double-blind placebo-controlled RCTs were performed, and both studies showed significant amelioration of psychosis without worsening of motor symptoms [71, 72]. One of them showed significant alleviation of VH [72]. However, in a 12-week open-label extension study of these RCTs, one withdrawal out of 108 patients due to leukocytopenia was registered [73, 74]. Clozapine leukocytopenia can be fatal, and weekly blood sampling is required for several months according to each country's regulation [75]. In addition, it may cause myocarditis and hyperglycemia [76, 77]. Therefore, clozapine is clinically useful but requires monitoring.

Quetiapine is possibly useful for VH in PD patients, but the evidence is insufficient [46]. Five double-blind placebo-controlled RCTs were performed [78–82]. No significant amelioration of psychiatric symptoms was demonstrated in four studies [78–81]. However, one study showed significant improvement of the clinical global impression scale and the hallucination item of the brief psychiatric rating scale scores [82]. In addition, two RCTs compared effects of quetiapine and clozapine, and both were almost equally effective on psychosis [83, 84]. No worsening of motor symptoms was seen in all of these studies. Quetiapine is possibly beneficial for PDD patients with VH. However, it should be used cautiously because it is associated with risks of arrhythmia and hyperglycemia [85, 86]. We have summarized the quetiapine studies in **Table 2**.

Pimavanserin is a serotonin 5-HT2A agonist without dopaminergic affinity [87]. A systematic review reported it effective in the treatment of PD psychosis [46], and it is the only drug that has FDA approval for the PD psychosis treatment. A double-blind, placebo-controlled RCT showed significantly better amelioration of VH and other psychiatric symptoms compared with that in the placebo group [88]. A subgroup analysis revealed that it was also efficacious and safe for cognitively impaired patients; therefore, it may be useful for PDD patients [89]. However, ten out of 105 experimental patients discontinued the treatment due to adverse events. Six of these patients experienced psychosis. In addition, pimavanserin may prolong the QT interval, and thus, it should not be used in patients with arrhythmias [90]. Pimavanserin administration requires caution and careful monitoring for psychiatric adverse events.

Other antipsychotic agents (e.g., olanzapine, risperidone, or aripiprazole) lack evidence of the beneficial effect on VH or other psychiatric symptoms. If other antipsychotic agents, especially typical ones, are required, they should be administered for as short a period as possible.

Authors	Year	Patients	Protocol	Main outcome
Morgante et al. [84]	2004	45 PD patients with psychosis	Randomized rater-blinded prospective comparison with clozapine	No significant difference
Ondo et al. [81]	2005	31 Non-demented PD patients with VH	Randomized double-blind, placebo-controlled, unforced titration parallel trial	No significant difference
Merims et al. [83]	2006	27 PD patients with psychosis	Randomized rater-blinded prospective comparison with clozapine	Significantly less delusions in clozapine group
Kurlan et al. [78]	2007	40 patients with DLB or PDD or AD	Randomized double-blind placebo-controlled trial	No significant difference
Rabey et al. [79]	2007	58 PD patients with psychosis	Randomized double-blind placebo-controlled trial	No significant difference
Shotbolt et al. [80]	2009	24 PD patients with psychosis	Randomized double-blind placebo-controlled trial	No significant difference
Fernandez et al. [82]	2009	16 PD patients with VH	Randomized double-blind placebo-controlled trial	Significantly better VH status in quetiapine group

The clinical evidence of quetiapine's beneficial effect on PD patients is not sufficient because most RCTs did not show preferable results.

Table 2.
Studies of quetiapine on PD patients.

4.5 Treatment strategy

In mild cases, the administration of cholinesterase inhibitors is the first option. When VH are troublesome, modification of dopaminergic agent is recommended. If VH are not controlled by dopaminergic agent modification and cholinesterase inhibitors, antipsychotic agents are recommended. We propose a treatment plan in light of these findings (**Figure 5**). The optimal treatment will be different for each patient and should be selected depending on the patient's condition.

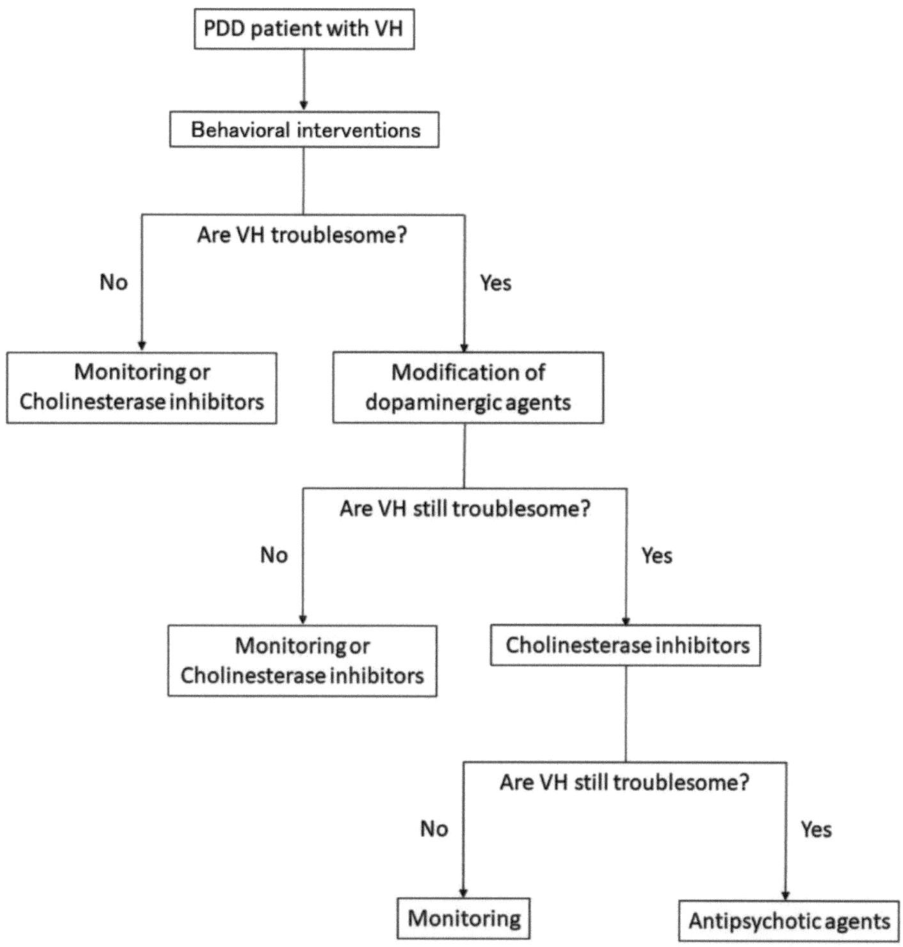

Figure 5.
Flowchart for management of PD patients with VH. Optimal education about VH can ameliorate the behavioral symptoms in some patients. The need for medical treatment depends on whether VH are troublesome after behavioral interventions. However, if VH do not cause problems, it can worsen in the disease course and must be monitored.

5. Conclusion

VH are a frequent symptom in PDD. The lifetime incidence was reported as 50% [8]. VH can cause delusions and violent behavior that can be a considerable burden on patients and their caregivers [4–6]; therefore, optimal treatments are indispensable.

The cause of VH is hypothesized to be linked to the overactivity of the DMN [3]. Dopaminergic or cholinergic dysfunction is associated with dysregulation of the DMN. It is reasonable to adjust dopaminergic agents and administer antidementia drugs to treat the VH of PDD patients.

Reducing dopaminergic drug dosage can ameliorate symptoms [2]. However, this frequently worsens motor symptoms. The administration of cholinesterase inhibitors is effective and rarely worsens parkinsonism [2].

Antipsychotic agents should be used in a minimal dose because of adverse events [45]. However, several studies have reported that clozapine and pimavanserin can ameliorate VH without worsening motor symptoms [46]. Although there is not sufficient evidence, quetiapine is possibly useful too [46].

An optimal treatment plan should be selected depending on the patient's condition.

Conflict of interest

The authors declare no conflict of interest.

Author details

Yuki Asahara*, Taiji Mukai, Machiko Suda and Masahiko Suzuki
Department of Neurology, The Jikei University Katsushika Medical Center, Tokyo, Japan

*Address all correspondence to: yuki.asahara.1988@jikei.ac.jp

References

[1] Walker Z, Possin KL, Boeve BF, Aarsland D. Lewy body dementias. Lancet. 2015;**386**(10004):1683-1697. DOI: 10.1016/s0140-6736(15)00462-6

[2] Kalia LV, Lang AE. Parkinson's disease. Lancet. 2015;**386**(9996):896-912. DOI: 10.1016/s0140-6736(14)61393-3

[3] Russo M, Carrarini C, Dono F, Rispoli MG, Di Pietro M, Di Stefano V, et al. The pharmacology of visual hallucinations in synucleinopathies. Frontiers in Pharmacology. 2019;**10**:1379. DOI: 10.3389/fphar.2019.01379

[4] Martinez-Martin P, Rodriguez-Blazquez C, Forjaz MJ, Frades-Payo B, Agüera-Ortiz L, Weintraub D, et al. Neuropsychiatric symptoms and caregiver's burden in Parkinson's disease. Parkinsonism & Related Disorders. 2015;**21**(6):629-634. DOI: 10.1016/j.parkreldis.2015.03.024

[5] Aarsland D, Brønnick K, Ehrt U, De Deyn PP, Tekin S, Emre M, et al. Neuropsychiatric symptoms in patients with Parkinson's disease and dementia: Frequency, profile and associated care giver stress. Journal of Neurology, Neurosurgery, and Psychiatry. 2007;**78**(1):36-42. DOI: 10.1136/jnnp.2005.083113

[6] Kulisevsky J, Pagonabarraga J, Pascual-Sedano B, García-Sánchez C, Gironell A. Prevalence and correlates of neuropsychiatric symptoms in Parkinson's disease without dementia. Movement Disorders. 2008;**23**(13):1889-1896. DOI: 10.1002/mds.22246

[7] Biglan KM, Holloway RG Jr, McDermott MP, Richard IH. Risk factors for somnolence, edema, and hallucinations in early Parkinson disease. Neurology. 2007;**69**(2):187-195. DOI: 10.1212/01.wnl.0000265593.34438.00

[8] Williams DR, Lees AJ. Visual hallucinations in the diagnosis of idiopathic Parkinson's disease: A retrospective autopsy study. Lancet Neurology. 2005;**4**(10):605-610. DOI: 10.1016/s1474-4422(05)70146-0

[9] Mishkin M, Ungerleider LG, Macko KA. Object vision and spatial vision: Two cortical pathways. Trends in Neurosciences. 1983;**6**:414-417. DOI: https://doi.org/10.1016/0166-2236(83)90190-X

[10] Raichle ME. The restless brain: How intrinsic activity organizes brain function. Philosophical Transactions of the Royal Society of London. Series B, Biological Sciences. 2015;**370**(1668):20140172. DOI: 10.1098/rstb.2014.0172

[11] Fox MD, Snyder AZ, Vincent JL, Corbetta M, Van Essen DC, Raichle ME. The human brain is intrinsically organized into dynamic, anticorrelated functional networks. Proceedings of the National Academy of Sciences of the United States of America. 2005;**102**(27):9673-9678. DOI: 10.1073/pnas.0504136102

[12] Blumenfeld H. Neuroanatomical basis of consciousness. In: The Neurology of Conciousness. Amsterdam: Elsevier; 2016. pp. 3-29

[13] Gallagher DA, Parkkinen L, O'Sullivan SS, Spratt A, Shah A, Davey CC, et al. Testing an aetiological model of visual hallucinations in Parkinson's disease. Brain 2011;**134**(Pt 11):3299-3309. DOI: 10.1093/brain/awr225

[14] Connolly BS, Lang AE. Pharmacological treatment of Parkinson disease: A review. Journal of the American Medical Association. 2014;**311**(16):1670-1683. DOI: 10.1001/jama.2014.3654

[15] Bilder RM, Volavka J, Lachman HM, Grace AA. The catechol-O-methyltransferase polymorphism: Relations to the tonic-phasic dopamine hypothesis and neuropsychiatric phenotypes. Neuropsycho pharmacology. 2004;**29**(11):1943-1961. DOI: 10.1038/sj.npp.1300542

[16] Meyer-Lindenberg A, Kohn PD, Kolachana B, Kippenhan S, McInerney-Leo A, Nussbaum R, et al. Midbrain dopamine and prefrontal function in humans: Interaction and modulation by COMT genotype. Nature Neuroscience. 2005;**8**(5):594-596. DOI: 10.1038/nn1438

[17] Williams GV, Goldman-Rakic PS. Modulation of memory fields by dopamine D1 receptors in prefrontal cortex. Nature. 1995;**376**(6541):572-575. DOI: 10.1038/376572a0

[18] Kroener S, Chandler LJ, Phillips PE, Seamans JK. Dopamine modulates persistent synaptic activity and enhances the signal-to-noise ratio in the prefrontal cortex. PLoS ONE. 2009;**4**(8):e6507. DOI: 10.1371/journal.pone.0006507

[19] Chudasama Y, Robbins TW. Dopaminergic modulation of visual attention and working memory in the rodent prefrontal cortex. Neuropsychopharmacology. 2004;**29**(9):1628-1636. DOI: 10.1038/sj.npp.1300490

[20] Kalaitzakis ME, Christian LM, Moran LB, Graeber MB, Pearce RK, Gentleman SM. Dementia and visual hallucinations associated with limbic pathology in Parkinson's disease. Parkinsonism & Related Disorders. 2009;**15**(3):196-204. DOI: 10.1016/j.parkreldis.2008.05.007

[21] Goetz CG, Fan W, Leurgans S, Bernard B, Stebbins GT. The malignant course of "benign hallucinations" in Parkinson disease. Archives of Neurology. 2006;**63**(5):713-716. DOI: 10.1001/archneur.63.5.713

[22] Stotz M, Thümmler D, Schürch M, Renggli JC, Urwyler A, Pargger H. Fulminant neuroleptic malignant syndrome after perioperative withdrawal of antiParkinsonian medication. British Journal of Anaesthesia. 2004;**93**(6):868-871. DOI: 10.1093/bja/aeh269

[23] Ong KC, Chew EL, Ong YY. Neuroleptic malignant syndrome without neuroleptics. Singapore Medical Journal. 2001;**42**(2):85-88

[24] Talati R, Baker WL, Patel AA, Reinhart K, Coleman CI. Adding a dopamine agonist to preexisting levodopa therapy vs. levodopa therapy alone in advanced Parkinson's disease: A meta analysis. International Journal of Clinical Practice. 2009;**63**(4):613-623. DOI: 10.1111/j.1742-1241.2009.02027.x

[25] Gerlach M, Double K, Arzberger T, Leblhuber F, Tatschner T, Riederer P. Dopamine receptor agonists in current clinical use: Comparative dopamine receptor binding profiles defined in the human striatum. Journal of Neural Transmission (Vienna). 2003;**110**(10): 1119-1127. DOI: 10.1007/s00702-003-0027-5

[26] Nirenberg MJ. Dopamine agonist withdrawal syndrome: Implications for patient care. Drugs & Aging. 2013;**30**(8):587-592. DOI: 10.1007/s40266-013-0090-z

[27] Rabinak CA, Nirenberg MJ. Dopamine agonist withdrawal syndrome in Parkinson disease. Archives of Neurology. 2010;**67**(1):58-63. DOI: 10.1001/archneurol.2009.294

[28] Pondal M, Marras C, Miyasaki J, Moro E, Armstrong MJ, Strafella AP, et al. Clinical features of dopamine agonist withdrawal syndrome in a movement disorders clinic. Journal of

Neurology, Neurosurgery, and Psychiatry. 2013;**84**(2):130-135. DOI: 10.1136/jnnp-2012-302684

[29] Cunnington A-L, White L, Hood K. Identification of possible risk factors for the development of dopamine agonist withdrawal syndrome in Parkinson's disease. Parkinsonism & Related Disorders. 2012;**18**(9):1051-1052. DOI: 10.1016/j.parkreldis.2012.05.012

[30] Mizuno Y, Takubo H, Mizuta E, Kuno S. Malignant syndrome in Parkinson's disease: Concept and review of the literature. Parkinsonism & Related Disorders. 2003;**9**(**Suppl 1**): S3-S9. DOI: 10.1016/s1353-8020(02)00125-6

[31] Suchowersky O. Parkinson's disease: Medical treatment of moderate to advanced disease. Current Neurology and Neuroscience Reports. 2002;**2**(4):310-316. DOI: 10.1007/s11910-002-0006-5

[32] Stinton C, McKeith I, Taylor JP, Lafortune L, Mioshi E, Mak E, et al. Pharmacological management of Lewy body dementia: A systematic review and meta-analysis. The American Journal of Psychiatry. 2015;**172**(8):731-742. DOI: 10.1176/appi.ajp.2015.14121582

[33] Satoh M, Ishikawa H, Meguro K, Kasuya M, Ishii H, Yamaguchi S. Improved visual hallucination by donepezil and occipital glucose metabolism in dementia with Lewy bodies: The Osaki-Tajiri project. European Neurology. 2010;**64**(6):337-344. DOI: 10.1159/000322121

[34] Ravina B, Putt M, Siderowf A, Farrar JT, Gillespie M, Crawley A, et al. Donepezil for dementia in Parkinson's disease: A randomised, double blind, placebo controlled, crossover study. Journal of Neurology, Neurosurgery, and Psychiatry. 2005;**76**(7):934-939. DOI: 10.1136/jnnp.2004.050682

[35] Mori E, Ikeda M, Kosaka K. Donepezil for dementia with Lewy bodies: A randomized, placebo-controlled trial. Annals of Neurology. 2012;**72**(1):41-52. DOI: 10.1002/ana.23557

[36] McKeith I, Del Ser T, Spano P, Emre M, Wesnes K, Anand R, et al. Efficacy of rivastigmine in dementia with Lewy bodies: A randomised, double-blind, placebo-controlled international study. Lancet. 2000;**356**(9247):2031-2036. DOI: 10.1016/s0140-6736(00)03399-7

[37] Litvinenko IV, Odinak MM, Mogil'naya VI, Emelin AY. Efficacy and safety of galantamine (reminyl) for dementia in patients with Parkinson's disease (an open controlled trial). Neuroscience and Behavioral Physiology. 2008;**38**(9):937-945. DOI: 10.1007/s11055-008-9077-3

[38] Leroi I, Brandt J, Reich SG, Lyketsos CG, Grill S, Thompson R, et al. Randomized placebo-controlled trial of donepezil in cognitive impairment in Parkinson's disease. International Journal of Geriatric Psychiatry. 2004;**19**(1):1-8. DOI: 10.1002/gps.993

[39] Emre M, Aarsland D, Albanese A, Byrne EJ, Deuschl G, De Deyn PP, et al. Rivastigmine for dementia associated with Parkinson's disease. The New England Journal of Medicine. 2004;**351**(24):2509-2518. DOI: 10.1056/NEJMoa041470

[40] Edwards K, Royall D, Hershey L, Lichter D, Hake A, Farlow M, et al. Efficacy and safety of galantamine in patients with dementia with Lewy bodies: A 24-week open-label study. Dementia and Geriatric Cognitive Disorders. 2007;**23**(6):401-405. DOI: 10.1159/000101512

[41] Dubois B, Tolosa E, Katzenschlager R, Emre M, Lees AJ, Schumann G, et al. Donepezil in

Parkinson's disease dementia: A randomized, double-blind efficacy and safety study. Movement Disorders. 2012;**27**(10):1230-1238. DOI: 10.1002/mds.25098

[42] Burn D, Emre M, McKeith I, De Deyn PP, Aarsland D, Hsu C, et al. Effects of rivastigmine in patients with and without visual hallucinations in dementia associated with Parkinson's disease. Movement Disorders. 2006;**21**(11):1899-1907. DOI: 10.1002/mds.21077

[43] Aarsland D, Laake K, Larsen JP, Janvin C. Donepezil for cognitive impairment in Parkinson's disease: A randomised controlled study. Journal of Neurology, Neurosurgery, and Psychiatry. 2002;**72**(6):708-712. DOI: 10.1136/jnnp.72.6.708

[44] Wang HF, Yu JT, Tang SW, Jiang T, Tan CC, Meng XF, et al. Efficacy and safety of cholinesterase inhibitors and memantine in cognitive impairment in Parkinson's disease, Parkinson's disease dementia, and dementia with Lewy bodies: Systematic review with meta-analysis and trial sequential analysis. Journal of Neurology, Neurosurgery, and Psychiatry. 2015;**86**(2):135-143. DOI: 10.1136/jnnp-2014-307659

[45] Ballard C, Isaacson S, Mills R, Williams H, Corbett A, Coate B, et al. Impact of current antipsychotic medications on comparative mortality and adverse events in people with Parkinson disease psychosis. Journal of the American Medical Directors Association. 2015;**16**(10):898.e891-897. DOI: 10.1016/j.jamda.2015.06.021

[46] Seppi K, Ray Chaudhuri K, Coelho M, Fox SH, Katzenschlager R, Perez Lloret S, et al. Update on treatments for nonmotor symptoms of Parkinson's disease-an evidence-based medicine review. Movement Disorders. 2019;**34**(2):180-198. DOI: 10.1002/mds.27602

[47] Seppi K, Weintraub D, Coelho M, Perez-Lloret S, Fox SH, Katzenschlager R, et al. The movement disorder society evidence-based medicine review update: Treatments for the non-motor symptoms of Parkinson's disease. Movement Disorders. 2011; **26 Suppl 3**(03):S42-S80. DOI: 10.1002/mds.23884

[48] Halliday GM, Leverenz JB, Schneider JS, Adler CH. The neurobiological basis of cognitive impairment in Parkinson's disease. Movement Disorders. 2014;**29**(5):634-650. DOI: 10.1002/mds.25857

[49] Bohnen NI, Kaufer DI, Hendrickson R, Ivanco LS, Lopresti BJ, Constantine GM, et al. Cognitive correlates of cortical cholinergic denervation in Parkinson's disease and parkinsonian dementia. Journal of Neurology. 2006;**253**(2):242-247. DOI: 10.1007/s00415-005-0971-0

[50] Kandiah N, Pai MC, Senanarong V, Looi I, Ampil E, Park KW, et al. Rivastigmine: The advantages of dual inhibition of acetylcholinesterase and butyrylcholinesterase and its role in subcortical vascular dementia and Parkinson's disease dementia. Clinical Interventions in Aging. 2017;**12**:697-707. DOI: 10.2147/cia.S129145

[51] Blesa R, Bullock R, He Y, Bergman H, Gambina G, Meyer J, et al. Effect of butyrylcholinesterase genotype on the response to rivastigmine or donepezil in younger patients with Alzheimer's disease. Pharmacogenetics and Genomics. 2006;**16**(11):771-774. DOI: 10.1097/01.fpc.0000220573.05714.ac

[52] Perry EK, Perry RH, Blessed G, Tomlinson BE. Changes in brain cholinesterases in senile dementia of Alzheimer type. Neuropathology and Applied Neurobiology. 1978;**4**(4):273-277. DOI: 10.1111/j.1365-2990.1978.tb00545.x

[53] Irwin DJ, Lee VM, Trojanowski JQ. Parkinson's disease dementia: Convergence of α-synuclein, tau and amyloid-β pathologies. Nature Reviews. Neuroscience. 2013;**14**(9):626-636. DOI: 10.1038/nrn3549

[54] Yang LP, Keating GM. Rivastigmine transdermal patch: In the treatment of dementia of the Alzheimer's type. CNS Drugs. 2007;**21**(11):957-965. DOI: 10.2165/00023210-200721110-00007

[55] Winblad B, Cummings J, Andreasen N, Grossberg G, Onofrj M, Sadowsky C, et al. A six-month double-blind, randomized, placebo-controlled study of a transdermal patch in Alzheimer's disease--rivastigmine patch versus capsule. International Journal of Geriatric Psychiatry. 2007;**22**(5):456-467. DOI: 10.1002/gps.1788

[56] Anand P, Singh B. A review on cholinesterase inhibitors for Alzheimer's disease. Archives of Pharmacal Research. 2013;**36**(4):375-399. DOI: 10.1007/s12272-013-0036-3

[57] Harvey AL. The pharmacology of galanthamine and its analogues. Pharmacology & Therapeutics. 1995;**68**(1):113-128. DOI: 10.1016/0163-7258(95)02002-0

[58] Asiri YA, Mostafa GA. Donepezil. Profiles of Drug Substances Excipients and Related Methodology. 2010;**35**:117-150. DOI: 10.1016/s1871-5125(10)35003-5

[59] Farlow MR. Clinical pharmacokinetics of galantamine. Clinical Pharmacokinetics. 2003;**42**(15):1383-1392. DOI: 10.2165/00003088-200342150-00005

[60] Herrmann N, Rabheru K, Wang J, Binder C. Galantamine treatment of problematic behavior in Alzheimer disease: Post-hoc analysis of pooled data from three large trials. The American Journal of Geriatric Psychiatry. 2005;**13**(6):527-534. DOI: 10.1176/appi.ajgp.13.6.527

[61] Johnson JW, Kotermanski SE. Mechanism of action of memantine. Current Opinion in Pharmacology. 2006;**6**(1):61-67. DOI: 10.1016/j.coph.2005.09.007

[62] Wilkinson D, Wirth Y, Goebel C. Memantine in patients with moderate to severe Alzheimer's disease: Meta-analyses using realistic definitions of response. Dementia and Geriatric Cognitive Disorders. 2014;**37**(1-2):71-85. DOI: 10.1159/000353801

[63] Reisberg B, Doody R, Stöffler A, Schmitt F, Ferris S, Möbius HJ. Memantine in moderate-to-severe Alzheimer's disease. The New England Journal of Medicine. 2003;**348**(14):1333-1341. DOI: 10.1056/NEJMoa013128

[64] McShane R, Areosa Sastre A, Minakaran N. Memantine for dementia. Cochrane Database Systematic Review. 2006;(2):Cd003154. DOI: 10.1002/14651858.CD003154.pub5

[65] Jiang J, Jiang H. Efficacy and adverse effects of memantine treatment for Alzheimer's disease from randomized controlled trials. Neurological Sciences. 2015;**36**(9):1633-1641. DOI: 10.1007/s10072-015-2221-2

[66] Doody RS, Tariot PN, Pfeiffer E, Olin JT, Graham SM. Meta-analysis of six-month memantine trials in Alzheimer's disease. Alzheimer's & Dementia. 2007;**3**(1):7-17. DOI: 10.1016/j.jalz.2006.10.004

[67] Aarsland D, Ballard C, Walker Z, Bostrom F, Alves G, Kossakowski K, et al. Memantine in patients with Parkinson's disease dementia or dementia with Lewy bodies: A double-blind, placebo-controlled, multicentre trial. Lancet Neurology. 2009;**8**(7):613-618. DOI: 10.1016/s1474-4422(09)70146-2

[68] Emre M, Tsolaki M, Bonuccelli U, Destée A, Tolosa E, Kutzelnigg A, et al. Memantine for patients with Parkinson's disease dementia or dementia with Lewy bodies: A randomised, double-blind, placebo-controlled trial. Lancet Neurology. 2010;**9**(10):969-977. DOI: 10.1016/s1474-4422(10)70194-0

[69] Leroi I, Overshott R, Byrne EJ, Daniel E, Burns A. Randomized controlled trial of memantine in dementia associated with Parkinson's disease. Movement Disorders. 2009;**24**(8):1217-1221. DOI: 10.1002/mds.22495

[70] Ridha BH, Josephs KA, Rossor MN. Delusions and hallucinations in dementia with Lewy bodies: Worsening with memantine. Neurology. 2005;**65**(3):481-482. DOI: 10.1212/01.wnl.0000172351.95783.8e

[71] Clozapine in drug-induced psychosis in Parkinson's disease. The French clozapine Parkinson study group. Lancet. 1999;**353**(9169): 2041-2042

[72] Parkinson Study Group. Low-dose clozapine for the treatment of drug-induced psychosis in Parkinson's disease. The New England Journal of Medicine. 1999;**340**(10):757-763. DOI: 10.1056/nejm1999031134
01003

[73] Pollak P, Tison F, Rascol O, Destée A, Péré JJ, Senard JM, et al. Clozapine in drug induced psychosis in Parkinson's disease: A randomised, placebo controlled study with open follow up. Journal of Neurology, Neurosurgery, and Psychiatry. 2004;**75**(5):689-695. DOI: 10.1136/jnnp.2003.029868

[74] Factor SA, Friedman JH, Lannon MC, Oakes D, Bourgeois K. Clozapine for the treatment of drug-induced psychosis in Parkinson's disease: Results of the 12 week open label extension in the PSYCLOPS trial. Movement Disorders. 2001;**16**(1):135-139. DOI: 10.1002/1531-8257(200101)16:1<135::aid-mds1006>3.0.co;2-q

[75] Nielsen J, Young C, Ifteni P, Kishimoto T, Xiang YT, Schulte PF, et al. Worldwide differences in regulations of clozapine use. CNS Drugs. 2016;**30**(2):149-161. DOI: 10.1007/s40263-016-0311-1

[76] Joshi RS, Singh SP, Panicker MM. 5-HT(2A) deletion protects against clozapine-induced hyperglycemia. Journal of Pharmacological Sciences. 2019;**139**(2):133-135. DOI: 10.1016/j.jphs.2018.11.015

[77] Bellissima BL, Tingle MD, Cicović A, Alawami M, Kenedi C. A systematic review of clozapine-induced myocarditis. International Journal of Cardiology. 2018;**259**:122-129. DOI: 10.1016/j.ijcard.2017.12.102

[78] Kurlan R, Cummings J, Raman R, Thal L. Quetiapine for agitation or psychosis in patients with dementia and parkinsonism. Neurology. 2007;**68**(17):1356-1363. DOI: 10.1212/01.wnl.0000260060.60870.89

[79] Rabey JM, Prokhorov T, Miniovitz A, Dobronevsky E, Klein C. Effect of quetiapine in psychotic Parkinson's disease patients: A double-blind labeled study of 3 months' duration. Movement Disorders. 2007;**22**(3):313-318. DOI: 10.1002/mds.21116

[80] Shotbolt P, Samuel M, Fox C, David AS. A randomized controlled trial of quetiapine for psychosis in Parkinson's disease. Neuropsychiatric Disease and Treatment. 2009;**5**:327-332. DOI: 10.2147/ndt.s5335

[81] Ondo WG, Tintner R, Voung KD, Lai D, Ringholz G. Double-blind, placebo-controlled, unforced titration parallel trial of quetiapine for

dopaminergic-induced hallucinations in Parkinson's disease. Movement Disorders. 2005;**20**(8):958-963. DOI: 10.1002/mds.20474

[82] Fernandez HH, Okun MS, Rodriguez RL, Malaty IA, Romrell J, Sun A, et al. Quetiapine improves visual hallucinations in Parkinson disease but not through normalization of sleep architecture: Results from a double-blind clinical-polysomnography study. The International Journal of Neuro science. 2009;**119**(12):2196-2205. DOI: 10.3109/00207450903222758

[83] Merims D, Balas M, Peretz C, Shabtai H, Giladi N. Rater-blinded, prospective comparison: Quetiapine versus clozapine for Parkinson's disease psychosis. Clinical Neuropharmacology. 2006;**29**(6):331-337. DOI: 10.1097/01.Wnf.0000236769.31279.19

[84] Morgante L, Epifanio A, Spina E, Zappia M, Di Rosa AE, Marconi R, et al. Quetiapine and clozapine in parkinsonian patients with dopaminergic psychosis. Clinical Neuropharmacology. 2004;**27**(4):153-156. DOI: 10.1097/01.wnf.0000 136891.17006.ec

[85] Aghaienia N, Brahm NC, Lussier KM, Washington NB. Probable quetiapine-mediated prolongation of the QT interval. Journal of Pharmacy Practice. 2011;**24**(5):506-512. DOI: 10.1177/0897190011415683

[86] Domon SE, Cargile CS. Quetiapine-associated hyperglycemia and hypertriglyceridemia. Journal of the American Academy of Child and Adolescent Psychiatry. 2002;**41**(5):495-496. DOI: 10.1097/00004583-200205000-00004

[87] Vanover KE, Weiner DM, Makhay M, Veinbergs I, Gardell LR, Lameh J, et al. Pharmacological and behavioral profile of N-(4-fluorophenylmethyl)-N-(1-methylpiperidin-4-yl)-N'-(4-(2-methylpropyloxy)phenylmethyl) carbamide (2R,3R)-dihydroxy butanedioate (2:1) (ACP-103), a novel 5-hydroxytryptamine(2A) receptor inverse agonist. The Journal of Pharmacology and Experimental Therapeutics. 2006;**317**(2):910-918. DOI: 10.1124/jpet.105.097006

[88] Cummings J, Isaacson S, Mills R, Williams H, Chi-Burris K, Corbett A, et al. Pimavanserin for patients with Parkinson's disease psychosis: A randomised, placebo-controlled phase 3 trial. Lancet. 2014;**383**(9916):533-540. DOI: 10.1016/s0140-6736(13)62106-6

[89] Cummings J, Ballard C, Tariot P, Owen R, Foff E, Youakim J, et al. Pimavanserin: Potential treatment for dementia-related psychosis. The Journal of Prevention of Alzheimer's Disease. 2018;**5**(4):253-258. DOI: 10.14283/jpad.2018.29

[90] Cruz MP. Pimavanserin (Nuplazid): A treatment for hallucinations and delusions associated with Parkinson's disease. P T. 2017;**42**(6):368-371

Chapter 3

Homocysteine and Dementia in Parkinson Disease

Jin Jun Luo, Lin Zhang and Nae J. Dun

Abstract

Parkinson disease (PD) and dementia are neurodegenerative disorders that can be frequently seen in the elderly. Homocysteine (Hcy) is an intermediary metabolite from methylation, which is highly relevant to body physiologic activities including DNA metabolism. Elevated plasma level of homocysteine (eHcy) is seen in normal aging individuals and patients with neurologic disorders such as PD or dementia. Although clinical observations confirm the finding that eHcy is prevalent in PD patients, the former is not a recognized etiology causing PD but rather, an adverse outcome related to the therapy of dopaminergic supplementation. Notably, eHcy may exacerbate various medical and neurologic conditions such as cardiovascular diseases, stroke, mild cognitive impairment, all of which are potential risks for dementia. This chapter discusses the concerns of eHcy relative to dementia in PD.

Keywords: dementia, homocysteine, neurodegeneration, Parkinson disease

1. Introduction

Parkinson disease (PD) is a progressive, neurodegenerative disorder caused by multifactorial including genetic and environmental influences [1, 2]. PD is the second most common neurodegenerative disorder after Alzheimer disease (AD), affecting approximately 1.5–2% of individuals over 65 years and 4% over 80 years of age. Incidence of PD is estimated ranging from 5 to >35 per 100,000 populations [3]. In an early population-based study with pathologically confirmed clinical diagnoses in Minnesota, USA, the incidence of PD was 21 cases per 100,000 person-years [4]. Onset of PD before 50 years of age is not common, but the incidence escalates 5–10-fold from the sixth to the ninth decade of life [2–6]. Noticeably, PD is twice as common in men than in women in most populations [5, 7], suggesting gender and/or age may play a role in the development of PD [8]. The exact cause for PD is not fully understood and much research has been directed the past 200 years toward the underlying etiology responsible for the development of PD.

2. Clinical features of PD

Clinical manifestations of PD include motor and non-motor symptoms. The classic motor features of PD are tremor, rigidity, akinesia/bradykinesia, and postural instability (mnemonic "TRAP") [9] although recent revision of the diagnostic criteria excludes postural instability as a fourth hallmark (**Figure 1**). PD has a wide variety of non-motor symptoms such as cognitive impairment, sleep disturbances,

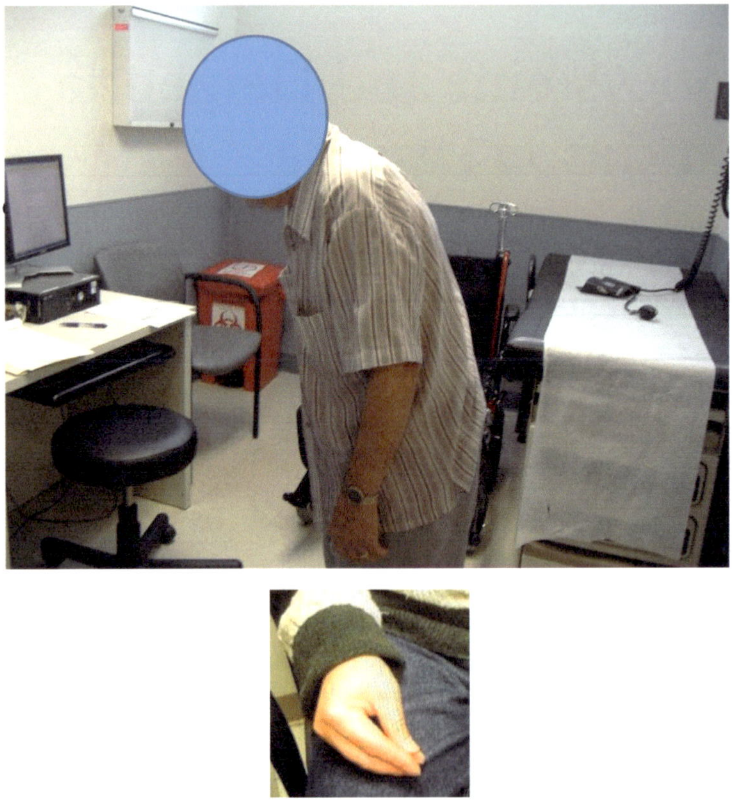

Figure 1.
Features of Parkinson disease.

depression, and hallucinations [10, 11]. The neuropathological hallmarks of PD are loss of dopaminergic neurons in the substantia nigra resulting in striatal dopamine deficiency and intracellular inclusions of Lewy body containing aggregates of α-synuclein. Loss of dopaminergic neurons in the substantia nigra is responsible for the inability to synthesize an adequate amount of the neurotransmitter dopamine in the brain. Treatment of PD usually includes pharmacological replacement of striatal dopamine, in addition to non-dopaminergic agents to treat both motor and non-motor symptoms, and surgical interventions such as deep brain stimulation for refractory motor symptoms.

3. Why dementia in PD?

Dementia is an acquired, irreversible neurodegenerative disorder manifesting progressive impairment in cognitive function and affecting the awareness of surroundings. It is caused by structural and/or functional disturbances in the cerebral cortex, its subcortical connections, or both. It may result from genetic and environmental influences. Dementia and cognitive impairment are the leading chronic disease contributors to disability and particularly, dependence among older people worldwide [12]. Many diseases including neurologic such as stroke, severe brain traumatic injury, and depression; and non-neurologic such as cardiovascular, toxic, malnutrition, systemic infection/inflammation can now be added to the list, particularly of health consequences of aging, causing initially cognitive decline, or mild cognitive impairment (MCI), and subsequently advancing to dementia.

Dementia has been estimated to affect 5–20% of populations older than 65 years [13, 14] and its incidence increases with age. A recent epidemiologic study [15] based on the database of System for the Development of Research in Primary Care (SIDIAP) in Spain enrolled with 1,035,046 subjects, mainly women (56.2%), from urban areas (80.9%) and 75.7 (7.9) years old on average disclosed that the estimated incidence of dementia was at 9.5/1000 person-years (95% CI 9.3–9.7), adjusted for gender at 9.3/1000 person-years (95% CI 9.0–9.6), age at 8.8/1000 person-years (95% CI 8.4–9.2), and combining age-and-gender at 8.6/1000 person-years (95% CI 8.0–9.3). Interestingly, women have a higher incidence than men, and the incidence increased with age: namely 25 times higher in the individuals of 90 years and older than in the 65–69 years [15]. Indeed, the incidence of dementia increases exponentially worldwide with increasing age; [16] particularly, early hallucinations and akinetic-dominant PD were associated with an increased risk of dementia [17]. Based on the available estimates for the global incidence of dementia dating from 2010, the incidence of dementia doubled with every 5.9-year increase in age, from 3.1/1000 person-years at age 60–64 to 175.0/1000 person-years at age 95+ [16]. The number of people living with dementia worldwide in 2015 was estimated to be at 47.47 million, reaching 75.63 million in 2030 and 135.46 million in 2050 [12, 18].

Dementia in PD (PDD) is a clinical syndrome with impaired attention, executive dysfunctions, and secondarily impaired memory. The most significant deficits are loss of cholinergic activities and the degrees of Lewy bodies in certain limbic and cortical areas in neuropathology, both of which correlate well with the clinical severity of dementia in PDD [19]. Clinical trials have shown cholinesterase inhibitors, which may be beneficial in PDD [19].

Notably, dementia in PD was not initially included in the article "*An Essay on the Shaking Palsy*" published in 1817 by James Parkinson [20–22], who first described the symptoms and signs of 6 patients, the differential diagnosis, etiology, and contemporary treatment in his monograph comprising 5 chapters and 66 pages. This eponymous disease was named after him. Importantly, many atypical clinical features of PD have been subsequently detailed over the past several decades. Among those non-motor symptoms of PD, dementia was not recognized until 3 decades ago and now is increasingly being recognized [23]. Robust clinical studies have been conducted on the epidemiology, clinical features, pathological correlations, and treatment of dementia in PD. The International PD and Movement Disorders Society published new clinical criteria for PD diagnosis in 2015 that manifestation of concomitant dementia is no longer as an exclusion criterion [21, 22]. The new diagnostic criteria accept the diagnosis of PD independent of when dementia arises (before or within the first year as well as after that) as long as the clinical criteria for PD are fulfilled. These diagnostic criteria have been validated subsequently by demonstrating high sensitivity and specificity compared with the gold standard, expert diagnosis with higher sensitivity and specificity [24]. It is now known that PDD represents one of the most significant non-motor symptoms, especially in more advanced PD [25, 26]. The prevalence of PDD has been reported ranging from 20 to more than 70% of PD patients depending on the diagnostic criteria employed and the nature of the study population conducted [19, 27]. An earlier study has reported the point prevalence of PDD to be approximately 30% [28], indicating that dementia is common in PD. Importantly, PDD is associated with increased mortality, impairments in well-being, caregiver strain with increased health care, and institutionalization costs [29–31]. Risks of developing dementia in PD have drawn intense interest and they are often an important topic for health workers, patients, and their families given its significant impact [32]. Searching for the risks, predictors, and measures of prevention for dementia in PD patients continues.

4. What is mild cognitive impairment?

Mild cognitive impairment (MCI) is a medical condition, encountered with normal aging, that clinically borders between early dementia and cognitive impairments. Individuals who experience MCI are still able to perform daily activities, but with evidence of a gradual decline in memory or other cognitive functions. MCI is divided into two subtypes: amnestic and nonamnestic, but neither type meets the diagnostic criteria for dementia. MCI is considered a prodrome to dementia as the rates of conversion from MCI to dementia are greater than that of normal cognition associated with aging [33]. Cognitive decline includes deficit in executive, visuospatial function, attention, and memory. Behavioral symptoms are frequent including apathy, visual hallucinations, and delusions. Notably, the most prominent pathology in PDD is the expression of Lewy body type of inclusions. Insofar as the biochemical deficit is concerned, a cholinergic hypoactivity has been documented. Placebo-controlled randomized trials with cholinesterase inhibitors have shown modest but significant benefits in cognition, behavioral symptoms, and global functions [27]. Clinical observations and laboratory animal studies have shown that homocysteine plays a role in MCI and dementia.

5. What is homocysteine?

Homocysteine (Hcy) is an intermediary metabolite during the transmethylation of the essential sulfur-containing amino acid methionine. Hcy can be either remethylated to methionine or converted to cysteine through the transsulfuration pathway (**Figure 2**). In remethylation, there are two different pathways. One is the 5-methyltetrahydrofolate (5-MTHF) pathway. 5-MTHF is an active form of folate serving the methyl donor in the methionine synthase reaction, which requires vitamin B12 as a cofactor. 5-MTHF is produced by a reaction catalyzed by

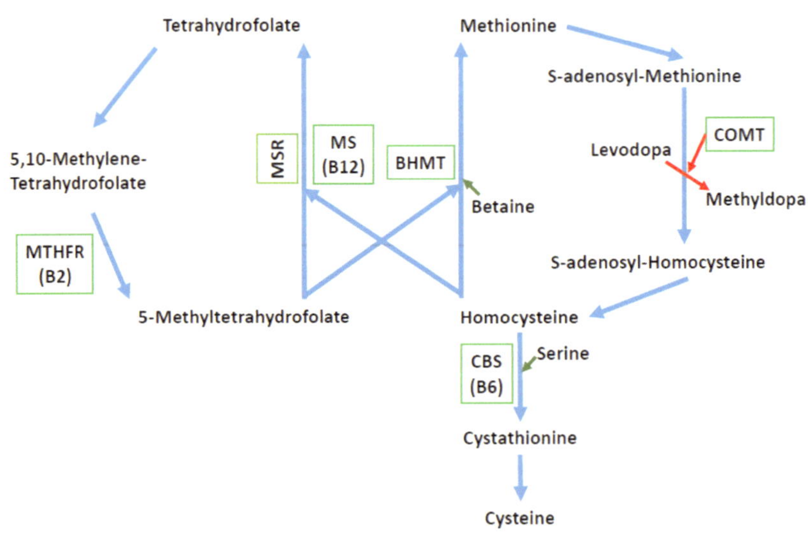

Figure 2.
Homocysteine metabolism. BHMT: *betaine-homocysteine methyltransferase;* CBS: *cystathionine beta-synthase; COMT: catechol-O-methyltransferase;* MTHFR: *5,10-methylene tetrahydrofolate reductase;* MS: *methionine synthase; MSR: methionine synthase reductase.* BHMT *is active in liver; CBS requires peridoxal phosphate (vitamin B6); MTHFR requires riboflavin* (B2)*; MS requires methylcobalamin* (B12)*;* MSR *is required for the reductive activation of MS. Methylation of levodopa and dopamine by COMT, that uses* S-adenosylmethionine *as a methyl donor to generate* S-*adenosylhomocysteine.*

5,10-methylenetetrahydrofolate reductase (MTHFR), which is a common, thermolabile enzyme. The methyl donor 5-MTHF is generated from 5,10-MTHF through the enzyme MTHFR. 5-MTHF is mainly synthesized in the liver and then distributed to various tissues and cells in the body where it acts as a methyl donor for transferring to Hcy *via* methionine synthase, which regenerates methionine. Mutations or polymorphisms of MTHFR may result in a decreased enzymatic activity, such as cytosine to thymidine substitution at the position 677 (C677T) or adenine to cytosine at 1298 (A1298C) of the MTHFR gene. Approximately 5% of the general population and 17% of patients with coronary artery disease are C677T homozygous. Polymorphism of A1298C is also linked with reduced enzymatic activity. Heterozygosity for both of these polymorphisms (C677T and A1298C) in pregnant women is associated with a greater risk of neural tube defects in newborns [33–40].

The second pathway whereby Hcy is methylated to methionine is by the enzyme betaine-homocysteine methyltransferase (BHMT). BHMT is also rich in the liver, whereas methionine synthase (MS, a B12-dependent enzyme) is present in all tissues and requires 5-methylene tetrahydrofolate as a methyl donor. The MS gene has several mutations and polymorphisms. Substitution of adenine to guanine at 2756 (A2756G) of MS has an allele frequency ranging from 8 to 32% in different populations; for example, mutation and polymorphisms occur in 8% of the population in West Bengal in India, 11% in East Asia, 17% in European, 18% in American, 28% in African, and 32% in South Asian populations [41]. The A2756G allele is associated with a moderate effect on Hcy levels [37]. Initially, this variant was thought to be associated with lower enzyme activity, causing elevated plasma level of homocysteine (eHcy) and DNA hypomethylation [42]. However, subsequent investigations suggested a modest inverse association between 2756GG polymorphism and Hcy levels, indicating increased enzymatic activity of the variant genotype with an effect to reduce Hcy levels [43].

Methionine synthase reductase (MSR) is critical for the reductive activation of MS. Mutation in the gene for MSR results in an autosomal recessive disorder of folate/cobalamin metabolism, leading to hyperhomocysteinemia, hypomethioninemia, and megaloblastic anemia. At least 11 mutations with defective MSR genes have been reported [44].

In the transsulfuration pathway, cystathionine beta-synthase (CBS), which requires vitamin B6 as a cofactor, converts Hcy to serine with the formation of cystathionine, which is subsequently cleaved to form cysteine by cystathionase. More than 150 mutations with a change in single amino acid have been reported in the CBS gene that causes eHcy and homocystinuria. The most common mutation substitutes the amino acid isoleucine with the amino acid threonine at position 278 in the enzyme. Another common mutation, which is the most frequent cause of homocystinuria in the Irish population, replaces the amino acid glycine with the amino acid serine at position 307, causing eHcy and homocystinuria [33, 34, 38, 40].

6. Why is Hcy a concern in PDD?

eHcy has been considered as a risk factor for various pathophysiologic conditions including normal aging, static lifestyle with lack of physical exercise, cigarette smoking, cardiovascular disorders, chronic kidney disease, hypertension, hyperlipidemia, etc. Earlier clinical observations revealed the presence of eHcy in PD patients, which was initially considered to be relevant to PD neurodegeneration [45]. However, subsequent studies showed a lack of convincing evidence that eHcy and PD were causally related; [46] rather, eHcy could be generated by the administration of dopaminergic agents, which was confirmed in patients in clinical [47–51] and animals in laboratory studies [52, 53].

eHcy may exert its neurotoxic effects *via* a direct and/or indirect intracellular action by stimulating free radical production, provoking oxidative stress response, increasing cytosolic calcium level, rendering hypersensitivity to excitotoxicity, interfering with mitochondrial function, depleting ATP reserve, impairing transmethylation of DNA, resulting in DNA breakage, and leading to neural cell death and apoptosis [33, 38, 54, 55].

The most common cause of eHcy is the deficiency of folate or vitamin B12, enzymatic derangements due to genetic mutation or polymorphisms, and/or environmental stress alone or in combination. However, the occurrence of eHcy in patients with PD has been proven not to be causally related to vitamin deficiency but an adverse effect of dopamine supplementation from methylation of levodopa and dopamine by catechol-O-methyltransferase (COMT), an enzyme that uses *S*-adenosylmethionine as a methyl donor to generate *S*-adenosylhomocysteine, which is rapidly converted to Hcy [51, 56].

eHcy is also a risk factor for vascular disease and potentially for dementia. eHcy is observed to be associated with the transition from being cognitively healthy to develop dementia [57–59]. Observations from a longitudinal clinical study over 6 years revealed that eHcy is an independent risk factor for the decline of cognitive performance in normal elderly subjects [60] and patients with AD; therefore, a negative role of eHcy in cognitive functions was proposed [13]. To support this claim, a study on the relationship between eHcy and hippocampal function or generalization performance was performed. The result demonstrated the role of eHcy in declining cognitive function in both healthy controls and patients with MCI [58]. Additionally, a double-blind, randomized controlled clinical study showed an association of the degrees of eHcy with the rates of brain atrophy in elderly with MCI [59]. Indeed, dopamine supplementation therapy with levodopa may render patients with PD at an increased risk for vascular disease by promoting eHcy and therefore, susceptible to becoming PDD [51] *via* the mechanism of COMT in levodopa therapy [51, 56]. However, controversy exists regarding the evidence for associations between MCI and eHcy [61–63] and dementia in long-term PD patients. A recent retrospective study [32] has investigated the frequency of PDD in a pooled 2327 PD patients across the UK and Australia. Of the PD participants, 36 with disease durations of 20 years or longer were identified. Among these 36 patients with long durations of PD, only 7 (19%) were recognized as probable PDD, and 34 (94%) manifested a non-tremor dominant phenotype. The authors concluded that the prevalence of dementia in long-term PD patients may be lower than anticipated and the trajectory of cognitive decline in PD patients can be different [32].

7. How should we deal with Hcy in PD?

As aforementioned, eHcy in patients with PD may result from the adverse effect of therapeutic dopamine supplementation with levodopa, rather than a vitamin deficiency [51, 64–66]. This observation has been confirmed in several independent studies showing that pharmacologic treatment of PD patients with levodopa therapy is associated with eHcy, which may irreversibly promote the occurrence of atherosclerotic vascular disease and stroke, both are risk factors for MCI and dementia [48, 67].

It is a standard practice to administer a peripheral-acting dopa decarboxylase inhibitor (DDCI; carbidopa) simultaneously with levodopa to treat PD patients, in which DDCI prevents levodopa from being metabolized into dopamine peripherally. However, co-administering a DDCI with levodopa results in increased metabolism of levodopa to 3-O-methyldopa via the enzyme COMT in peripheral tissues [68]. Apparently, COMT activity requires S-adenosyl-L-methionine (SAM) as the methyl donor, leading to the formation of the by-product, S-adenosyl-L-homocysteine (SAH), which can be further hydrolyzed to homocysteine leading to eHcy [53]. Indeed, eHcy has been detected in PD patients treated with levodopa, compared to age- and sex-matched controls, and to non-levodopa treated PD patients, and also has been replicated in laboratory animals [52, 53]. The increase in the blood level of Hcy after administering a single dose of levodopa can be reduced with co-administering a COMT inhibitor, such as entacapone [53, 69], suggesting that a COMT inhibitor can prevent levodopa-induced eHcy via the COMT mechanism and bears potential therapeutic benefits in reducing the risk of eHcy-related vascular diseases [69].

It is noteworthy levodopa, the most effective drug known in the treatment of PD, has been shown to be able to induce eHcy in PD patients [47, 49–52, 56, 66, 70–72]. This increase is even more pronounced in patients with polymorphisms of the enzyme MTHFR, such as C677T [49, 72].

Clinical observations revealed that eHcy may be involved with various neurologic conditions, including MCI, dementia, epilepsy, stroke, and neurodevelopmental disorders [33]. In addition, eHcy-induced neurotoxicity has been demonstrated, causing hippocampal neuronal death [55], which may be associated with cognitive decline leading to dementia. Hcy can be marked in humans by radiological evidence of white matter lesions as well as silent brain infarcts and atrophy of the cerebral cortex and hippocampus [73], even in healthy, middle-aged adults [74].

Epidemiologic studies have shown that eHcy is an independent risk factor for cardiovascular diseases and responsible for about 10% of total risk [75], even in the youths [76]. eHcy may cause vascular endothelial cell dysfunction leading to hypercoagulation, atherosclerosis, and stroke [77], which may, in turn, play a role in the pathogenesis of neurodegeneration, causing MCI and dementia [38]. The estimated hierarchy of eHcy relevant to the risk of cardiovascular diseases and stroke was proposed as 7 μM, low; 8–11 μM, moderate; 12–16 μM, high; >16 μM, very high [78]. Laboratory studies showed that eHcy potentiates Aβ neurotoxicity in cultured neurons [79], which is relevant to the development of AD and dementia. In organotypic cultures, both Hcy and its metabolites exhibit excitotoxic potency by interaction with various glutamate receptor subtypes [79, 80].

Evidence from clinical and preclinical studies has shown that eHcy is a risk factor for stroke, coronary artery and cardiovascular disease, and dementia [39, 40, 73, 81–85]. Levodopa therapy, rather than the course of PD, was proposed to cause eHcy in PD patients. The deficiency of folate or vitamin B12 does not fully explain eHcy in these patients [51]. Collectively, findings of levodopa associated with eHcy [47, 49–52, 56, 66, 70–72] suggested a disconcerting possibility that levodopa therapy may cause eHcy and subsequently increase the risk of dementia and other medical conditions such as atherosclerotic cardiovascular disease, stroke, and MCI [33, 67, 86]. Notably, the mean plasma Hcy levels in patients with PD were 31% higher in levodopa-treated patients, which was as a consequence of levodopa methylation by COMT [51], and eHcy in PD patients treated with levodopa is observed to be associated with a nearly twofold increased prevalence of coronary artery diseases [51]. A treatment aiming to decrease the formation of eHcy in PD patients may bear the potential beneficial and remote effects for patients with PD. [33, 67, 86]

Additionally, eHcy was considered as a strong and independent risk factor for osteoporotic fracture of the hip in the elderly [87, 88], particularly for elderly women [88]. Patients with homocystinuria are frequently associated with skeletal deformities, including osteoporosis. Importantly, eHcy also has been documented as an independent risk for peripheral neuropathy [89–93]. Collectively, eHcy may play a role in promoting adversely effects on daily living in PD patients.

Currently, no effective therapy to cure neurodegeneration is clinically available. The best approach in clinical practice is primarily prevention through the modification of acquired risk factors [33, 67, 86]. As aforementioned, eHcy may play a role in promoting the early onset of various medical and neurologic conditions even during normal aging [60], potentially accelerates neurodegeneration, and exacerbates symptoms of those ailments, and prophylactic treatment of eHcy may be beneficial. In fact, generation of eHcy from levodopa administration is associated with a greater reduction in Hcy from co-administration of a COMT inhibitor and entacapone [56, 94]. Clinically, administration of vitamin B-complex with folate to reduce eHcy is inexpensive, potentially effective, and devoid of significant adverse effects, therefore, having an exceptionally favorable therapeutic index [75, 95, 96]. Well-designed prospective randomized placebo-controlled clinical trials may be warranted to evaluate the efficacy of co-administering vitamin B-complex with folate to patients with eHcy in order to delay the onset or mitigate the severity of neurologic disorders [67, 86]. Of course, elimination of the occurrence of atherosclerotic cardiovascular disease or MCI and dementia should not be expected even when folate status is kept sufficiently high and in B-complex regimen. Similarly, improvements in folate status may not eliminate cognitive decline in patients with PDD. Administration of B-complex with folate is inexpensive and with an exceptionally favorable benefit/risk ratio. However, direct evidence of eHcy as a therapeutic target in order to prevent dementia is currently not available. The therapeutic efficacy of lowering eHcy to prevent PDD remains to be firmly established [78].

8. Summary

PD is a progressive, neurodegenerative disorder. The high prevalence of PDD is the most common manifestation of non-motor symptoms of PD. eHcy can be seen in many pathologic and physiologic conditions such as normal aging, deficiency of vitamin B12 or folic acid, enzymatic deviation due to genetic polymorphisms, concomitant chronic diseases, or dopamine supplementary therapy. eHcy has been considered as an independent risk factor for many medical and neurological conditions including atherosclerotic cardiovascular diseases, stroke, and MCI, all of which are potential risks for the development of dementia in PD. Additionally, eHcy may cause osteoporosis, hip fracture, and peripheral neuropathy, which may worsen daily living and compromise the quality of life in patients with PDD. Treatment with COMT inhibitor and B-complex together with folate to prevent or reduce eHcy in PD patients may prove to be a potentially valuable and cost-effective approach to exerting therapeutic efficacy of reducing eHcy.

Conflict of interest

All authors reported no conflict of interest.

Author details

Jin Jun Luo[1,3]*, Lin Zhang[2] and Nae J. Dun[3]

1 Neurology, Lewis Katz School of Medicine at Temple University, Philadelphia, PA, USA

2 Neurology, University of California Davis, Sacramento, CA, USA

3 Pharmacology, Lewis Katz School of Medicine at Temple University, Philadelphia, PA, USA

*Address all correspondence to: jin.jun.luo@temple.edu

References

[1] Kouli ATK, Kuan WL. Parkinson's Disease: Etiology, Neuropathology, and Pathogenesis. Brisbane, Australia: Codon Publications; 2018

[2] Poewe W, Seppi K, Tanner CM, et al. Parkinson disease. Nature Reviews Disease Primers. 2017;**3**:17013

[3] Twelves D, Perkins KS, Counsell C. Systematic review of incidence studies of Parkinson's disease. Movement Disorders. 2003;**18**(1):19-31

[4] Savica R, Grossardt BR, Bower JH, Ahlskog JE, Rocca WA. Incidence and pathology of synucleinopathies and tauopathies related to parkinsonism. JAMA Neurology. 2013;**70**(7):859-866

[5] Van Den Eeden SK, Tanner CM, Bernstein AL, et al. Incidence of Parkinson's disease: Variation by age, gender, and race/ethnicity. American Journal of Epidemiology. 2003;**157**(11):1015-1022

[6] Pringsheim T, Jette N, Frolkis A, Steeves TD. The prevalence of Parkinson's disease: A systematic review and meta-analysis. Movement Disorders. 2014;**29**(13):1583-1590

[7] Baldereschi M, Di Carlo A, Rocca WA, et al. Parkinson's disease and parkinsonism in a longitudinal study: Two-fold higher incidence in men. ILSA Working Group. Italian Longitudinal Study on Aging. Neurology. 2000;**55**(9):1358-1363

[8] Luo JJ, Dun NJ. Estrogen and Parkinson's disease. Current Trends in Neurology. 2011;**5**:49-57

[9] Jankovic J. Parkinson's disease: Clinical features and diagnosis. Journal of Neurology, Neurosurgery, and Psychiatry. 2008;**79**(4):368-376

[10] Chaudhuri KR, Healy DG, Schapira AH. Non-motor symptoms of Parkinson's disease: Diagnosis and management. Lancet Neurology. 2006;**5**(3):235-245

[11] Sauerbier A, Jenner P, Todorova A, Chaudhuri KR. Non motor subtypes and Parkinson's disease. Parkinsonism & Related Disorders. 2016;**22**(Suppl 1):S41-S46

[12] WHO. The Epidemiology and Impact of Dementia: Current State and Future Trends. WHO/MSD/MER/15.3. 2015. pp. 01-04. https://www.who.int/mental_health/neurology/dementia/dementia_thematicbrief_epidemiology.pdf. Accessed on January 31, 2021

[13] Annerbo S, Wahlund LO, Lokk J. The significance of thyroid-stimulating hormone and homocysteine in the development of Alzheimer's disease in mild cognitive impairment: A 6-year follow-up study. American Journal of Alzheimer's Disease and Other Dementias. 2006;**21**(3):182-188

[14] Postiglione A, Milan G, Ruocco A, Gallotta G, Guiotto G, Di Minno G. Plasma folate, vitamin B(12), and total homocysteine and homozygosity for the C677T mutation of the 5,10-methylene tetrahydrofolate reductase gene in patients with Alzheimer's dementia. A case-control study. Gerontology. 2001;**47**(6):324-329

[15] Ponjoan A, Garre-Olmo J, Blanch J, et al. Epidemiology of dementia: Prevalence and incidence estimates using validated electronic health records from primary care. Clinical Epidemiology. 2019;**11**:217-228

[16] WHO. Dementia: A Public Health Priority. World Health Organization; 2012

[17] Aarsland D, Andersen K, Larsen JP, Lolk A, Kragh-Sorensen P. Prevalence and characteristics of dementia in Parkinson disease: An 8-year

prospective study. Archives of Neurology. 2003;**60**(3):387-392

[18] Government. Policy Brief for G8 Heads of Government. The Global Impact of Dementia 2013-2050. London: Alzheimer's Disease International; 2013.

[19] Emre M. Dementia in Parkinson's disease: Cause and treatment. Current Opinion in Neurology. Aug 2004;**17**(4): 399-404

[20] Parkinson J. An essay on the shaking palsy. 1817. The Journal of Neuropsychiatry and Clinical Neurosciences. 2002;**14**(2):223-236. discussion 222

[21] Postuma RB, Berg D, Stern M, et al. MDS clinical diagnostic criteria for Parkinson's disease. Movement Disorders. 2015;**30**(12):1591-1601

[22] Rizzo G, Copetti M, Arcuti S, Martino D, Fontana A, Logroscino G. Accuracy of clinical diagnosis of Parkinson disease: A systematic review and meta-analysis. Neurology. 2016;**86**(6):566-576

[23] Meireles J, Massano J. Cognitive impairment and dementia in Parkinson's disease: Clinical features, diagnosis, and management. Frontiers in Neurology. 2012;**3**:88

[24] Postuma RB, Poewe W, Litvan I, et al. Validation of the MDS clinical diagnostic criteria for Parkinson's disease. Movement Disorders. 2018; **33**(10):1601-1608

[25] Braak H, Rub U, Jansen Steur EN, Del Tredici K, de Vos RA. Cognitive status correlates with neuropathologic stage in Parkinson disease. Neurology. 2005;**64**(8):1404-1410

[26] Emre M, Aarsland D, Brown R, et al. Clinical diagnostic criteria for dementia associated with Parkinson's disease. Movement Disorders. 2007;**22**(12): 1689-1707. quiz 1837

[27] Hanagasi HA, Tufekcioglu Z, Emre M. Dementia in Parkinson's disease. Journal of the Neurological Sciences. 2017;**374**:26-31

[28] Aarsland D, Zaccai J, Brayne C. A systematic review of prevalence studies of dementia in Parkinson's disease. Movement Disorders. 2005;**20**(10): 1255-1263

[29] Levy G, Tang MX, Louis ED, et al. The association of incident dementia with mortality in PD. Neurology. 2002;**59**(11):1708-1713

[30] Vossius C, Larsen JP, Janvin C, Aarsland D. The economic impact of cognitive impairment in Parkinson's disease. Movement Disorders. 2011;**26**(8):1541-1544

[31] Aarsland D, Bronnick K, Ehrt U, et al. Neuropsychiatric symptoms in patients with Parkinson's disease and dementia: Frequency, profile and associated care giver stress. Journal of Neurology, Neurosurgery, and Psychiatry. 2007;**78**(1):36-42

[32] Szeto JYY, Walton CC, Rizos A, et al. Dementia in long-term Parkinson's disease patients: A multicentre retrospective study. npj Parkinson's Disease. 2020;**6**(1):2

[33] Ansari R, Mahta A, Mallack E, Luo JJ. Erratum: Hyperhomocysteinemia and neurologic disorders: A review. Journal of Clinical Neurology. 2015;**11**(1):106

[34] Luft FC. Who's afraid of homocysteine? Journal of Molecular Medicine (Berlin, Germany). 2000;**78**(3):119-120

[35] Greene ND, Stanier P, Copp AJ. Genetics of human neural tube defects. Human Molecular Genetics. 2009;**18**(R2):R113-R129

[36] Mishra PR, Barik M, Mahapatra AK. Molecular genetics involved in neural

tube defects: Recent advances and future prospective for molecular medicine. Neurology India. 2020;**68**(5):1144-1150

[37] Laraqui A, Allami A, Carrie A, et al. Influence of methionine synthase (A2756G) and methionine synthase reductase (A66G) polymorphisms on plasma homocysteine levels and relation to risk of coronary artery disease. Acta Cardiologica. 2006;**61**(1):51-61

[38] Mattson MP, Shea TB. Folate and homocysteine metabolism in neural plasticity and neurodegenerative disorders. Trends in Neurosciences. 2003;**26**(3):137-146

[39] Kelly PJ, Rosand J, Kistler JP, et al. Homocysteine, MTHFR 677C-->T polymorphism, and risk of ischemic stroke: Results of a meta-analysis. Neurology. 2002;**59**(4):529-536

[40] Schnyder G, Roffi M, Flammer Y, Pin R, Hess OM. Effect of homocysteine-lowering therapy with folic acid, vitamin B12, and vitamin B6 on clinical outcome after percutaneous coronary intervention: The Swiss Heart study: A randomized controlled trial. JAMA. 2002;**288**(8):973-979

[41] Sadhukhan S, Paul S, Bankura B, Munian D, Ghosh S, Das M. Genetic analysis of MTR and MTRR gene polymorphisms in healthy mothers from Eastern part of India. International Journal of Research and Development in Pharmacy & Life Sciences. 2017;**7**(1):2881-2885

[42] Matsuo K, Suzuki R, Hamajima N, et al. Association between polymorphisms of folate- and methionine-metabolizing enzymes and susceptibility to malignant lymphoma. Blood. 2001;**97**(10):3205-3209

[43] Goode EL, Potter JD, Bigler J, Ulrich CM. Methionine synthase D919G polymorphism, folate metabolism, and colorectal adenoma risk. Cancer Epidemiology, Biomarkers & Prevention. 2004;**13**(1):157-162

[44] Wilson A, Leclerc D, Rosenblatt DS, Gravel RA. Molecular basis for methionine synthase reductase deficiency in patients belonging to the cblE complementation group of disorders in folate/cobalamin metabolism. Human Molecular Genetics. 1999;**8**(11):2009-2016

[45] Bialecka M, Robowski P, Honczarenko K, Roszmann A, Slawek J. Genetic and environmental factors for hyperhomocysteinaemia and its clinical implications in Parkinson's disease. Neurologia i Neurochirurgia Polska. 2009;**43**(3):272-285

[46] Martignoni E, Tassorelli C, Nappi G, Zangaglia R, Pacchetti C, Blandini F. Homocysteine and Parkinson's disease: A dangerous liaison? Journal of the Neurological Sciences. 2007;**257**(1-2):31-37

[47] Kuhn W, Roebroek R, Blom H, et al. Elevated plasma levels of homocysteine in Parkinson's disease. European Neurology. 1998;**40**(4):225-227

[48] Muller T, Werne B, Fowler B, Kuhn W. Nigral endothelial dysfunction, homocysteine, and Parkinson's disease. Lancet. 1999;**354**(9173):126-127

[49] Yasui K, Nakaso K, Kowa H, Takeshima T, Nakashima K. Levodopa-induced hyperhomocysteinaemia in Parkinson's disease. Acta Neurologica Scandinavica. 2003;**108**(1):66-67

[50] Miller JW, Selhub J, Nadeau MR, Thomas CA, Feldman RG, Wolf PA. Effect of L-dopa on plasma homocysteine in PD patients: Relationship to B-vitamin status. Neurology. 2003;**60**(7):1125-1129

[51] Rogers JD, Sanchez-Saffon A, Frol AB, Diaz-Arrastia R. Elevated

plasma homocysteine levels in patients treated with levodopa: Association with vascular disease. Archives of Neurology. 2003;**60**(1):59-64

[52] Allain P, Le Bouil A, Cordillet E, Le Quay L, Bagheri H, Montastruc JL. Sulfate and cysteine levels in the plasma of patients with Parkinson's disease. Neurotoxicology. 1995;**16**(3):527-529

[53] Miller JW, Shukitt-Hale B, Villalobos-Molina R, Nadeau MR, Selhub J, Joseph JA. Effect of L-Dopa and the catechol-O-methyltransferase inhibitor Ro 41-0960 on sulfur amino acid metabolites in rats. Clinical Neuropharmacology. 1997;**20**(1):55-66

[54] Ho PI, Ortiz D, Rogers E, Shea TB. Multiple aspects of homocysteine neurotoxicity: Glutamate excitotoxicity, kinase hyperactivation and DNA damage. Journal of Neuroscience Research. 2002;**70**(5):694-702

[55] Kruman II, Culmsee C, Chan SL, et al. Homocysteine elicits a DNA damage response in neurons that promotes apoptosis and hypersensitivity to excitotoxicity. Journal of Neuroscience. 2000;**20**(18):6920-6926

[56] Muller T, Kuhn W. Tolcapone decreases plasma levels of S-adenosyl-L-homocysteine and homocysteine in treated Parkinson's disease patients. European Journal of Clinical Pharmacology. 2006;**62**(6):447-450

[57] Blasko I, Jellinger K, Kemmler G, et al. Conversion from cognitive health to mild cognitive impairment and Alzheimer's disease: Prediction by plasma amyloid beta 42, medial temporal lobe atrophy and homocysteine. Neurobiology of Aging. 2008;**29**(1):1-11

[58] Moustafa AA, Hewedi DH, Eissa AM, Myers CE, Sadek HA. The relationship between associative learning, transfer generalization, and homocysteine levels in mild cognitive impairment. PLoS ONE. 2012;7(9):e46496

[59] Smith AD, Smith SM, de Jager CA, et al. Homocysteine-lowering by B vitamins slows the rate of accelerated brain atrophy in mild cognitive impairment: A randomized controlled trial. PLoS One. 2010;**5**(9):e12244

[60] Elias MF, Sullivan LM, D'Agostino RB, et al. Homocysteine and cognitive performance in the Framingham offspring study: Age is important. American Journal of Epidemiology. 2005;**162**(7):644-653

[61] Blasko I, Hinterberger M, Kemmler G, et al. Conversion from mild cognitive impairment to dementia: Influence of folic acid and vitamin B12 use in the VITA cohort. The Journal of Nutrition, Health & Aging. 2008;**16**(8):687-694

[62] Kim G, Kim H, Kim KN, et al. Relationship of cognitive function with B vitamin status, homocysteine, and tissue factor pathway inhibitor in cognitively impaired elderly: A cross-sectional survey. Journal of Alzheimer's Disease. 2013;**33**(3):853-862

[63] Reitz C, Tang MX, Miller J, Green R, Luchsinger JA. Plasma homocysteine and risk of mild cognitive impairment. Dementia and Geriatric Cognitive Disorders. 2009;**27**(1):11-17

[64] O'Suilleabhain PE, Sung V, Hernandez C, et al. Elevated plasma homocysteine level in patients with Parkinson disease: Motor, affective, and cognitive associations. Archives of Neurology. 2004;**61**(6):865-868

[65] Miller JW. Homocysteine, folate deficiency, and Parkinson's disease. Nutrition Reviews. 2002;**60**(12):410-413

[66] Blandini F, Fancellu R, Martignoni E, et al. Plasma

homocysteine and l-dopa metabolism in patients with Parkinson disease. Clinical Chemistry. 2001;**47**(6):1102-1104

[67] Postuma RB, Lang AE. Homocysteine and levodopa: Should Parkinson disease patients receive preventative therapy? Neurology. 2004;**63**(5):886-891

[68] Mannisto PT, Kaakkola S. New selective COMT inhibitors: Useful adjuncts for Parkinson's disease? Trends in Pharmacological Sciences. 1989;**10**(2):54-56

[69] Nissinen E, Nissinen H, Larjonmaa H, et al. The COMT inhibitor, entacapone, reduces levodopa-induced elevations in plasma homocysteine in healthy adult rats. Journal of Neural Transmission (Vienna). 2005;**112**(9):1213-1221

[70] Muller T, Woitalla D, Fowler B, Kuhn W. 3-OMD and homocysteine plasma levels in parkinsonian patients. Journal of Neural Transmission (Vienna). 2002;**109**(2):175-179

[71] Muller T, Woitalla D, Hauptmann B, Fowler B, Kuhn W. Decrease of methionine and S-adenosylmethionine and increase of homocysteine in treated patients with Parkinson's disease. Neuroscience Letters. 2001;**308**(1):54-56

[72] Yasui K, Kowa H, Nakaso K, Takeshima T, Nakashima K. Plasma homocysteine and MTHFR C677T genotype in levodopa-treated patients with PD. Neurology. 2000;**55**(3):437-440

[73] den Heijer T, Vermeer SE, Clarke R, et al. Homocysteine and brain atrophy on MRI of non-demented elderly. Brain. 2003;**126**(Pt 1):170-175

[74] Seshadri S, Wolf PA, Beiser AS, et al. Association of plasma total homocysteine levels with subclinical brain injury: Cerebral volumes, white matter hyperintensity, and silent brain infarcts at volumetric magnetic resonance imaging in the Framingham Offspring Study. Archives of Neurology. 2008;**65**(5):642-649

[75] Stanger O, Herrmann W, Pietrzik K, et al. Clinical use and rational management of homocysteine, folic acid, and B vitamins in cardiovascular and thrombotic diseases. Zeitschrift für Kardiologie. 2004;**93**(6):439-453

[76] Akar N, Akar E, Ozel D, Deda G, Sipahi T. Common mutations at the homocysteine metabolism pathway and pediatric stroke. Thrombosis Research. 2001;**102**(2):115-120

[77] Hankey GJ, Eikelboom JW. Homocysteine and stroke. Current Opinion in Neurology. 2001;**14**(1):95-102

[78] Toole JF, Malinow MR, Chambless LE, et al. Lowering homocysteine in patients with ischemic stroke to prevent recurrent stroke, myocardial infarction, and death: The Vitamin Intervention for Stroke Prevention (VISP) randomized controlled trial. JAMA. 2004;**291**(5):565-575

[79] Ho PI, Collins SC, Dhitavat S, et al. Homocysteine potentiates beta-amyloid neurotoxicity: Role of oxidative stress. Journal of Neurochemistry. 2001;**78**(2):249-253

[80] Flott-Rahmel B, Schurmann M, Schluff P, et al. Homocysteic and homocysteine sulphinic acid exhibit excitotoxicity in organotypic cultures from rat brain. European Journal of Pediatrics. 1998;**157**(Suppl 2):S112-S117

[81] Klerk M, Verhoef P, Clarke R, Blom HJ, Kok FJ, Schouten EG. MTHFR 677C-->T polymorphism and risk of coronary heart disease: A meta-analysis. JAMA. 2002;**288**(16):2023-2031

[82] Collaboration HS. Homocysteine and risk of ischemic heart disease and stroke: A meta-analysis. JAMA. 2002;**288**(16):2015-2022

[83] Seshadri S, Beiser A, Selhub J, et al. Plasma homocysteine as a risk factor for dementia and Alzheimer's disease. New England Journal of Medicine. 2002; **346**(7):476-483

[84] Vermeer SE, van Dijk EJ, Koudstaal PJ, et al. Homocysteine, silent brain infarcts, and white matter lesions: The Rotterdam Scan Study. Annals of Neurology. 2002;**51**(3):285-289

[85] Dufouil C, Alperovitch A, Ducros V, Tzourio C. Homocysteine, white matter hyperintensities, and cognition in healthy elderly people. Annals of Neurology. 2003;**53**(2): 214-221

[86] Luo JJ, Dun NJ. Should homocysteine be a therapetutic target for neurological disorders? Brain Disorders & Therapy. 2013;**2**:e107

[87] van Meurs JB, Dhonukshe-Rutten RA, Pluijm SM, et al. Homocysteine levels and the risk of osteoporotic fracture. New England Journal of Medicine. 2004;**350**(20):2033-2041

[88] McLean RR, Jacques PF, Selhub J, et al. Homocysteine as a predictive factor for hip fracture in older persons. New England Journal of Medicine. 2004;**350**(20):2042-2049

[89] Muller T, Renger K, Kuhn W. Levodopa-associated increase of homocysteine levels and sural axonal neurodegeneration. Archives of Neurology. 2004;**61**(5):657-660

[90] Luo JJ, Sivaraaman K, Nouh A, Dun NJ. Elevated plasma level of homocysteine is an independent risk factor for peripheral neuropathy. British Journal of Medicine and Medical Research. 2014;**4**(1):161-169

[91] Shandal V, Luo JJ. Clinical manifestations of isolated elevated homocysteine-induced peripheral neuropathy in adults. Journal of Clinical Neuromuscular Disease. 2016;**17**(3):106-109

[92] Luo JJ, Dun NJ. Causes of neuropathy in patients referred as "idiopathic neuropathy". Muscle & Nerve. 2016;**54**(5):983

[93] Hsu RT, Bumanlag F, Mehta AK, et al. Homocysteine and peripheral neuropathy. Journal of Neurology and Experimental Neuroscience. 2020;**6**(2):58-61

[94] Zesiewicz TA, Wecker L, Sullivan KL, Merlin LR, Hauser RA. The controversy concerning plasma homocysteine in Parkinson disease patients treated with levodopa alone or with entacapone: Effects of vitamin status. Clinical Neuropharmacology. 2006;**29**(3):106-111

[95] Clarke R, Armitage J. Vitamin supplements and cardiovascular risk: Review of the randomized trials of homocysteine-lowering vitamin supplements. Seminars in Thrombosis and Hemostasis. 2000;**26**(3):341-348

[96] Cockroft DL. Vitamin deficiencies and neural-tube defects: Human and animal studies. Human Reproduction. 1991;**6**(1):148-157

Section 2

Diagnostic Principles and Practices

Chapter 4

Diagnosis of Dementia with Lewy Bodies: Fluctuations, Biomarkers, and Beyond

John M. Olichney, Wentao Li, Yasmine Gharbaoui, Alison P. Kwok and Jade E. Jenkins

Abstract

Dementia with Lewy bodies (DLB), the second most common cause of dementia, remains a difficult condition to accurately diagnose and manage. Variable involvement of motor and cognitive functions, plus psychiatric and behavioral symptoms, contributes to the difficulty in managing DLB. Additionally, DLB can cause severe sleep disruption through REM sleep behavior disorder, autonomic symptoms, disruptions of olfaction/taste and mood, hallucinations, and more. In this chapter, advances and remaining challenges in the diagnosis of DLB are discussed, including a review of the current consensus criteria for DLB. The spectrum of disorders with Lewy bodies (LBs) are described including their wide-range of clinical presentations and overlap with Alzheimer's disease (AD) and Parkinson's disease with and without dementia. Particular consideration is given to advancements in quantification of cognitive fluctuations through improved clinical instruments, EEG, and other advanced biomarkers. Detection of DLB has improved, but establishing the "primary" pathology in cases with concomitant LB andd AD remains difficult. Likelihood of a clinical DLB syndrome is thought to be a function of distribution of LBs and severity of AD-type pathology. Further work is needed to better understand LB disease subtypes and the underlying pathophysiological mechanisms to allow for more targeted and comprehensive therapies.

Keywords: dementia, Lewy body, quantitative EEG, cognitive fluctuations

1. Introduction

1.1 Background

Dementia with Lewy bodies (DLB) is now generally accepted to be the second most common cause of dementia [1–4] accounting for approximately 20% of cases in the Western world, second in prevalence to only Alzheimer's disease (AD) (which is usually accompanied by some degree of cerebrovascular disease) [5]. Yet, it remains a difficult condition to accurately diagnose and manage. Highly sensitive and specific biomarkers from blood or cerebrospinal fluid (CSF) have been elusive and lag behind recent progress in AD. Management is challenging due to variable involvement of motor and cognitive function plus psychiatric and behavioral symptoms. Optimal management of motor parkinsonism is a very complex topic, worthy of textbook-length discussion, and DLB patients are generally not responsive (or only mildly responsive) to dopaminergic therapies. On top of this, DLB can cause severe disruption of sleep with REM sleep behavior disorder (RBD), autonomic symptoms, disruptions of olfaction/taste and mood, hallucinations, and more. Furthermore, these patients often have adverse effects of medications such as neuroleptic sensitivity, even to atypical antipsychotics, worsening of orthostatic hypotension by L-Dopa, and behavioral disinhibition to clonazepam and other benzodiazepines taken to treat RBD.

After reviewing the composition and regional distribution of Lewy bodies, this chapter will focus on the advances and remaining challenges in the diagnosis of DLB, rather than therapies and management, for which the reader is referred to other chapters in this volume. The spectrum of disorders with Lewy bodies will be described, with their wide range of clinical presentations and overlap with AD, as well as Parkinson's disease (PD) with and without dementia.

1.2 Scope and methods

This chapter reviews current consensus diagnosis criteria for dementia with Lewy bodies (DLB). This diagnosis can be challenging, especially if reliant on clinical criteria alone. Differentiation from PD with dementia (or without dementia) can be challenging and vague. Diagnosis in the setting of centers that focus on Alzheimer's disease or memory loss is particularly difficult as diagnostic criteria are less sensitive in these cohorts and some dementia cases with superimposed Lewy body (LB) pathology may only have a hint of the typical DLB or PD phenotype, or sometimes no attributable symptoms to their LB pathology. The 2017 DLB diagnostic criteria advanced the field by adding a category of "indicative biomarkers," and these are assigned equal diagnostic weight to the four core clinical features (fluctuating cognition, recurrent visual hallucinations, REM sleep behavior disorder (RBD), one or more cardinal features of parkinsonism).

This chapter will review the wide range of clinical presentations seen in Lewy body disease (motor, cognitive, and behavioral/psychiatric). The 2017 DLB diagnostic criteria will be reviewed in detail and the validation of these criteria and previous diagnostic criteria, for which there is greater neuropathological validation in the literature, will be critically reviewed. Advances in diagnosis will be reviewed, particularly in the areas of better quantification of fluctuations (made possible by electrophysiologic EEG studies and improved clinical instruments) and advanced biomarkers (including radionuclear imaging studies, polysomnography, CSF, and other biospecimens).

1.2.1 Literature search methods

This chapter was outlined by JMO. All coauthors participated in English literature searches conducted on PubMed and Google Scholar in January–February 2021. Search terms included: "incidence of Parkinson's disease," "prevalence of Parkinson's disease," "dementia with Lewy bodies epidemiology," "dementia with Lewy bodies REM sleep behavior disorder," "alpha-synucleinopathy," "dementia with Lewy bodies neuropathology," "dementia with Lewy bodies diagnosis," "Parkinson's disease dementia diagnosis," "dementia with Lewy bodies vs. Parkinson's disease dementia," "dementia with Lewy bodies clinical course," "serum and CSF biomarkers in synucleinopathy," "genetics of dementia with Lewy bodies," "dementia with Lewy bodies phenocopies," "imaging in dementia with Lewy bodies," and "electrophysiology and EEG in dementia with Lewy bodies."

1.3 Lewy bodies: What? Where? Why?

In 1912, Frederic Lewy described eosinophilic neuronal inclusion bodies in cases of "paralysis agitans" or idiopathic PD [6]. Lewy bodies (LBs) were initially found in a restricted distribution involving primarily the substantia nigra, locus caeruleus, dorsal vagus motor nucleus, and substantia innominata. Recent advances have shown that neocortical LBs are also commonly present in PD, as well as in other neurological disorders associated with cognitive and behavioral abnormalities. This family of disorders is now considered "synucleinopathies" but commonly overlaps with AD pathology, particularly among cases presenting with dementia or cognitive impairment.

Lewy bodies are intracytoplasmic eosinophilic inclusions that have slightly different appearances in the brain stem and basal forebrain ("classical" or brain stem–type LBs) than in the cerebral neocortex. The brain stem or classical-type LBs typically are large (>15 μm diameter) and have an eosinophilic core surrounded by a less densely staining peripheral halo. These LBs are usually single and round. Ultrastructurally, brain stem LBs have a dense osmiophilic core of granular and vesicular material and a concentric rim of radially or haphazardly arranged 8- to 10-nm diameter fibrils [7–10]. These fibrils are composed of abnormally phosphorylated neurofilament proteins aggregated with ubiquitin and α-synuclein (αS) [11]. The classical LB has been described in monoaminergic and cholinergic neurons [12, 13].

Neocortical LBs, in contrast, are smaller and more difficult to discern on hematoxylin and eosin staining than those found in the brain stem. They are more homogenous with no distinct core and have comparatively loosely arranged fibrils and granular material [14–18]. In the 1980s, identification of neocortical LBs was greatly facilitated by immunohistochemical staining with antiubiquitin antibodies [16]. Advances in the 1990s resulted in the development of antibodies that stain αS [19], which are now the gold standard for identifying LBs and other synuclein pathology such as Lewy neurites. αS is expressed in a number of neuronal and nonneuronal cell types such as cortical neurons, dopaminergic neurons, noradrenergic neurons, endothelial cells, and platelets. Its functions have been found to include the binding of fatty acids, the regulation of certain enzymes and transporters, the modulation of synaptic plasticity, and the production and regulation of neurotransmitter vesicles, including those for dopamine and acetylcholine [20, 21]. The filamentous ultrastructural character of the LB and its immunohistochemical profile suggest that disturbed neurofilament metabolism or transportation is important in LB formation [22].

Braak described an orderly progression of LBs and alpha-synuclein pathology in PD [23] from olfactory and brain stem to subcortical motor to cortical regions, with cortical involvement in the later stages 5 and 6. Most, but not all, cases follow this orderly progression, but some dementia series find cases that seem to skip the more primitive brain regions and instead can have cortical or limbic predilection, where other neurodegenerative pathology is also usually present. The overlap of LBs with AD pathology (senile plaques and neurofibrillary tangles) is particularly common, especially in cases of "plaque-predominant" AD, who usually have only intermediate Braak stage tau pathology [24, 25]. Cortical LBs have a predilection for the cingulate gyrus, insular, and frontotemporal cortex, a distribution that correlates with mesolimbic dopaminergic projections [25–27].

1.4 Epidemiology

The epidemiology of PD is much better understood than that of DLB. The prevalence of PD reaches ~1% in the U.S. by age 70 in males and 75 in females [28].

This prevalence then roughly doubles with every 10 years of aging and is expected to rise by ~25% in the U.S. population over the next 10 years. Criteria to diagnose DLB have shifted over the last two decades. Both clinical and biomarker indices have been reassigned and refined. Epidemiological studies of DLB are rare and difficult to distinguish from PD with dementia (discussed below under Clinical Presentations). The literature of the last 40 years has used a plethora of terms to refer to the spectrum of patients with Lewy body disease. These terms have included "senile dementia of the Lewy body type" [29], "Lewy body variant of Alzheimer's disease" [30], "diffuse Lewy body disease, common form, with plaques and/or tangles" [31], "Alzheimer's disease with Lewy bodies" [32], and "Parkinson's disease in Alzheimer's disease" [33] to refer to patients with dementia and/or concomitant AD pathology. Other terms such as "diffuse Lewy body disease, pure form" or "idiopathic PD" have been used to describe those without AD pathology. "Dementia with Lewy bodies" is now the preferred term, and current diagnostic criteria are discussed below. However, the neuropathology in these patients is heterogeneous. Also, one should keep in mind that DLB prevalence underestimates how common Lewy body pathology is with advanced aging, as it does not include those with mild cognitive impairment (MCI), pure motor parkinsonism, or Parkinson's disease with dementia. The clinical phenotypic heterogeneity and evolving diagnostic criteria further complicate the epidemiological study of DLB. Studies, especially community based with autopsy verification, are few and far between. Most studies of DLB prevalence have been based on selected dementia cohorts and are discussed under Pathological Validation below. In a longitudinal cohort of Olmsted, Minnesota, of 542 cases of parkinsonism, prevalence was 11.8% for DLB and 8.5% for PDD [34]. To truly reflect DLB prevalence, more population-based studies with diagnostic standardization are needed. The prevalence of subcortical LBs with aging is even higher, reported to be about 5–10% in "normal" older subjects over 50 years old, and appears to rise with increasing age [35]. When neurological or psychiatric symptoms are rigorously excluded, prevalence of LBs appears to still be ~4% in those above 70 years old [36].

1.4.1 Age of onset and survival

DLB primarily affects the elderly, with nearly all cases presenting at 60 years of age and older. In contrast, ~4% of PD cases present before age 50 and many of the "diffuse Lewy body disease (DLBD), pure form" cases described by Kosaka and colleagues had juvenile parkinsonism for decades before developing dementia [37]. Mean age of onset in a representative clinically diagnosed DLB cohort was 75.8 years (female = 77.2, male = 72.4) with mean survival time of only 5.5 years from symptom onset [38]. Cases with "Lewy body variant" (AD + LB pathology) had a mean survival of 7.7 years from onset of cognitive symptoms, ~1.5 years shorter than AD cases in an ADRC-autopsied cohort [39]. Clinicopathological studies of Lewy body density did not find correlations with age of onset, or with various other clinical features such as presence/absence of cognitive fluctuations, visual hallucinations, delusions, recurrent falls, or parkinsonism [40]. Age of onset is significantly later in DLB and PDD, relative to PD without dementia [41].

2. Clinical presentations

Diagnosing DLB often presents a particular challenge given the disease's wide range of symptomatology and high rate of comorbidity with AD and cerebrovascular disease (CVD). Associated signs and symptoms include various combinations of motor, cognitive, and psychiatric changes as described below. The common overlap of some of the most frequent symptoms (specifically visual hallucinations (VH), extrapyramidal signs (EPS), and RBD) is well illustrated in Mayo Clinic's DLB sample (see **Figure 1**, adapted from Ferman et al. [42]).

2.1 Cognition

As in other types of dementias, the diagnosis of DLB requires cognitive decline to be sufficiently severe as to prevent the ability to function independently. Current DSM-V criteria for dementia require "evidence of significant cognitive decline from a previous level of performance" that "interfere[s] with independence in everyday activities" most often described clinically as a loss of independence with instrumental activities of daily living such as paying bills or managing medications. Though previous editions of the DSM required a clear decline in at least two cognitive domains, this is no longer the case and DLB (along with other types of dementias) may be diagnosed based on decline in a single domain (along with functional decline). This represents an advance in the diagnosis of frontal and subcortical dementias, which typically present with dysexecutive deficits. When frontal-executive functions are significantly impaired, there is usually an impact on social, occupational, or independent function and a "single domain dementia" is therefore an appropriate diagnosis. Although patients with DLB often present with memory complaints and are frequently misdiagnosed with AD [43], neuropsychological testing tends to uncover relatively more pronounced impairments in attention, executive function, and visual processing in these patients compared with those with AD and normal cohorts. Patients with DLB tend to perform more poorly on tests of processing speed, divided attention, and perceptual discrimination than their counterparts with AD, who typically have more difficulty with short-term memory and object naming [44].

One of the core features of DLB is frequent fluctuations in cognition and/or alertness, which is discussed further below. Fluctuations can be particularly difficult to recognize, however, and can mimic seizures, delirium, and other transient alterations of alertness. Other cognitive differences between DLB and AD may be subtle and tend to be lost as the diseases progress. This increases the need to assess for motor and psychiatric changes, as well as the judicious deployment of biomarker testing (discussed below). Of note, functional limitations due to cognitive decline in patients who present with parkinsonism may be difficult to tease out from the downstream effects of motor changes.

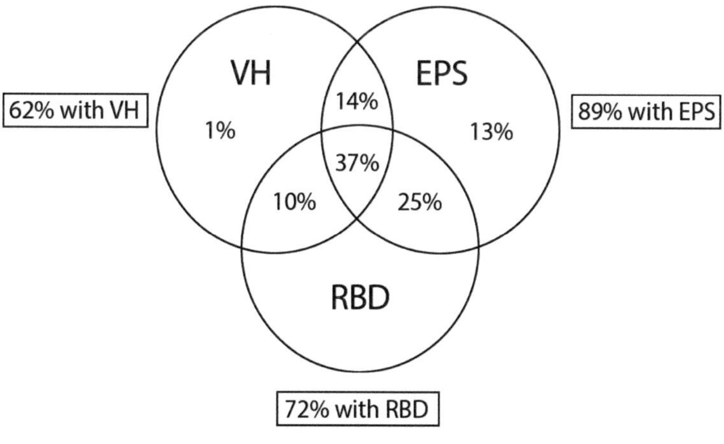

Figure 1.
Frequency of clinical features. Adapted from Ferman et al. [42] Neurology.

Contrary to James Parkinson's original description of the "senses and intellects" being "uninjured" [45], dementia is now recognized to occur fairly commonly in PD. The reported frequency of dementia in PD has varied widely—from 8% [46] to 81% [47] in early studies, owing largely to different populations, methodologies, and criteria for "dementia" [48]. Although mild cognitive impairment is very common in PD (and has been demonstrated in over 90% of PD patients [49]), many are unlikely to satisfy criteria for dementia. Most studies that required functional decline due to cognitive deficits have found dementia prevalence in PD to be between ~25 and 40% [47, 50].

2.2 Motor

The presence of Lewy bodies is associated with motor changes in both idiopathic Parkinson's disease and DLB. In contrast to idiopathic PD in which patients present with motor changes that precede significant cognitive decline, patients with DLB experience cognitive decline around the same time as motor symptoms/changes. Both conditions present with EPS, though DLB patients more often have "atypical" parkinsonian features such as a lack of resting tremor. The presence of one or more "cardinal" signs of parkinsonism (bradykinesia, rest tremor, or rigidity) is considered a core feature of DLB [51]. Other parkinsonian features are considered supportive for the diagnosis of DLB; these include postural instability, shuffling gait, frequent falls, dysautonomia, hypersomnia, and hyposmia. It has been long known that among PD patients, those with prominent postural instability and gait disorder (PIGD) have greater risk of cognitive deterioration than those with a tremor-dominant pattern of motor parkinsonism. Severity of motor impairment also predates dementia risk in PD [52]. In patients with possible CVD and atypical parkinsonism, neuroimaging is useful to rule out vascular causes of parkinsonism such as lacunar infarcts in the basal ganglia, or severe white matter lesions affecting motor tracts, speed, and balance.

2.3 Sleep

Another core clinical feature of DLB is the presence of REM sleep behavior disorder (RBD), which may begin years before the onset of other DLB symptoms. In RBD, patients recurrently manifest abnormal movements and/or vocalizations during REM sleep due to loss of atonia, which can be confirmed by polysomnogram. These episodes are often associated with a subjective experience of being chased or attacked within the dream and may result in injuries to self or bed partner. Caregivers, especially bed partners, will often report sleep disturbances and sleep-related injuries, as a consequence of DLB patients acting out their dreams [53]. Parkinsonism may arise at onset of RBD, or later in the course of the disease. RBD may precede diagnosis of DLB by several years or even decades. RBD should be differentiated from similar sleep disturbances in elderly patients such as confusional awakenings, periodic limb movements, and obstructive sleep apnea, which can be done via polysomnography. A wide range of sleep disturbances have been associated with PD, including reduced sleep spindle density, which appears to confer on increased risk of developing dementia [54–56].

2.4 Psychiatric

Compared to those with AD, DLB patients are particularly prone to depression and apathy that occurs earlier in the disease and is associated with increased caregiver burden and decreased quality of life [57]. It is not unusual to have primary psychiatric presentations of DLB, which may account for ~10–15% of cases [37]. Note that parkinsonian features such as masked facies and bradykinesia may initially be thought to represent a dysthymic affect and psychomotor retardation and attributed to a depressive disorder. While it is important to address psychiatric issues in this population, the lack of specificity of these symptoms makes this less useful clinically for the diagnosis of DLB. Notably, however, the development of recurrent, well-formed visual hallucinations [58] is a rather specific core feature of DLB. In fact, a patient with dementia who develops recurrent, detailed visual hallucinations (not due to delirium or other known causes) makes a strong case for the diagnosis of DLB. Less specific, but still suggestive of DLB, are nonvisual hallucinations and systematized delusions, including Capgras syndrome. Besides increasing caregiver burden, the neuropsychiatric symptoms accompanying DLB increase medical care expenses [59]. Psychiatric symptomatology in DLB is thought to cause lower quality of life and self-sufficiency [60].

Importantly, patients with Lewy body disorders tend to exhibit significant neuroleptic sensitivity and are at higher risk of extrapyramidal side effects. With the increasingly common use of atypical antipsychotics over conventional ones, this criterion has become less sensitive but remains an important consideration when managing a patient with agitation or psychotic features who may have an underlying Lewy body disorder. The management of such changes is best achieved through behavioral and environmental manipulations, such as verbal de-escalation and reassurance, setting a daily routine, regulating sleep, and regular exercise. Other nonpharmacological interventions include sensory and cognitive stimulation therapies such as acupressure, music therapy, and animal-assisted therapy, but these are less well understood in the DLB population. Nonpharmacological interventions have shown mixed results in their effectiveness but remain the first line of treatment given their low risk of adverse effects and their potential cost-effectiveness [61]. There is evidence that such interventions improve quality of life of dementia patients and their caregivers [62]. If behavioral symptoms are still not adequately controlled, a trial of low-dose atypical antipsychotic such as quetiapine or olanzapine may be appropriate with close monitoring of side effects including dystonia, orthostatic hypotension, and fall risks. It is also worth noting that the use of cholinesterase inhibitors (donepezil or rivastigmine) is associated with improvement in both cognitive and neuropsychiatric symptoms [63] and should be prioritized in the long term with the goal of minimizing administration of antipsychotics.

3. Current diagnostic criteria

The clinical diagnosis of DLB relies first on the presence of dementia as defined in the Cognition section of Clinical Presentations (adapted from McKeith et al. [51]). There are four identified "core" clinical features: (1) fluctuating cognition; (2) recurrent visual hallucinations; (3) RBD; and (4) at least one spontaneous cardinal feature of parkinsonism (bradykinesia, rest tremor, or rigidity). Two of these core features are sufficient to diagnose "probable" DLB. If only one core feature is present, probable DLB can be diagnosed with at least one of three indicative biomarkers: (1) reduced dopamine transporter uptake in basal ganglia on SPECT or PET, (2) low uptake of 123iodine-MIBG in myocardial scintigraphy, or (3) confirmation of REM sleep without atonia on polysomnography. These are discussed in the Section 5. In the absence of any core features, the presence of an indicative biomarker fulfills the criterion for diagnosing "possible" DLB. Possible DLB can also be diagnosed when a single core feature is present without any indicative biomarkers. "Supportive" clinical features and supportive biomarkers are consistent with DLB and may help with diagnostic evaluation but are of unclear diagnostic specificity. Supportive clinical features may include neuroleptic sensitivity, postural instability, frequent falls, severe autonomic dysfunction, urinary incontinence, hyposmia, and other psychiatric symptoms. Supportive biomarkers can be evaluated with CT/MRI (relative preservation of medial temporal lobe structures, indicating a higher likelihood of AD pathology), SPECT/PET (abnormal generalized uptake with reduced occipital activity), as well as EEG (prominent posterior slow-wave activity with fluctuations). Biomarkers are further described below. In patients who present with dementia and parkinsonism, the 1-year rule is recommended to differentiate between DLB and PDD. Cognitive decline in DLB should precede (or occur within 1 year of) motor changes. When dementia begins at least 1 year after motor changes, PDD is thought to be more likely. This rule is rather arbitrary and generally more useful in research settings. As mentioned above, Lewy body diseases are likely on a continuum rather than distinct subtypes, and there is a lack of neuropathological data to support the arbitrary distinction of the 1-year rule [3, 64], or a separation of DLB from PDD.

3.1 Differential diagnosis

It should be noted that historically, lower specificity has been found for cases meeting criteria for "Possible DLB" [65]. To reduce the false diagnosis of DLB, clinicians should be cautious when the only core feature is atypical parkinsonism. Careful history is critical to exclude prior exposure to phenothiazines (including prochlorperazine and metoclopramide) as atypical antipsychotics, which are sometimes tried liberally to control behavioral symptoms in dementia. Furthermore, the differential diagnosis of other dementias with atypical parkinsonism needs to be considered closely including vascular parkinsonism, corticobasal degeneration (CBD), progressive supranuclear palsy (PSP), multiple system atrophy (MSA), Hallervorden-Spatz (now termed PKAN), Fahr's disease, and other disorders affecting the basal ganglia and its connections.

Other dementias to consider in the differential diagnosis include Alzheimer's disease, vascular dementia, and "mixed" AD/vascular dementia, which has been the most common reason for false-positive diagnoses of DLB in the UC Davis ADRC's multiethnic cohort. False-positive diagnoses can occasionally be made in the setting of delirium, which may mimic symptoms of DLB (e.g., fluctuations in alertness and psychosis). The classic triad of cognitive decline, urinary incontinence, and gait disorder in normal-pressure hydrocephalus (NPH) may be present as features of DLB. Notably absent from patients with NPH are the psychotic manifestations typical of DLB. Finally, Creutzfeldt-Jakob disease can also present similar to DLB with prominent visual disturbances and motor changes, but generally with very rapid progression.

4. Fluctuations

4.1 Clinical instruments and studies

Cognitive fluctuations (CF) are spontaneous episodes of impaired attention and reduced arousal [66]. CF have been designated as a core clinical feature since the earliest consensus diagnostic criteria in 1996 [67] and remain a core clinical criterion in the current (Fourth consensus report of the DLB Consortium) diagnostic criteria discussed below [51]. Despite their importance, CF are difficult to operationalize and detect on clinical history. While some U.K. studies have found prevalences of up to 90% in DLB [68], many U.S. centers have reported much lower prevalences [69, 70], especially among cases with concomitant AD [71]. Many caregivers report day-to-day fluctuations (e.g., "bad days") and some do not seem to detect subtler episodes of mildly reduced attention. Differentiating CF from delirium caused by infection or concurrent medical conditions, or from the effects of sedating medications, can prove difficult in clinical populations. Ferman et al. [42] found that the presence of three symptoms of neuropsychiatric fluctuation including daytime drowsiness, daytime sleep of 2 hours or more, staring episodes, or episodes of disorganized speech was found in 63% of DLB patients (n = 70) [42]. Thus, asking about "excessive daytime sleepiness" can often be more fruitful than asking about "fluctuations in alertness," which can be overly vague and difficult to discriminate normal vs. excessive changes in alertness. Walker and colleagues have introduced two clinical scales designed to quantify such issues: the One Day Fluctuation Assessment Scale and the Clinician Assessment of Fluctuation (CAF). The CAF has been well validated and is commonly used in clinical trial assessments of CF. It should be scored by an experienced clinician with significant exposure to DLB or PD patients, which poses a barrier to its more widespread use in the community, primary care, or general neurology practices. Biomarkers that can quantify CF would clearly be of value by: (1) increasing our sensitivity to CF, and thereby improving diagnostic sensitivity; (2) allowing insights into the physiological mechanisms that underlie CF, as this could point the way toward treatments that reduce CF and their associated disability; (3) reducing the need for specialized raters; and (4) objective measures could be used across cultures and reduce the subjective aspects of current clinical rating scales.

4.2 Electrophysiological studies

Electroencephalography (EEG), a time-honored technique used in the assessment of alertness, level of consciousness, and the stages of sleep, has also showed much promise in the assessment of CF. EEG is a noninvasive, inexpensive, and widely available technology with unsurpassed temporal resolution. It offers high signal-to-noise ratio and portability and is more easily tolerated by dementia patients than MRI or PET scanning. Walker et al. [68] found DLB patients to have significantly greater CF than AD or vascular dementia patients, and the EEG also showed greater variation in the mean frequency and increased fluctuations over time, apparent even on a second-to-second basis within 90-second samples of EEG data. Further work with quantitative EEG (qEEG) has suggested several biomarkers for DLB, as well as for PD dementia. Bonanni and colleagues [72] found slower dominant frequency over the posterior scalp in DLB (n = 36) and PD dementia patients with CF (n = 16). A follow-up study by this group [73] showed reduced dominant frequency and increased dominant frequency variability can be detected before the diagnosis of DLB, when patients are in the MCI stage, and these EEG patterns confer an increased risk for conversion from MCI to dementia, that is, the loss of functional independence. Stylianou et al. have added to this literature by showing abnormalities in theta activity in DLB, with more variability in theta range dominant frequency and greater prevalence of slow theta activity [74]. This body of work has led to the Consensus DLB Diagnostic Criteria adding EEG as a supportive biomarker in 2017 particularly when "prominent posterior slow-wave activity with periodic fluctuations in the pre-alpha/theta range" is present. A prealpha dominant frequency intermixed with alpha/theta/delta activities in pseudoperiodic patterns may have >90% predictive value in differentiating DLB from AD [75].

5. Biomarkers

Direct biomarker evidence of Lewy body pathology is not yet clinically available for the diagnosis of DLB. In 2017, the fourth consensus report of the DLB consortium categorized available biomarkers into "indicative" and "supportive" categories based on available evidence and diagnostic specificity [51]. Below, we discuss the validity and potential pitfalls of these tests as well as future biomarkers still under development.

5.1 Indicative biomarkers

Indicative biomarkers include (1) reduced dopamine transporter (DAT) uptake in the basal ganglia demonstrated by SPECT or PET; (2) abnormal (low) 123iodine-MIBG uptake on myocardial scintigraphy; and (3) Polysomnographic (PSG) confirmation of REM sleep without atonia.

Reduced nigrostriatal DAT uptake by SPECT or PET imaging is reflective of dopaminergic neuron dysfunction due to αS deposition and has a specificity of 90% and sensitivity of 78% in distinguishing DLB from AD [76]. However, parkinsonism and reduced DAT uptake may also be seen in disorders such as PSP, MSA, CBD, and frontotemporal dementia; therefore, caution must be exercised in diagnosing dementia patients with probable DLB when parkinsonism is the only core clinical feature present. Occasionally, normal DAT uptake may also be seen in autopsy-confirmed DLB due to limited nigral neuron loss or a balanced loss of dopamine across the whole striatum [77].

Evaluation of imaging biomarkers typically relies on visual interpretations and manual selection of regions of interest and can leave it susceptible to interrater and intrarater variability. The advent of automated imaging processing software such as GE Healthcare's DaTQUANT potentially increases the predictive yield over that of manual DAT-SPECT interpretation and combining with the use of two other imaging modalities (MRI and FDG-PET) has been shown to increase the concordance (c-statistic) rate of predicting DLB to 0.996 [78].

Low 123Iodine-MIBG myocardial scintigraphy uptake has a specificity of 87% and sensitivity of 69% in discriminating probable DLB from probable AD. Abnormal MIBG uptake results from reduced postganglionic sympathetic cardiac innervation due to αS deposition, as such other causes of peripheral neuropathies, including diabetes mellitus, and cardiac conditions such as heart failure and recent ischemic heart disease, and certain medications such as labetalol and tricyclic antidepressants may also reduce MIBG uptake [79].

REM sleep behavior disorder is a parasomnia characterized by a loss of normal skeletal muscle atonia during REM sleep with prominent motor activity during dreaming, including punching, kicking, talking, and moving purposefully. Onset is typically after the age of 50 and can precede the manifestation of a neurodegenerative syndrome by years or decades. PSG confirmation of REM sleep without atonia, along with a history of dementia and RBD, has a predictive accuracy of 98% for the presence of a synucleinopathy. Rarely, PSG-confirmed cases may be associated with nonsynucleinopathies such as AD or CBD (3 cases out of 82 total patients) [80].

5.2 Supportive biomarkers

Supportive biomarkers include (1) relative preservation of medial temporal lobe (MTL) structures on CT/MRI scan; (2) generalized low uptake on SPECT/PET perfusion/metabolism scan with reduced occipital activity and/or the "cingulate island sign" on FDG-PET imaging; and (3) prominent posterior slow-wave activity on EEG with periodic fluctuations in the prealpha/theta range.

DLB patients demonstrate less MTL atrophy compared to AD. Absent or minimal medial temporal atrophy on MRI has a sensitivity of 64% and specificity of 68% for separating AD from DLB [81]. For clear DLB cases, concurrent MTL atrophy may signal additional AD pathology and predict a more rapid clinical course.

On FDG-PET, DLB patients demonstrate occipital hypometabolism and relative preservation of posterior cingulate metabolism compared to AD, the latter has been coined the "cingulate island sign." Occipital hypometabolism in DLB has a sensitivity of 70% and specificity of 74% in distinguishing DLB from AD [82]. Relative preservation of cingulate island metabolism on FDG-PET has been associated with lower Braak tangle stage at autopsy and predicted better clinical trajectory in DLB [83].

Quantitative EEG analysis of DLB patients using multiple methods has been shown to reliably identify DLB with a correct classification rate of 90%. Posterior slow-wave activity and the presence of prealpha- (5.5–7.5 Hz) or theta- (>4 Hz–8 Hz) dominant frequencies are associated with DLB [75].

In an anonymous survey of 22 DLB center of excellence investigators, MRI and DAT-SPECT were the most ordered biomarkers (90% and 86.4%, respectively). Myocardial scintigraphy and EEG use were the rarest (13.6% and 9.1%, respectively). Insurance coverage of DAT-SPECT is variable among U.S. insurers; some consider the use "investigational" for the indication of distinguishing DLB from AD, while others cover it for the indication of clinically uncertain DLB [84]. MIBG compounds for diagnosis of neurological indications is considered off-label use in the U.S. by the FDA but are more widely available in Europe [85].

5.3 Future biomarkers (in development)

Genetic testing and peripheral tissue and CSF biomarkers for the diagnosis of DLB are an area of ongoing research. Genome-wide association studies (GWAS) in DLB have demonstrated variations in glucocerebrosidase (GBA) and α-synuclein gene (SNCA) alleles as risk factors for DLB and PD, while APOE E4 is a shared risk allele in DLB and AD [86, 87]. Common genetic variants including the H1G haplotype of microtubule-associated protein (MAPT) and in the scavenger receptor class B member 2 (SCARB2) loci confer a higher risk of DLB compared to controls, whereas the H2 MAPT haplotype and a common variant in the butyrylcholinesterase (BuChE) loci have been associated with a decreased risk of DLB. Additional genetic variants such as the parkin (PARK2), PTEN-induced putative kinase 1 (PINK1), granulin (GRN), triggering receptor expressed on myeloid cells 2 (TREM2), and SNCB alleles have also been associated with DLB but are often of unclear pathogenicity [88]. At the current time, the Fourth Consensus Report suggests that it is premature to recommend genetic testing in a clinical setting, either for confirmation of diagnosis or for prediction of disease [51].

Direct assays of alpha-synuclein (αS) oligomers are being developed for CSF and peripheral nerve biopsies. In the CSF, abnormal αS aggregates can be measured taking advantage of the seeding-nucleation process of αS aggregation, where misfolded oligomers seed the polymerization of monomeric proteins. One such process uses a combination of protein misfolding cyclic amplification assays (PMCA) and thioflavin (ThT) fluorescence; in this method, DLB and PD result in the highest levels of ThT fluorescence and reliably differentiates these diseases from MSA (100% sensitivity and 93% specificity) and healthy controls [89]. Plasma and serum αS levels have been demonstrated to reliably differentiate between PD and normal controls with a c-statistic of 0.992 (plasma) and 0.917 (serum) with regard to the clinical diagnosis. Its diagnostic capacity for diagnosing DLB remains to be seen [90]. Studies of cutaneous αS aggregation in the skin nerve fibers using skin biopsies and in gastrointestinal specimens using colonic biopsies are also under investigation [91].

Alternative fluid biomarkers under development include CSF levels of DJ-1, a ubiquitous protein involved in inhibition of αS aggregation; mutations in the DJ-1 gene (PARK7) can also cause early-onset PD [92]. Results have been mixed: one study demonstrated CSF DJ-1 levels were lower in PD compared to AD and normal controls and had a sensitivity of 90% and specificity of 70% in distinguishing PD from controls [93]. Another demonstrated higher CSF DJ-1 levels in MSA compared to PD and normal controls, with a sensitivity and specificity of 78% in distinguishing MSA from PD [94]. Others include β-glucocerebrosidase activity, CSF neurofilament light chain (NF-L), and combination testing with AD biomarkers amyloid and tau [92].

6. Pathological validation

Initial criteria for the pathologic diagnosis of DLB required the presence of brain stem or cortical Lewy bodies; this was subsequently expanded to include five subtypes based on the region of LB deposition, including diffuse neocortical, limbic (or transitional), amygdala-predominant, brain stem–predominant, and olfactory bulb-only variants [95]. In one prospective study, 84% of patients with clinically probable DLB (n = 43) had diffuse cortical LB, 14% demonstrated the limbic/transitional subtype at autopsy, and the one remaining patient had mixed PSP/AD pathology [96].

Over 50% of DLB cases have concurrent Alzheimer's pathology (neocortical tau and β-amyloid) on autopsy. Diffuse, rather than neuritic, plaques make up the preponderance of amyloid burden in DLB [97], and the presence of amyloid could contribute to faster progression of dementia [98]. The presence of neocortical tangles affects the phenotypic expression of DLB; combined diffuse Lewy body disease (DLBD) and neocortical tangles were associated with comparable memory-naming impairment but worse baseline attention-visual processing than AD. Dementia trajectory was also the fastest for this combined pathology group, compared to transitional LBD without neocortical tangles, which had the slowest progression of the clinical DLB patients. In general, a clinical diagnosis of DLB was highly likely when the distribution of αS pathology was greater than tau and less likely when the distribution of tau pathology was greater than αS [99]. In an ADRC series of cases autopsied within 3 years of last cognitive assessment, both the presence of Lewy bodies and advanced Braak neurofibrillary tangle stage were associated with more severe dementia [100]. Lewy bodies appeared to be a major determinant of dementia severity in "Lewy body variant" cases with milder AD pathology (Braak III–IV), but not in those with severe AD pathology (Braak V–VI; see **Figure 2**). It may be that advanced AD-related neurodegeneration facilitates LB formation and, reciprocally, that neocortical LBs promote secondary beta-amyloid deposition and AD pathology.

Illustrating the spectrum of Lewy body disorders, coexistence of LB pathology in AD patients results in higher Unified Parkinson's Disease Rating Scale (UPDRS) scores compared to pure AD patients [101]. Matching cases diagnosed with DLB, AD, and LBV in the NACC database on MMSE scores, Kaur et al. found UPDRS scores increased with cognitive impairment in all three patient groups. Thus, total UPDRS scores may be useful for indicating likelihood of dual pathology in dementia cohorts [102]. On qEEG measures, DLB and AD copathology also demonstrates

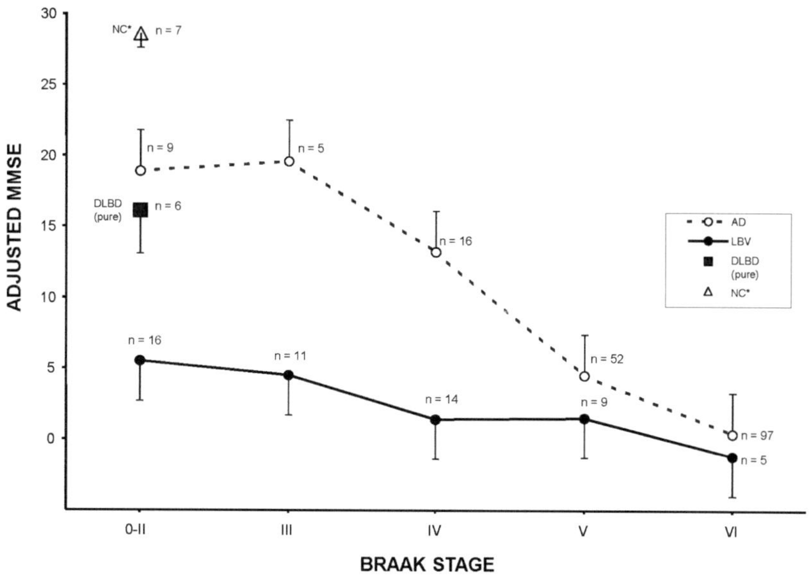

Figure 2.
Dementia severity by Braak stage in AD and LBV. NC—normal controls; last MMSE (unadjusted) plotted. Mean age = 82.9 years. Excluded if met NIA or CERAD neuropathological criteria for possible AD. All other groups (AD, LBV, pure DLBD) had MMSE adjusted using 3 pt/yr correction estimate.*

greater reduction of posterior alpha, beta, and gamma frequencies compared to pure AD cases but is similar to the qEEG findings in pure DLB [103].

In summary, the likelihood of a clinical DLB syndrome is thought to be a function of both the distribution of Lewy bodies and the severity of AD-type pathology; this probability is positively correlated with LBs and negatively correlated with NIA-Alzheimer's Association Braak staging of neurofibrillary tangles (i.e., higher Braak stages were associated with a lower probability of clinical DLB in diffuse cortical and transitional LB pathology, and vice versa). Brain stem, amygdala-predominant, and olfactory bulb-only subtypes had a low probability of clinical DLB regardless of Braak staging [104, 105]. A separate research criteria for the diagnosis of prodromal DLB have been proposed, compatible with current criteria of other prodromal neurodegenerative disorders including AD and PD; further validation studies are underway [106].

7. Conclusions and future directions

In conclusion, this chapter has attempted to summarize the recent advances in both clinical diagnostic criteria and biomarkers with higher sensitivity or specificity to DLB. It should be noted that these advances have improved in the detection of DLB, but the attribution of which disease process is "primary" remains difficult in cases with concomitant LB and AD pathology. Clinical criteria alone have good specificity but limited sensitivity to many of these cases, where the AD phenotype may be more evident in the so-called LBV of AD cases. Adding biomarkers has increased sensitivity further, but the specificity of the biomarkers may be less than the specificity of clinical criteria.

Further work is clearly needed to parse the "mixed" dementias, both among neurodegenerative diseases where "quadruple proteinopathy" cases are increasingly recognized [107], plus the common coexistence of cerebral vascular disease, which makes AD with CVD arguably the most common dementia in the U.S. [108].

Another limitation of DLB criteria is that while it captures well a subgroup of patients with poor prognosis and who need the most care, it does not capture the full spectrum of phenotypes attributable to LBs. The validation of prodromal DLB criteria is a current important focus of the field, and the capture of PD dementia cases in population-based studies with comparisons to DLB prevalence is important for an understanding of this relative impact on the public health. Further advances may be possible with better detection of olfactory deficits (anosmia being common in PD, DLB, and LBV), autonomic dysfunction, and subclinical motor dysfunction.

We have emphasized recent advances in the detection of CF both with clinical instruments and qEEG. Further applications and work in this area are needed, as CF are disabling and the electrophysiological mechanisms may be treatment-responsive. In this digital age, advances in EEG analytic methods, for example, statistical pattern recognition (SPR) [109, 110], artificial intelligence, and machine learning with support vector machine EEG classifiers [111], hold promise in detecting LBs, perhaps independent of clinical presentation (PD, DLB, LBV), or alternatively as a "digital fingerprint" for disease subtypes. Future investigations are encouraged to characterize the physiological abnormalities using more comprehensive biomarker approaches (e.g., biofluids, PSG, EEG, PET, autonomic and olfactory testing), while capturing a broader range of phenotypes. Further neuropathologic studies to validate the disease subtypes are also needed, for which careful phenotyping will allow increased ability to detect less widespread LB disease (e.g., olfactory and brain stem) and ultimately stage patients accurately during life. One recent clinicopathologic study found different clinical phenotypes in transitional Lewy body disease (TLBD) than in DLBD, and neurofibrillary tangles were associated with faster decline and less sensitivity of the consensus criteria (48–70% vs. 87–96% in LB disease cases without tangles) [99].

We expect that, as in any disease, a better understanding of its subtypes and underlying pathophysiological mechanisms will allow future treatments for DLB and the other synucleinopathies that are more targeted and comprehensive. While symptomatic treatments for PD and DLB are quite well developed and tested, future advances will increasingly address prevention and presymptomatic treatments that are disease-modifying. Such advances would have a truly major impact on the public health of our elderly population.

Author details

John M. Olichney[1*], Wentao Li[2], Yasmine Gharbaoui[1], Alison P. Kwok[1,3] and Jade E. Jenkins[3]

1 Department of Neurology, School of Medicine, University of California, Davis, Sacramento, California, USA

2 Department of Neurology, Mayo Clinic, Rochester, MN, USA

3 Center for Mind and Brain, University of California, Davis, Davis, CA, USA

*Address all correspondence to: jmolichney@ucdavis.edu

References

[1] Heidebrink JL. Is dementia with Lewy bodies the second most common cause of dementia? Journal of Geriatric Psychiatry and Neurology 2002;15(4):182-187.

[2] Hogan DB, Fiest KM, Roberts JI, Maxwell CJ, Dykeman J, Pringsheim T, et al. The prevalence and incidence of dementia with Lewy bodies: A systematic review. The Canadian Journal of Neurological Sciences 2016;43(S1):S83–S95.

[3] Jellinger KA. Dementia with Lewy bodies and Parkinson's disease-dementia: Current concepts and controversies. Journal of Neural Transmission 2018;125(4):615-650.

[4] Perry R, Irving D, Blessed G, Perry E, Fairbairn A. Clinically and neuropathologically distinct form of dementia in the elderly. The Lancet. 1989;333(8630):166.

[5] Schneider JA, Wilson RS, Bienias JL, Evans DA, Bennett DA. Cerebral infarctions and the likelihood of dementia from Alzheimer disease pathology. Neurology 2004;62(7):1148-1155.

[6] Lewy F. Paralysis agitans. I. Pathologische anatomie. In: Lewandowsky M, editor. Handbuch der Neurologie. Berlin: Springer; 1912. p. 920-933.

[7] Duffy PE, Tennyson VM. Phase and electron microscopic observations of Lewy bodies and melanin granules in the substantia Nigra and locus Caeruleus in Parkinson's disease. Journal of Neuropathology and Experimental Neurology 1965;24(3):398-414.

[8] Forno LS. The Lewy body in Parkinson's disease. Advances in Neurology 1987;45:35-43.

[9] Galloway PG, Mulvihill P, Perry G. Filaments of Lewy bodies contain insoluble cytoskeletal elements. The American Journal of Pathology 1992;140(4):809-822.

[10] Hill WD, Lee VM-Y, Hurtig HI, Murray JM, Trojanowski JQ. Epitopes located in spatially separate domains of each neurofilament subunit are present in parkinson's disease lewy bodies. Journal of Comparative Neurology 1991;309(1):150-160.

[11] McKeith IG. Dementia with Lewy bodies. The British Journal of Psychiatry 2002;180(2):144-147.

[12] Ohama E, Ikuta F. Parkinson's disease: Distribution of Lewy bodies and monoamine neuron system. Acta Neuropathologica 1976;34(4):311-319.

[13] Zweig RM, Jankel WR, Hedreen JC, Mayeux R, Price DL. The pedunculopontine nucleus in Parkinson's disease. Annals of Neurology 1989;26(1):41-46.

[14] Bergeron C, Pollanen M. Lewy bodies in Alzheimer disease—One or two diseases? Alzheimer Disease and Associated Disorders 1989;3(4):197-204.

[15] Dickson DW, Crystal H, Mattiace LA, Kress Y, Schwagerl A, Ksiezak-Reding H, et al. Diffuse Lewy body disease: Light and electron microscopic immunocytochemistry of senile plaques. Acta Neuropathologica 1989;78(6):572-584.

[16] Kuzuhara S, Mori H, Izumiyama N, Yoshimura M, Ihara Y. Lewy bodies are ubiquitinated. A light and electron microscopic immunocytochemical study. Acta Neuropathologica 1988;75(4):345-353.

[17] Schmidt ML, Murray J, Lee VM, Hill WD, Wertkin A, Trojanowski JQ.

Epitope map of neurofilament protein domains in cortical and peripheral nervous system Lewy bodies. The American Journal of Pathology 1991;139(1):53-65.

[18] Tiller-Borcich JK, Forno LS. Parkinson's disease and dementia with neuronal inclusions in the cerebral cortex: Lewy bodies or pick bodies. Journal of Neuropathology and Experimental Neurology 1988;47(5):526-535.

[19] Galvin JE, Uryu K, Lee VM-Y, Trojanowski JQ. Axon pathology in Parkinson's disease and Lewy body dementia hippocampus contains α-, β-, and γ-synuclein. Proceedings of the National Academy of Sciences 1999;96(23):13450-13455.

[20] Dev KK, Hofele K, Barbieri S, Buchman VL, van der Putten H. Part II: α-Synuclein and its molecular pathophysiological role in neurodegenerative disease. Neuropharmacology 2003;45(1):14-44.

[21] Krüger R, Schulz JB. The α-synuclein pathway to neurodegeneration. In: Tolosa E, Schulz B, McKeith IG, editors. Neurodegenerative Disorders Associated with α-Synuclein Pathology. Barcelona, Spain: Ars Medica; 2002. p. 11-22.

[22] Pollanen MS, Dickson DW, Bergeron C. Pathology and biology of the Lewy body. Journal of Neuropathology and Experimental Neurology 1993;52(3):183-191.

[23] Braak H, Tredici KD, Rüb U, de Vos RAI, Jansen Steur ENH, Braak E. Staging of brain pathology related to sporadic Parkinson's disease. Neurobiology of Aging 2003;24(2):197-211.

[24] Galvin JE, Lee VM, Schmidt M, Tu P-H, Iwatsubo T, Trojanowski JQ. Pathobiology of the Lewy body. Advances in Neurology 1999;80:313-324.

[25] Mosimann UP, McKeith IG. Dementia with lewy bodies—Diagnosis and treatment. Swiss Medical Weekly 2003;133(9-10):131-142.

[26] De Keyser J, Herregodts P, Ebinger G. The mesoneocortical dopamine neuron system. Neurology 1990;40(11):1660-1660.

[27] Eggertson DE, Sima AAF. Dementia with cerebral Lewy bodies: A mesocortical dopaminergic defect? Archives of Neurology 1986;43(5):524-527.

[28] Marras C, Beck JC, Bower JH, Roberts E, Ritz B, Ross GW, et al. Prevalence of Parkinson's disease across North America. NPJ Parkinson's Disease 2018;4(1):21.

[29] Perry RH, Irving D, Blessed G, Fairbairn A, Perry EK. Senile dementia of Lewy body type: A clinically and neuropathologically distinct form of Lewy body dementia in the elderly. Journal of the Neurological Sciences 1990;95(2):119-139.

[30] Hansen L, Salmon D, Galasko D, Masliah E, Katzman R, DeTeresa R, et al. The Lewy body variant of Alzheimer's disease: A clinical and pathologic entity. Neurology 1990;40(1):1-1.

[31] Kosaka K. Diffuse Lewy body disease in Japan. Journal of Neurology 1990;237(3):197-204.

[32] Hansen LA, Masliah E, Quijada-Fawcett S, Rexin D. Entorhinal neurofibrillary tangles in Alzheimer disease with Lewy bodies. Neuroscience Letters 1991;129(2):269-272.

[33] Ditter SM, Mirra SS. Neuropathologic and clinical features of Parkinson's disease in Alzheimer's disease patients. Neurology 1987;37(5):754-754.

[34] Savica R, Grossardt BR, Bower JH, Boeve BF, Ahlskog JE, Rocca WA. Incidence of dementia with Lewy bodies and Parkinson disease dementia. JAMA Neurology 2013;70(11):1396.

[35] Gibb W, Lees A. The relevance of the Lewy body to the pathogenesis of idiopathic Parkinson's disease. Journal of Neurology, Neurosurgery, and Psychiatry 1988;51(6):745-752.

[36] Perry RH, Irving D, Tomlinson BE. Lewy body prevalence in the aging brain: Relationship to neuropsychiatric disorders, Alzheimer-type pathology and catecholaminergic nuclei. Journal of the Neurological Sciences 1990;100(1-2):223-233.

[37] Kosaka K, Iseki E, Odawara T, Yamamoto T. Cerebral type of Lewy body disease. Neuropathology 1996;16(1):32-35.

[38] Walker Z, Allen RL, Shergill S, Mullan E, Katona CLE. Three years survival in patients with a clinical diagnosis of dementia with Lewy bodies. International Journal of Geriatric Psychiatry 2000;15(3):267-273.

[39] Olichney JM, Galasko D, Salmon DP, Hofstetter CR, Hansen LA, Katzman R, et al. Cognitive decline is faster in Lewy body variant than in Alzheimer's disease. Neurology 1998;51(2):351-357.

[40] Gomez-Tortosa E, Newell K, Irizarry MC, Albert M, Growdon JH, Hyman BT. Clinical and quantitative pathologic correlates of dementia with Lewy bodies. Neurology 1999;53(6):1284-1284.

[41] Outeiro TF, Koss DJ, Erskine D, Walker L, Kurzawa-Akanbi M, Burn D, et al. Dementia with Lewy bodies: An update and outlook. Molecular Neurodegeneration 2019;14(1):5.

[42] Ferman TJ, Smith G, Boeve BF, Ivnik R, Petersen RC, Knopman D, et al. DLB fluctuations: Specific features that reliably differentiate DLB from AD and normal aging. Neurology 2004;62(2):181-187.

[43] Palmqvist S, Hansson O, Minthon L, Londos E. Practical suggestions on how to differentiate dementia with Lewy bodies from Alzheimer's disease with common cognitive tests. International Journal of Geriatric Psychiatry 2009;24(12):1405-12.

[44] Salmon DP, Galasko D, Hansen LA, Masliah E, Butters N, Thal LJ, et al. Neuropsychological deficits associated with diffuse Lewy body disease. Brain and Cognition 1996;31(2):148-165.

[45] Parkinson J. An Essay on the Shaking Palsy Whittingham and Rowland for Sherwood, Neely, and Jones, London. 1817;325. DOI: 10.1016/s0140-6736(85)90986-9

[46] Lees A. Parkinson's disease and dementia. Lancet 1985;325 434-434. DOI: 10.1016/s0140-6736(85)90986-9

[47] Martin WE, Loewenson RB, Resch JA, Baker AB. Parkinson's disease: Clinical analysis of 100 patients. Neurology 1973;23(8):783-783.

[48] Brown R, Marsden C. How common is dementia in Parkinson's disease? The Lancet. 1984;324(8414):1262-1265.

[49] Pirozzolo FJ, Hansch EC, Mortimer JA, Webster DD, Kuskowski MA. Dementia in Parkinson disease: A neuropsychological analysis. Brain and Cognition 1982;1(1):71-83.

[50] Mayeux R, Denaro J, Hemenegildo N, Marder K, Tang M-X, Cote LJ, et al. A population-based investigation of Parkinson's disease with and without dementia: Relationship to age and gender. Archives of Neurology 1992;49(5):492-497.

[51] McKeith IG, Boeve BF, Dickson DW, Halliday G, Taylor J-P, Weintraub D, et al.

Diagnosis and management of dementia with Lewy bodies: Fourth consensus report of the DLB consortium. Neurology 2017;89(1):88-100.

[52] Ebmeier KP, Calder SA, Crawford JR, Stewart L, Besson JA, Mutch WJ Clinical features predicting dementia in idiopathic Parkinson's disease: A follow-up study. Neurology 1990;40(8):1222-1222.

[53] Chan, P.-C., Lee, H.-H., Hong, C.-T., Hu, C.-J., Wu, D., 2018. REM Sleep Behavior Disorder (RBD) in Dementia with Lewy Bodies (DLB). Behavioural Neurology 2018, 1-10. https://doi.org/10.1155/2018/9421098

[54] Christensen JAE, Nikolic M, Warby SC, Koch H, Zoetmulder M, Frandsen R, et al. Sleep spindle alterations in patients with Parkinson's disease. Frontiers in Human Neuroscience. 2015;9.233 Available from: https://www.ncbi.nlm.nih.gov/pmc/articles/PMC4416460/

[55] Latreille V, Carrier J, Lafortune M, Postuma RB, Bertrand J-A, Panisset M, et al. Sleep spindles in Parkinson's disease may predict the development of dementia. Neurobiology of Aging 2015;36(2):1083-1090.

[56] Stefani A, Högl B. Sleep in Parkinson's disease. Neuropsychopharmacology 2020;45(1):121-128.

[57] van de Beek M, van Steenoven I, van der Zande JJ, Barkhof F, Teunissen CE, van der Flier WM, et al. Prodromal dementia with Lewy bodies: Clinical characterization and predictors of progression. Movement Disorders, An Official Journal of the International Parkinson and Movement Disorder Society 2020;35(5):859-867.

[58] Hickey C, Chisholm T, Passmore M, O'Brien J, Johnston J. Differentiating the dementias. Revisiting Synucleinopathies and Tauopathies. Current Alzheimer Research 2008;5(1):52-60.

[59] Boström F, Jönsson L, Minthon L, Londos E. Patients with Lewy body dementia use more resources than those with Alzheimer's disease. International Journal of Geriatric Psychiatry 2007;22(8):713 719.

[60] Boström F, Jönsson L, Minthon L, Londos E. Patients with dementia with Lewy bodies have more impaired quality of life than patients with alzheimer disease: Alzheimer Disease and Associated Disorders. 2007;21(2):150-154.

[61] Magierski R, Sobow T, Schwertner E, Religa D. Pharmacotherapy of behavioral and psychological symptoms of dementia: State of the art and future progress. Frontiers in Pharmacology 2020;11:1168.

[62] Olazarán J, Reisberg B, Clare L, Cruz I, Peña-Casanova J, Del Ser T, et al. Nonpharmacological therapies in Alzheimer's disease: A systematic review of efficacy. Dementia and Geriatric Cognitive Disorders 2010;30(2):161-178.

[63] Stinton C, McKeith I, Taylor J-P, Lafortune L, Mioshi E, Mak E, et al. Pharmacological management of Lewy body dementia: A systematic review and meta-analysis. The American Journal of Psychiatry 2015;172(8):731-742.

[64] McKeith I, Mintzer J, Aarsland D, Burn D, Chiu H, Cohen-Mansfield J, et al. Dementia with Lewy bodies. Lancet Neurology 2004;3(1):19-28.

[65] Doody RS, Stevens J, Beck C, Dubinsky R, Kaye J, Gwyther L, et al. Practice parameter: Management of dementia (an evidence-based review): Report of the Quality Standards Subcommittee of the American Academy of Neurology. Neurology 2001;56(9):1154-1166.

[66] Matar E, Shine JM, Halliday GM, Lewis SJG. Cognitive fluctuations in Lewy body dementia: Towards a pathophysiological framework. Brain: A Journal of Neurology 2020;143(1):31-46.

[67] McKeith IG, Galasko D, Kosaka K, Perry EK, Dickson DW, Hansen LA, et al. Consensus guidelines for the clinical and pathologic diagnosis of dementia with Lewy bodies (DLB): Report of the consortium on DLB international workshop. Neurology 1996;47(5):1113-1124.

[68] Walker MP, Ayre GA, Cummings JL, Wesnes K, McKeith IG, O'Brien JT, et al. Quantifying fluctuation in dementia with Lewy bodies, Alzheimer's disease, and vascular dementia. Neurology 2000;54(8):1616-1625.

[69] Hohl U, Tiraboschi P, Hansen LA, Thal LJ, Corey-Bloom J. Diagnostic accuracy of dementia with Lewy bodies. Archives of Neurology 2000;57(3):347.

[70] Lopez OL, Litvan I, Catt KE, Stowe R, Klunk W, Kaufer DI, et al. Accuracy of four clinical diagnostic criteria for the diagnosis of neurodegenerative dementias. Neurology 1999;53(6):1292-1292.

[71] Verghese J, Crystal HA, Dickson DW, Lipton RB. Validity of clinical criteria for the diagnosis of dementia with Lewy bodies. Neurology 1999;53(9):1974-1974.

[72] Bonanni L, Thomas A, Tiraboschi P, Perfetti B, Varanese S, Onofrj M. EEG comparisons in early Alzheimer's disease, dementia with Lewy bodies and Parkinson's disease with dementia patients with a 2-year follow-up. Brain 2008;131(3):690-705.

[73] Bonanni L, Perfetti B, Bifolchetti S, Taylor J-P, Franciotti R, Parnetti L, et al. Quantitative electroencephalogram utility in predicting conversion of mild cognitive impairment to dementia with Lewy bodies. Neurobiology of Aging 2015;36(1):434-445.

[74] Stylianou M, Murphy N, Peraza LR, Graziadio S, Cromarty R, Killen A, et al. Quantitative electroencephalography as a marker of cognitive fluctuations in dementia with Lewy bodies and an aid to differential diagnosis. Clinical Neurophysiology 2018;129(6):1209-1220.

[75] Bonanni L, Franciotti R, Nobili F, Kramberger MG, Taylor J-P, Garcia-Ptacek S, et al. EEG markers of dementia with Lewy bodies: A multicenter cohort study. Journal of Alzheimer's Disease 2016;54(4):1649-1657.

[76] McKeith I, O'Brien J, Walker Z, Tatsch K, Booij J, Darcourt J, et al. Sensitivity and specificity of dopamine transporter imaging with 123I-FP-CIT SPECT in dementia with Lewy bodies: A phase III, multicentre study. Lancet Neurology 2007;6(4):305-313.

[77] Ogawa T, Fujii S, Kuya K, Kitao SI, Shinohara Y, Ishibashi M, et al. Role of neuroimaging on differentiation of Parkinson's disease and its related diseases. 61, Yonago Acta Medica. Tottori University Faculty of Medicine; 2018. p. 145-155.

[78] Miyagawa T, Przybelski SA, Maltais D, Min HK, Jordan L, Lesnick TG, et al. The value of multimodal imaging with 123I-FP-CIT SPECT in differential diagnosis of dementia with Lewy bodies and Alzheimer's disease dementia. Neurobiology of Aging 2021;99:11-18.

[79] Yoshita M, Arai H, Arai H, Arai T, Asada T, Fujishiro H, et al. Diagnostic accuracy of 123I-meta-iodobenzylguanidine myocardial scintigraphy in dementia with lewy bodies: A multicenter study. PLoS ONE 2015 10(3);e0120540.

[80] Boeve BF, Silber MH, Ferman TJ, Lin SC, Benarroch EE, Schmeichel AM, et al. Clinicopathologic correlations in 172 cases of rapid eye movement sleep behavior disorder with or without a coexisting neurologic disorder. Sleep Medicine 2013;14(8):754-762.

[81] Harper L, Fumagalli GG, Barkhof F, Scheltens P, O'Brien JT, Bouwman F, et al. MRI visual rating scales in the diagnosis of dementia: Evaluation in 184 post-mortem confirmed cases. Brain 2016;139(4):1211-1225.

[82] O'Brien JT, Firbank MJ, Davison C, Barnett N, Bamford C, Donaldson C, et al. 18F-FDG PET and perfusion SPECT in the diagnosis of Alzheimer and Lewy body dementias. Journal of Nuclear Medicine 2014;55(12):1959-1965.

[83] Graff-Radford J, Lesnick TG, Savica R, Chen Q, Ferman TJ, Przybelski SA, et al. 18F-fluorodeoxyglucose positron emission tomography in dementia with Lewy bodies. Brain Communications 2020 1;2(1).

[84] Armstrong MJ, Irwin DJ, Leverenz JB, Gamez N, Taylor A, Galvin JE. Biomarker use for dementia with Lewy body diagnosis: Survey of US experts. Alzheimer Disease and Associated Disorders 2020;35. DOI: 10.1097/WAD.0000000000000414

[85] Capouch SD, Farlow MR, Brosch JR. A review of dementia with lewy bodies' impact, diagnostic criteria and treatment. Neurology and Therapy. 2018;7(2):249-263.

[86] Galasko D, Saitoh T, Xia Y, Thai LJ, Katzman R, Hill LR, et al. The apolipoprotein E allele epsi;4 is overrepresented in patients with the Lewy body variant of Alzheimer's disease. Neurology 1994; 44(10):1950-1950.

[87] Orme T, Guerreiro R, Bras J. The genetics of dementia with Lewy bodies: Current understanding and future directions. Current Neurology and Neuroscience Reports. 2018;18(10):67

[88] Vergouw LJM, van Steenoven I, van de Berg WDJ, Teunissen CE, van Swieten JC, Bonifati V, et al. An update on the genetics of dementia with Lewy bodies. Parkinsonism & Related Disorders 2017;43:1-8.

[89] Singer W, Schmeichel AM, Shahnawaz M, Schmelzer JD, Boeve BF, Sletten DM, et al. Alpha-synuclein oligomers and neurofilament light chain in spinal fluid differentiate multiple system atrophy from Lewy body Synucleinopathies. Annals of Neurology 2020;88(3):503-512.

[90] Chang CW, Yang SY, Yang CC, Chang CW, Wu YR. Plasma and serum alpha-Synuclein as a biomarker of diagnosis in patients with Parkinson's disease. Frontiers in Neurology 2020 21;10.

[91] Kim JY, Illigens BMW, McCormick MP, Wang N, Gibbons CH. Alpha-synuclein in skin nerve fibers as a biomarker for alpha-synucleinopathies. J Clin Neurol Korea. 2019;15(2):135-142.

[92] Farotti L, Paciotti S, Tasegian A, Eusebi P, Parnetti L. Discovery, validation and optimization of cerebrospinal fluid biomarkers for use in Parkinson's disease. Expert Review of Molecular Diagnostics. 2017;17(8):771-780

[93] Hong Z, Shi M, Chung KA, Quinn JF, Peskind ER, Galasko D, et al. DJ-1 and α-synuclein in human cerebrospinal fluid as biomarkers of Parkinson's disease. Brain 2010;133(3):713-726.

[94] Herbert MK, Eeftens JM, Aerts MB, Esselink RAJ, Bloem BR, Kuiperij HB, et al. CSF levels of DJ-1 and tau distinguish MSA patients from PD patients and

controls. Parkinsonism & Related Disorders 2014;20(1):112-115.

[95] Beach TG, Adler CH, Lue LF, Sue LI, Bachalakuri J, Henry-Watson J, et al. Unified staging system for Lewy body disorders: Correlation with nigrostriatal degeneration, cognitive impairment and motor dysfunction. Acta Neuropathologica 2009;117(6):613-634.

[96] Fujishiro H, Ferman TJ, Boeve BF, Smith GE, Graff-Radford NR, Uitti RJ, et al. Validation of the neuropathologic criteria of the third consortium for dementia with lewy bodies for prospectively diagnosed cases. Journal of Neuropathology and Experimental Neurology 2008;67(7):649-656.

[97] Kantarci K, Lowe VJ, Chen Q, Przybelski SA, Lesnick TG, Schwarz CG, et al. β-Amyloid PET and neuropathology in dementia with Lewy bodies. Neurology 2020;94(3): e282–e291.

[98] Edison P, Rowe CC, Rinne JO, Ng S, Ahmed I, Kemppainen N, et al. Amyloid load in Parkinson's disease dementia and Lewy body dementia measured with [11C]PIB positron emission tomography. Journal of Neurology, Neurosurgery, and Psychiatry 2008;79(12):1331-1338.

[99] Ferman TJ, Aoki N, Boeve BF, Aakre JA, Kantarci K, Graff-Radford J, et al. Subtypes of dementia with Lewy bodies are associated with α-synuclein and tau distribution. Neurology 2020;95(2):E155–E165.

[100] Olichney J, Hansen L, Hofstetter C, Cho M, Thal L. Neuropathologic Determinants of Dementia Severity in Lewy Body Variant: P02. 133. Neurology. 2004;62(7) A160.

[101] Savica R, Beach TG, Hentz JG, Sabbagh MN, Serrano GE, Sue LI, et al. Lewy body pathology in Alzheimer's disease: A clinicopathological prospective study. Acta Neurologica Scandinavica 2019;139(1):76-81.

[102] Kaur B, Harvey DJ, DeCarli CS, Zhang L, Sabbagh MN, Olichney JM. Extrapyramidal signs by dementia severity in Alzheimer disease and dementia with Lewy bodies. Alzheimer Disease and Associated Disorders 2013;27(3):226-232.

[103] van der Zande JJ, Gouw AA, van Steenoven I, Scheltens P, Stam CJ, Lemstra AW. EEG characteristics of dementia with Lewy Bodies, Alzheimer's Disease and mixed pathology. Frontiers in Aging Neuroscience. 2018;10190

[104] Fujishiro H, Tsuboi Y, Lin WL, Uchikado H, Dickson DW. Co-localization of tau and α-synuclein in the olfactory bulb in Alzheimer's disease with amygdala Lewy bodies. Acta Neuropathologica 2008;116(1):17-24.

[105] Uchikado H, Lin WL, Delucia MW, Dickson DW. Alzheimer disease with amygdala lewy bodies: A distinct form of α-synucleinopathy. Journal of Neuropathology and Experimental Neurology 2006;65(7):685-697.

[106] McKeith IG, Ferman TJ, Thomas AJ, Blanc F, Boeve BF, Fujishiro H, et al. Research criteria for the diagnosis of prodromal dementia with Lewy bodies. Neurology. 2020;94(17):743-55.

[107] Karanth S, Nelson PT, Katsumata Y, Kryscio RJ, Schmitt FA, Fardo DW, et al. Prevalence and clinical phenotype of quadruple misfolded proteins in older adults. JAMA Neurology 2020;77(10):1299.

[108] Schneider, J.A., Arvanitakis, Z., Bang, W., Bennett, D.A., 2007. Mixed brain pathologies account for most dementia cases in community-dwelling older persons. Neurology 69, 2197-2204. https://doi.org/10.1212/01.wnl.0000271090.28148.24

[109] Engedal K, Snaedal J, Hoegh P, Jelic V, Bo Andersen B, Naik M, et al. Quantitative EEG applying the statistical recognition pattern method: A useful tool in dementia diagnostic workup. Dementia and Geriatric Cognitive Disorders 2015;40(1-2):1-12.

[110] Snaedal J, Johannesson GH, Gudmundsson TE, Blin NP, Emilsdottir AL, Einarsson B, et al. Diagnostic accuracy of statistical pattern recognition of electroencephalogram registration in evaluation of cognitive impairment and dementia. Dementia and Geriatric Cognitive Disorders 2012;34(1):51-60.

[111] Garn H, Coronel C, Waser M, Caravias G, Ransmayr G. Differential diagnosis between patients with probable Alzheimer's disease, Parkinson's disease dementia, or dementia with Lewy bodies and frontotemporal dementia, behavioral variant, using quantitative electroencephalographic features. Journal of Neural Transmission 2017;124(5):569-581.

Chapter 5

Perspectives of Cognitive Impairment and Behavioral Disturbances in Parkinson's Disease Dementia

Beatriz Munoz Ospina, Valentina Quintana-Peña, Daniela Alvarez, Jaime A. Valderrama, Yuri Takeuchi and Jorge L. Orozco

Abstract

Parkinson's disease dementia is a critical stage of the disease because that has a negative impact on the quality of life and functional independence in activities daily living. How the cognition progress to dementia is a key to be explored. The cognitive impairment shows two profiles: cortical (memory encoding, visuospatial abilities, and language) and subcortical, with a dysexecutive syndrome that includes deficits in recognition memory, attention processes, and visual perception as well as visual hallucinations and cognitive fluctuations. Behavioral problems such as apathy, anxiety, depression, and impulse control disorders take a significant part in the loss of autonomy and progression of the disease. To detect the risk of Parkinson's disease dementia development, the integral evaluation of patients in all stages of the disease should consider the interplay of genetic and epigenetic factors, motor subtypes, and non-motor symptoms (NMS) in order to implement different therapeutics and supportive strategies when they are likely to have efficacy.

Keywords: Parkinson's disease, biomarkers, cognitive impairment, dementia, personalized medicine

1. Introduction

Parkinson's disease (PD) is the second most common neurodegenerative disease worldwide after Alzheimer's disease (AD). Nowadays, PD is considered a pandemic and the projection in the next years exhibited a fast growing of the disease. Estimating the high prevalence of cognitive impairment in the course of the disease, we must encourage the research and increase of health policies to reduce the impact of quality of life and its costs to the health care system.

There is a new and necessary perspective to understand the multicausality of the neurodegenerative diseases that most affect the population. By making available clinical, biological, genetic, and functional brain imaging markers in an individual-centered clinical practice, it will allow an approach to the principle of precision medicine. This can contribute to optimization of the selection of pharmacological management or non-pharmacological strategies of symptomatic or preventive treatment for cognitive impairment even at early stages of PD. Therefore, identifying patients with potential risk of dementia could guarantee proper treatment and strategies to support the functional impact. We are beginning to understand the conceptual and therapeutic overlap by reclassifying the shared pathogenic mechanisms and therapeutic targets.

The integral and multidisciplinary approach of the motor symptoms (MS) and non-motor symptoms (NMS) through the natural history of the disease allows to provide a specific treatment and improve the quality of life.

2. Epidemiology

PD produces a considerable epidemiological burden associated with high rates of disability [1]. Due to the world population's aging and other unclear factors, PD prevalence and incidence are dramatically increasing, even surpassing the growth of AD [2]. Epidemiological data on PD are highly variable across countries. These differences can be explained by the variability in the diagnostic criteria, changes in population age distribution and the access to health care services, including the opportunity to consult with trained doctors and specialists [3–5].

According to the Global Burden of Disease study, 6.2 million patients live with PD and this frequency will double by 2040. In 2015, the country with the highest age-adjusted PD prevalence was China with 136.34 cases per 100,000 inhabitants (CI 11.56–165.55) and the lowest was Tanzania with 72.19 (CI 59.86–87.82) [5, 6]. Since 1990 until 2017, PD had a small but significant increase in the age-standardized rates of incidence (21.9% [UI, 11.2–14.6%]), prevalence (16.2% [UI, 2.7–31%]), mortality (33.1% [UI, -4.6–41.7%]), and DALY (24.8% [UI, -5.2–32.9%]) [6].

People living with PD often have other comorbidities, which contribute to their prognosis related to the quality of life, and mortality [7]. Xin Wang et al., in a large retrospective study in China, collected and quantified PD comorbidity burden by the Elixhauser Comorbidity Index (ECI) and Charlson Comorbidity Index (CCI). The comorbidity spectrum differed between PD and parkinsonism patients. The most frequent comorbidities for the PD patients were cerebrovascular disease (42.53%), hypertension (33.17%), diabetes (10.60%), chronic pulmonary disease (6.98%), and paralysis (5.53%). For the parkinsonism patients, cerebrovascular disease (53.22%), hypertension (39.00%), diabetes (11.66%), paralysis (11.06%), and dementia (7.05%) were more common. Parkinsonism patients more frequently had cerebrovascular disease, dementia, paralysis, hypertension, weight loss, and drug abuse than patients with PD, but they had a lower prevalence of solid tumor without metastasis and mild liver disease [8, 9].

Dementia occurs as part of the neurodegenerative process, which directly leads to a decrease in the quality of life of PD and parkinsonism patients. A systematic review showed that the prevalence of dementia in patients with PD (PDD) ranges from 17.4 to 31.5%, with an average of 24.5%, which is higher than that in our cohort. The prevalence of dementia in our Colombian cohort is 4.9% for all patients and 6.9% for patients aged 65 years and older, which is considerably higher than the prevalence of 5.14% observed in the general Chinese population aged 65 years and older [4, 10].

In addition, a recent meta-analysis shows that the pooled prevalence of mild cognitive impairment associated with PD was 40% more frequent for multiple domain subtype. Currently, it is considered that mild cognitive impairment is a risk factor for the development of dementia [11, 12]. The prevalence of mild cognitive impairment (PD-MCI) in patients with PD is in a range of 20–50%, and these patients are at high risk of developing dementia [13]. In a recent review on cognitive impairment in patients with PD, it was reported that in the long term the progression of the disease can generate dementia in more than 75% of patients, which is closely linked to the disease duration of 10 years or more [14]. Finally, PDD and PC-MCI have a great impact on quality of life in patients, and their caregivers [15]. Thus, it is necessary to understand deeply and broadly the motor and non-motor spectrum of the disease in order to find novel therapeutics and preventive approaches.

3. Pathophysiology

The clinical and pathological changes associated with PPD are complex. The following section summarizes the genetic and histological changes associated with the pathophysiology of dementia in these patients.

3.1 Genetics of PD dementia

Although the genetic risk factors for PD have been investigated, much less is known about the genetic factors associated with the development of dementia in PD. According to some studies, the prevalence of PDD is lower in patients with genetic PD. However, this will depend on the gene variant and other comorbidities that predispose the development of cognitive disorders. Some of the most important genes are discussed below:

- PARK1: patients with duplication or triplication of alpha-synuclein gene (α-Syn) have more severe motor progression and worse cognitive prognosis [16] compared to those without the mutation. Although the evidence suggests that the higher the number of replications, the lower the age of onset of cognitive impairment. Of all genes, this seems to be the most related to dementia. More studies are needed to confirm these findings [17].

- PARK2: according to some case series, mutations in PARK2 do not seem to cause cognitive decline [18].

- PARK14: PLA2G6 mutation could show heterogeneous phenotype including dementia.

- DJ-1: due to its low prevalence, there is no clear relationship between DJ-1 and a particular PD cognitive phenotype. There are some reports of dementia within the clinical spectrum of DJ-1 mutations. In a large population-based survey, there was no evidence for an increased risk of dementia in carriers of DJ-1 deletion [19].

- LRRK-2: there is conflicting evidence between this mutation and the development of dementia. In a large Algerian cohort of 106 patients (34 mutated), there was no relationship between the presence of mutations and cognitive abnormalities [20, 21].

- PINK1: due to its low prevalence, there is conflictive evidence on the relation between PINK1 and PD dementia or cognitive decline [22].

- APOE4: the presence of Aβ plaques and neurofibrillary tau tangles (NFT) are characteristic of cognitive impairment in AD. But, in PD patients, therefore, the APOE ε4 genotype is an additional risk factor to converse to PDD.

Although, some large cohort studies suggest there is no increased risk for developing dementia in carriers [23].

- GBA (glucocerebrosidase): this gene encodes a lysosomal membrane protein that cleaves the beta-glycosidic linkage of glycosylceramide, an intermediate in glycolipid metabolism [24]. Some studies suggest worse cognitive performance in patients with mutations in this gene. Even in some cohorts, it has been considered an independent risk factor for the development of dementia. Mutations in glucocerebrosidase are a major genetic risk factor for PD and increase susceptibility to dementia in a Flanders-Belgian cohort [25].

3.2 Histological changes in patients with PD dementia

Genetic and environmental factors lead to protein misfolding, aggregation, and finally, the neural loss that is reflected in histological changes as mentioned below.

The pathologic findings for PDD include Lewy bodies (LBs), AD pathology, and cerebrovascular disease, among others. Apparently, the inclusions type and the brain localization influence the severity and type of cognitive impairment. LBs and Lewy related pathology (LRP: Lewy neurites) localized in neocortex and limbic areas are related to the risk of suffering dementia with a rapid progression and lower scores in all cognitive domains [26]. On the other hand, limbic distribution is associated with visuospatial skills impairment [27]. LB densities in the temporal lobe were significantly higher in cases with PDD, compared to PD without dementia [28]. Furthermore, concomitant aggregation of b-amyloid (AD pathology) with LRP is associated with PDD. There is evidence in cell models that α-synuclein contributes to deposition of tau and b-amyloid, leading to a summative effect over the risk of PDD [29, 30].

The association of PDD and small vessel disease and cerebral amyloid angiopathy remains elusive because these are also common findings in brains of elderly people [26].

4. Biomarkers of Parkinson's disease dementia

Recent research is focused on the study of molecules or biomarkers related to the pathophysiological mechanisms of PD that can contribute in clinical practice to the diagnosis, prognosis, and monitoring of the progression of neurological diseases.

The most promising results have been obtained from neurofilament light chain protein (NFL), α-synuclein species, lysosomal enzyme activities, and classic AD biomarkers such as amyloid beta peptide 1–42 (Aβ42) and tau protein. An important innovation for diagnostic is the identification of forms of α-synuclein prone to aggregation in early stages of PD [31]. Furthermore, the highest diagnostic accuracies to identify PD patients have been obtained from the combination of different biomarkers (**Figure 1**) [32]. However, these studies require further validation for clinical practice [33–35].

4.1 Cerebrospinal fluid and serum

Prediction of cognitive decline and progression to dementia in PD patients could be a promising tool in clinical practice. Some biomarkers used for AD in cerebrospinal fluid (CSF) have shown that low concentrations of Aβ42 in CSF are associated with worse cognitive scores and could predict cognitive impairment in patients with PD [36, 37].

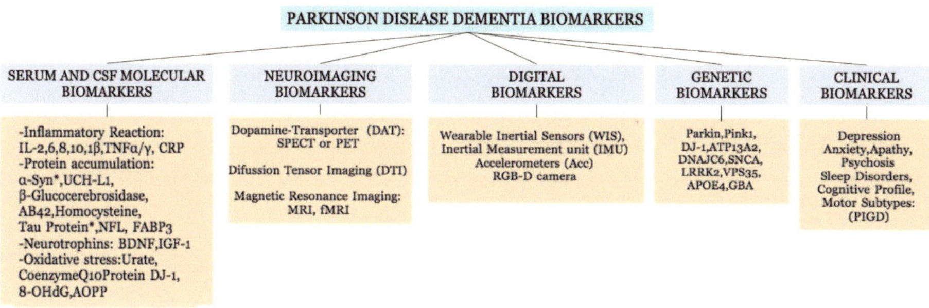

Figure 1.
*Main biomarkers of PD. Figure 1 summarizes the serum, imaging, digital evaluation, and genetic and clinical biomarkers associated with the pathophysiology and course of dementia in Parkinson's disease. TNF: tumor necrosis factor; CRP: C reactive protein; α-Syn: α-synuclein; UCH-L1: ubiquitin C-terminal hydrolase-L1; AB42: amyloid β peptide 1–42; NFL: neurofilament light chain; FABP3: heart-like fatty acid binding protein; BDNF: brain-derived neurotrophic factor; IGF-1: insulin-like growth factor-1; AOPP: advanced oxidation protein products; 8-OHdG: 8-hydroxy-2`-deoxyguanosine; MRI: magnetic resonance imaging; DAT: dopamine transporter; TCS: transcranial sonography; PET: positron emission tomography; SPECT: single photon emission computed tomography; WIS: wearable inertial sensors; and IMU: inertial measurement unit. *Includes species.*

The performance and prognostic value of CSF Aβ42 improved when combined with other biomarkers of CSF. CSF Aβ42 levels <626 ng/L was associated with a hazard ratio (HR) of 2.8 (95% CI 1.4 to 5.8) for the development of dementia within 5–9 years of follow-up. When the ratio of CSF NFL, FABP3, and Aβ42 is more than 2.1, the HR values increased to 11.8 (95% CI 3.3–42.1) [38]. In addition, if the clinical characteristics are analyzed with CSF Aβ42 levels, its prognostic value is further improved [39]. Thus, it has also been determined that low Aβ42 values could predict early psychosis in PD patients within 3–4 years of follow-up [40].

Both, total α-synuclein and homocysteine (Hcy) in CSF have shown contradictory results as a predictor of cognitive impairment [31, 32, 41, 42]. Some neuroinflammatory reaction molecules such as interleukin 8 (IL-8) and C-reactive protein (CRP) levels in CSF are related to decreased MOCA scores in PD patients and PDD patients, respectively [43–45].

It has recently been determined that the blood neurofilament (NFL) can discriminate between (PD) and atypical parkinsonian disorders (APD) with the same precision as in CSF, which would facilitate its use in the differential diagnosis of parkinsonian disorders, and would also allow to correlate the severity and progression of the motor and cognitive functions of PD [46].

Progression in motor disability in PD patients was associated with α-synuclein species concentrations [31]. Both the combination of ratio of phosphorylated tau to Aβ42 and CSF total tau have been found to have a correlation with a faster decline of performance in total unified Parkinson's disease rating scale (MDS-UPDRS) over time. Tau pathology, as assessed by CSF phosphorylated tau, seems to have a role in accelerating motor progression [47]. Some studies suggested that there is a positive correlation between DJ-1, advanced oxidation protein products (AOPP), and 8-OHdG levels, and a greater severity of the disease [32, 42, 48–50].

4.2 Neuroimaging

Advances in neuroimaging allow the identification of non-invasive biomarkers to confirm the diagnosis and possibly know the severity of the disease and also determine the functional prognosis. The Braak progression model does not respond precisely to the behavior of the clinical profiles or to the progression of parkinsonism in a real scenario, where epigenetic variables will be related to the evidence of overlapping between different protein aggregations and alterations of the midbrain-striatal-cortical loop.

Dopamine transporter single photon emission tomography (DAT-SPECT) provides a semi-quantitative assessment of striatal dopaminergic deafferentation. This PD biomarker has a strong correlation between the amount of dopamine transporters in the striatum and the number of dopaminergic neurons in substantia nigra [51, 52].

The combined analysis of various imaging techniques will allow characterizing the baseline alterations related to the disease using DAT-SPECT, DTI, and MRI [53–55]. Functional MRI (fMRI) can show variation of connectivity functional network by detecting oxygenated hemoglobin and deoxyhemoglobin content in brain regions in PD patients [7, 56]. These changes can be present before motor symptoms, and can detect PD patients from normal individuals with a sensitivity of 100% and a specificity of 89.5% [57, 58].

The combined blood and imaging biomarkers such as MR planimetric measurements and NFL serum levels, provided accurate differentiation of PD versus multiple system atrophy (MSA) and progressive supranuclear palsy (PSP) patients. The combined overall diagnostic yield was an accuracy of 83.7% (95% CI 69.8–90.8%) [59].

4.3 Digital data

Ecological and objective measurements made with wearable technology in patients' homes are a reality. The analysis of gait domains in PD patients and its changes over time is a promising biomarker to track normal aging and the progression of the disease as the response to treatment [60].

Considering the functional interdependence of cognition and gait, objective analysis of gait and changes in certain gait domains may be a sensitive marker of the risk of cognitive impairment in patients with PD, observing greater asymmetry and variability in stride time, swing time, and posture compared to AD and Lewy body dementia (LBD) [61].

New technologies applied to the objective measurement of neurological symptoms or diseases will have to be subjected to an adequate scientific validation process.

5. Clinical approach: the continuum of cognitive impairment and dementia in PD

It has been reported that PD patients may have normal cognition at the onset of the disease, although some patients present PD-MCI in the early stage of the disease and it is more frequent with the increment of years of the disease and older age [62]. In 2019, the International Parkinson and Movement Disorders Society (MDS) concluded that the diagnosis of level I PD-MCI is a risk factor to PDD while taking into account variables like age, sex, education, PD motor sign severity, and depression [63].

The most frequent alterations suggest that there are heterogeneous profiles that can be amnesic and non-amnesic. In general, it has been described that the most frequent deficits involve executive dysfunction, decreased attention, and visuospatial dysfunction, as well as in global cognition. However, it is recognized that the PDD extends beyond dysexecutive syndrome to include deficits in recognition memory [64] and visual perception, as well as visual hallucinations and cognitive fluctuations [65]. These findings would indicate that cognitive problems could occur in patients in prodromal stages, which would be in line with the evidence

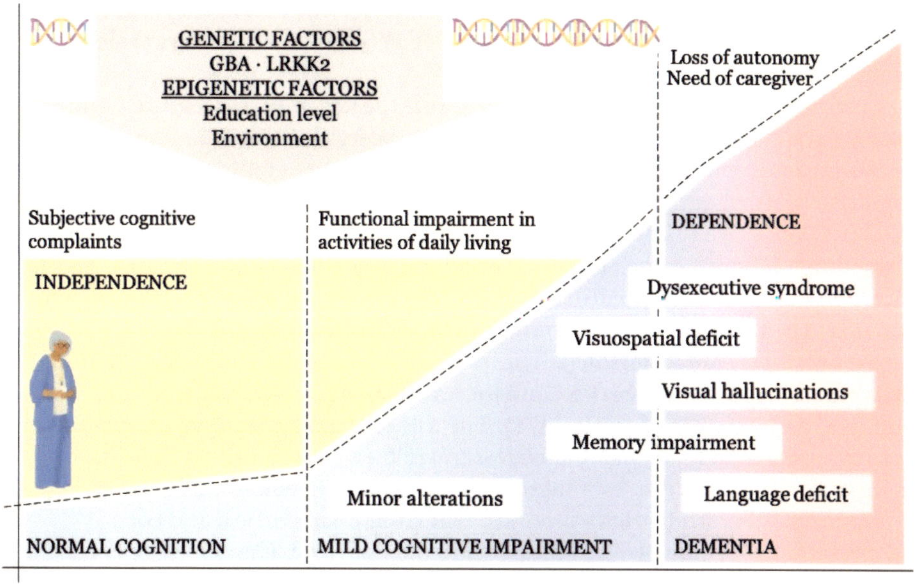

Figure 2.
The continuum of cognitive impairment in PD patients. Figure 2 shows the relationship between genetic and epigenetic factors in the natural course of cognitive decline in Parkinson's disease.

in favor of newly diagnosed or early stage patients already exhibiting deficits in cognition (**Figure 2**) [66].

The main cognitive domains that underlie the presence of PDD have been widely described, however, the compartmentalization is given to understand the complexity of clinical heterogeneity since neural networks interact and they overlap each other to finally define a cognitive function that is influenced by distributed individual actions [67]. Likewise, the existence of a "dual hypothesis" regarding the cognitive component has suggested that the PD-MCI could be a dopamine-dependent profile closely related to the executive and working memory deficit, while the PDD could be a superordinal stage that it would imply the presence of other neurotransmission systems, which generate a picture of rapid progression exhibiting deficits in learned movements (apraxia), in recognition (agnosia), and in language (aphasia) in these patients [68].

Executive impairments in PD are due to the damage of connections between dorsolateral and ventrolateral frontal cortices with the globus pallidus internus and head of the caudate, as well as degeneration of mesocortical pathways with hypometabolism and atrophy prefrontal, insular, and cingulate cortices. Attention problems detected in the early stage of PD and PDD are related to frontal-parietal networks. Memory complaints are common even at the early stage of PD, although subjective memory complaints (SMC) at that point are more related with attentional deficits. However, with the progression of PD-MCI to PDD dementia, memory impairments are similar to those found in AD, in relation to the difficulties with recalling and recognition, which are associated in PDD patients with medial temporal lobe atrophy. Further neuropsychological research is needed to make a proper association on this [67].

Visuospatial and visuoperceptive alterations are prominent of PDD, explained by deterioration in occipito-parietal connections (dorsal and ventral pathway related with spatial location and object recognition, respectively). Visual hallucinations are a hallmark of PDD, and a relevant symptom which suggests the interrelationship with LBD. Different networks are implicated in the visual hallucinations such as middle occipital, inferior parietal lobule, nucleus basalis Meynert (NBM), and dysfunctional sleep-wake cycling with REM (rapid eye movement) sleep behavioral disorder (RBD) [67, 69].

Since it is well established, dopamine loss is the key of motor features, and the cornerstone of the PD treatment. However, acetylcholine, noradrenalin, and serotonin are responsible for the presence of non-motor symptoms, especially cognitive impairment. Loss of cholinergic neurons in NBM is found in 54–70% of PDD patients as well as 40% loss of neurons in brainstem cholinergic nucleus and the pedunculopontine nucleus [70]. The cholinergic diffused afference to cerebral cortex disrupts focused attention, memory encoding, and visual discrimination, and it is implicated in the generation of visual hallucinations [67, 69, 71].

Furthermore, noradrenalin deficit from locus coeruleus involving outputs to the thalamus, amygdala, and cortex contributes to damage in executive control, attention, and maintenance of arousal [71]. The role of the serotonin system has been less investigated in PDD than the neurotransmitters exposed above. It is known there is a reduction in the serotonergic transmission to caudate nucleus [69].

Neuroimaging studies have reported that frontal-subcortical and cortical circuits could be involved in the development of PDD. The heterogeneous profile exhibits a decrease in dopaminergic frontal-striatal networks as well as a wide decrease in cholinergic cortical networks and a degeneration in the limbic-paralimbic system [72]. On the other hand, studies that combine cognitive measures with neurophysiological markers have demonstrated that posterior and frontal-executive cognitive task performance were associated with high risk of conversion to PDD [73].

The identification of PD-MCI is a critical point to management and potential clinical trials of pharmacological therapies. Moreover, the correct diagnosis of PD-MCI and PDD depends of the use of recommended cognitive tests for PD patients [74]. PD-MCI criteria include level I based on a screening evaluation to global cognition and level II based on comprehensive neuropsychological assessment [75]. The MDS Task Force recommends three global screening scales for use when it is not possible to do a comprehensive neuropsychological testing; the scales are the following: Montreal Cognitive Assessment (MoCA), Mattis Dementia Rating Scale, and Parkinson's Disease-Cognitive Rating Scale (PD-CRS) [76].

Because cognitive impairment in PD is beyond cognition, it is useful to ask to the patient and caregiver about subjective complaints, behavioral changes, and quality of life (**Table 1**). In addition, for the diagnosis of PDD, it is important to evaluate the functional independence in activity daily life (ADL) with questionnaires or scales recommended: Parkinson Disease Cognitive Functional Rating Scale (PD-CFRS), Functional assessment questionnaire, and the pill questionnaire [77].

Table 1 summarizes the affected neural networks and their effect on the patient's cognitive domains with the neuropsychological tests recommended for their evaluation.

5.1 The cognitive impairment, non-motor symptoms, and motor subtypes

Interplay between motor and non-motor symptoms has been described with the objective to explore the relationship with different neurotransmitters systems related in the disease progression. Depression, anxiety, apathy, psychosis, fatigue, and sleep problems are common in PDD or even PD-MCI [78].

Also, the different clinical phenotypes of PD can relate the motor symptoms (MS) to non-motor symptoms (NMS). Factors that could contribute to the progression of the disease are also related to advanced age, the severity of motor symptoms, as well as the postural instability gait disorder (PIGD) subtype, the presence of

Neural networks	Cognitive domains	Neuropsychological tests
Nigrostriatal dopamine network	Executive function Decision making/ reversal learning	• Wisconsin card sorting test (WCST)
Mesocortical dopamine network	Executive function Inhibitory control	• Stroop test; frontal assessment battery (FAB)
	Working memory	• Phonological verbal fluency • Trail making test part B (TMT-B) • WAIS-IV digit span
Noradrenergic network	Orientation	• WMS-IV orientation
	Executive attention	• Trail making test part A (TMT-A)
Cholinergic network	Visuoperceptual deficits	• Judgment of line orientation (JLO) Visual object and space perception (VOSP) battery WAIS-IV block design
	Memory deficits	• Hopkins verbal learning test (HVLT); Rey auditory verbal learning test (RAVLT) Wechsler memory scale (WMS-IV): logical memory, designs and visual reproduction Testt Rey-Osterrieth complex figure test (RCFT)
Mesial-frontal network Orbitofrontal cortex network Basal ganglia and dorsolateral prefrontal cortex network	Psychological status	• Beck depression inventory (BDI-II)
	Behavioral disturbance	• Beck anxiety inventory (BAI-II) • Frontal systems behavioral rating Scale (FrSB) • Neuropsychiatric inventory questionnaire (NPI-Q)
	Quality of life	• Parkinson disease questionnaire-39 (PDQ-39)

Table 1.
Neural networks affected in PDD.

visual hallucinations, and associated cognitive deficits to the cortical-posterior profile. Some NMS such as depression and anxiety have been related to specific motor subtypes, and it has been reported that poorer NMS profile are associated with PIGD subtype [79], besides history of falls and motor complications as an effect of pharmacological therapy [80].

Furthermore, PDD is more frequent among PIGD subtypes, and balance and gait disorders predict other non-motor symptoms (NMS) like hallucinations, urinary problems, and daytime sleepiness (12); whereas the alterations of attention and executive domain, which are related to frontostriatal deficits, could be considered a more stable profile [68]. Moreover, other studies have found that progression to PDD would also be associated with poor performance in executive tasks such as verbal fluency as well as other tests associated with cognitive flexibility, inhibition, and concept formation (commonly evaluated using the trail making test (TMT) part B, Wisconsin Card Sorting Test (WCST), and Stroop test) [81, 82].

The importance of detecting individual variables, as well as biomarkers for the heterogeneity of progression to PDD, then becomes useful information to contribute to the clarification of the pathophysiological mechanisms of cognitive impairment in patients with PD [83].

In PD patients, the loss of dopaminergic neurons in the substantia nigra impacts the connections with the prefrontal cortex, which has suggested that it may attenuate the cognitive component in these patients, as well as compromise the ability to cognitively compensate for the deficit in gait. Additionally, acetylcholine is related with attentional processes of the prefrontal cortex and has been strongly associated with a decrease in gait speed. In some patients with PD, this relationship may be exacerbated by freezing gait episodes, since it has been reported that this subgroup of patients has a worse performance in visuospatial skills tasks compared to those who have not, which could be related to a decrease in gray matter in posterior cortical areas [84].

In studies carried out with different motor subtypes and patients with PD-MCI, it has been suggested that scores in the visuospatial domain are correlated with the stability factor, while the executive domain does not correlate with any factor, probably suggesting a more general role of executive functions. The processing of visual information is important during the planning and the control of locomotion in patients with PD. Additionally, low scores in stability factor was inversely associated with advanced stages on the Hoehn and Yahr scale, worse scores in MDS-UPDRS part III, suggesting that there is a specific relationship between motor progression, instability, and visuospatial alteration [85].

The relationship between the different aspects of balance and gait with the cognitive domains suggests that they are mediated by multiple neural pathways. Degeneration in the dopaminergic systems could contribute to cognitive deficits and the PIGD subtype, while degeneration within the cholinergic system has been proposed as a factor that contributes to cognitive and axial symptoms in PD patients. Hypofunction of the cholinergic system has been implicated in impaired executive functioning as well as a greater slowdown in gait speed in patients with PD [86].

6. Treatment

So far, there are no available treatments to cure or stop the progression of the synucleinopathies; hence, offering the best balance in the control of motor and non-motor symptoms of the PD must be a main clinical objective. Due to the multisystemic and progressive nature of neurodegeneration, it is necessary to periodically update the inventory of cognitive, behavioral, and affective symptoms, alongside the motor and general health status, and also to determine the functional impact in daily life activities as well as on the social and working environment [87–89].

It is important to identify and strengthen the support network of caregivers to diagnose and give an appropriate support to the symptomatic complexity of each patient by a multidisciplinary team, which aims to improve their quality of life, reduce disability and health care costs, as well all risks mainly related to cognition and social behavior.

The adequate identification of high-risk clusters would allow the development of subtype specific therapeutic objectives. Moreover, recognizing the non-motor symptoms of high impact of quality of life such as mood disorders, sleep or eating disorders, and behavioral and social behaviors disorders could allow to define an appropriate clinical care [90].

Behind a specific symptom, there are brain areas or hypoactive or overactive functional associative networks with altered neurotransmitter systems such as dopaminergic, cholinergic, serotonergic, glutamatergic, or noradrenergic [26, 65]. For this reason, the analysis and functional neuroanatomical correlation on the temporal course of the disease as well as the cognitive profile is necessary for the

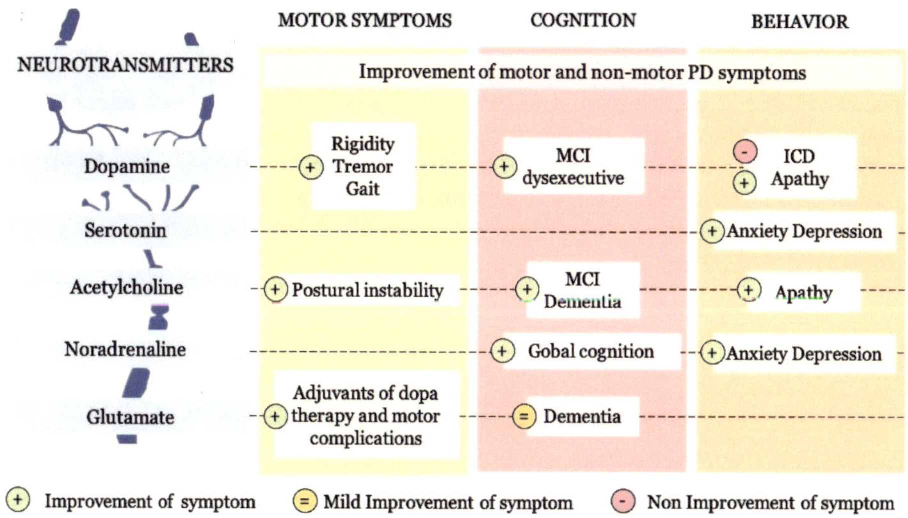

Figure 3.
Neurotransmitters systems related with motor and non-motor symptoms in PD. Figure 3 shows the interaction between neurotransmitters and PD symptoms with the estimated response in each category based on clinical experience.

therapeutic selection and to reestablish, as far as possible or partially, the neurochemical and functional balance (**Figure 3**).

Dopaminergic stimulation can cause some cognitive benefits on frontal executive functions, however, when the patient has motor complications, it could facilitate the appearance of some affective and cognitive fluctuations and could exert a negative effect on cognition [91].

Cholinergic denervation through different mechanisms affects cognition in patients with PD. For that reason, from cholinesterase inhibitors, Rivastigmine is the one with the best evidence of clinical efficacy and safety by improving some cognitive and neuropsychiatric domains. Such evidence is not similar for mild cognitive impairment, which is common in the disease [87, 92]. A possible application of the cholinesterase inhibitors is to improve some gait domains and reduce the risk of fall, by increasing the cholinergic stimuli in the brain areas related to motor and cognitive control of gait [93].

Despite finding a glutamatergic hyperactivity that causes the progression of cognitive deficit in PD, memantine, an N-methyl-D-aspartate (NMDA) antagonist has shown a weak efficacy in improving cognitive functions [94].

The use of atomoxetine, a selective norepinephrine reuptake inhibitor (SNRI), was not effective for the treatment of depressive symptoms in PD, but was associated with improvement in global cognitive performance and daytime sleepiness; however, there is insufficient evidence on new indications for this drug [95].

Likewise, the use of transcranial direct-current stimulation (t-DCS) as well as repetitive transcranial magnetic stimulation (r-TMS) to improve the cognitive impairment has not reached enough evidence and recommendation in order to be recommended [96].

Both the interactions and the potential side effects can aggravate the cognitive state and also produce psychosis, starting with the medicines used in the control of motor symptoms such as anticholinergics trihexyphenidyl, biperiden or benztropine, dopamine antagonist, and amantadine. It is important to monitor daily the interactions of medicines used in treatment of symptoms or concomitant chronic diseases and the potential interactions with the indicated medicines for the control of neurological symptoms. Especially with benzodiazepines, anticholinergics/antimuscarinics used in gastrointestinal or bladder disorders, tricyclic antidepressants, or antipsychotic drugs, several observational studies have shown an association between exposure to anticholinergic drugs and the risk of cognitive impairment [97].

Rehabilitation as well as cognitive stimulation, whose objective is to develop strategies to improve or maintain functionality in daily activities, must be customized according to the phenotype or the cognitive profile in each patient's context [98, 99].

7. Conclusion

PDD is a rising, broad, and complex spectrum disorder with a high burden to patients and their caregivers. The prompt recognition of PD patients with red flags to progress to PDD is crucial to early enrollment in a multidisciplinary and therapeutic approach to diminish disease load. Nowadays, therapeutic options are limited. However, the advent of molecular, cellular, and technological advances creates a promissory future to specific treatment, allowing truly improvement in the patient's and caregiver's quality of life.

Author details

Beatriz Munoz Ospina[1*], Valentina Quintana-Peña[2], Daniela Alvarez[3,4], Jaime A. Valderrama[1,4], Yuri Takeuchi[1] and Jorge L. Orozco[1]

1 Fundación Valle del Lili Cali, Colombia

2 Centro de Investigaciones Clínicas, Fundación Valle del Lili Cali, Colombia

3 Grupo de Investigación i2T Cali, Colombia

4 Universidad Icesi Cali, Colombia

*Address all correspondence to: beatriz.munoz@fvl.org.co

References

[1] Pringsheim T, Jette N, Frolkis A, Steeves TDL. The prevalence of Parkinson's disease: A systematic review and meta-analysis. Movement Disorders. 2014;**29**(13):1583-1590. DOI: 10.1002/mds.25945

[2] Partridge L, Deelen J, Slagboom PE. Facing up to the global challenges of ageing. Nature. 2018;**561**(7721):45-56. DOI: 10.1038/s41586-018-0457-8

[3] de Rijk MC et al. Prevalence of parkinsonism and Parkinson's disease in Europe: The EUROPARKINSON Collaborative Study. European Community Concerted Action on the Epidemiology of Parkinson's disease. Journal of Neurology, Neurosurgery & Psychiatry. 1997;**62**(1):10-15. DOI: 10.1136/jnnp.62.1.10

[4] Orozco JL et al. Parkinson's disease prevalence, age distribution and staging in Colombia. Neurology International. 2020;**12**(1):9-14. DOI: 10.4081/ni.2020.8401

[5] Muangpaisan W, Mathews A, Hori H, Seidel D. A systematic review of the worldwide prevalence and incidence of Parkinson's disease. Journal of the Medical Association of Thailand. 2011;**94**(6):749-755

[6] GBD 2017 US Neurological Disorders Collaborators, et al., "Burden of neurological disorders across the US from 1990-2017: A global burden of disease study," JAMA Neurology, Nov. 2020, 78(2):165-176. doi: 10.1001/jamaneurol.2020.4152.

[7] Macleod AD, Goddard H, Counsell CE. Co-morbidity burden in Parkinson's disease: Comparison with controls and its influence on prognosis. Parkinsonism & Related Disorders. 2016;**28**:124-129. DOI: 10.1016/j.parkreldis.2016.05.013

[8] Wang X et al. Comorbidity burden of patients with Parkinson's disease and Parkinsonism between 2003 and 2012: A multicentre, nationwide, retrospective study in China. Scientific Reports. 2017;**7**(1):1671. DOI: 10.1038/s41598-017-01795-0

[9] Lenka A, Padmakumar C, Pal PK. Chapter fourteen—Treatment of older Parkinson's disease. In: Bhatia KP, Chaudhuri KR, Stamelou M, editors. International Review of Neurobiology. Vol. 132. Academic Press; 2017. pp. 381-405

[10] Mayeux R, et al. The Frequency of idiopathic Parkinson's disease by age, ethnic group, and sex in Northern Manhattan, 1988-1993. American Journal of Epidemiology. 1995;**142**(8):820-827. DOI: 10.1093/oxfordjournals.aje.a117721

[11] Goldman JG, Litvan I. Mild cognitive impairment in Parkinson's disease. Minerva Medica. 2011;**102**(6):441-459

[12] Baiano C, Barone P, Trojano L, Santangelo G. Prevalence and clinical aspects of mild cognitive impairment in Parkinson's disease: A meta-analysis. Movement Disorders. 2020;**35**(1):45-54. DOI: 10.1002/mds.27902.

[13] Obi T et al. Clinicopathologic study of A SNCA gene duplication patient with Parkinson disease and dementia. Neurology. 2008;**70**(3):238-241. DOI: 10.1212/01.wnl.0000299387.59159.db.

[14] Fuchs J et al. Phenotypic variation in a large Swedish pedigree due to SNCA duplication and triplication. Neurology. 2007;**68**(12):916-922. DOI: 10.1212/01.wnl.0000254458.17630.c5.

[15] Leroi I, McDonald K, Pantula H, Harbishettar V. Cognitive impairment in Parkinson disease: Impact on quality of

life, disability, and caregiver burden. Journal of Geriatric Psychiatry and Neurology. 2012;**25**(4):208-214. DOI: 10.1177/0891988712464823

[16] Khan NL et al. Parkin disease: A phenotypic study of a large case series. Brain. 2003;**126**(6):1279-1292. DOI: 10.1093/brain/awg142.

[17] Annesi G et al. DJ-1 mutations and parkinsonism-dementia-amyotrophic lateral sclerosis complex. Annals of Neurology. 2005;**58**(5):803-807. DOI: 10.1002/ana.20666.

[18] Williams DR, Hadeed A, Al-Din ASN, Wreikat A-L, Lees AJ. Kufor Rakeb disease: Autosomal recessive, levodopa-responsive parkinsonism with pyramidal degeneration, supranuclear gaze palsy, and dementia. Movement Disorders. 2005;**20**(10):1264-1271. DOI: 10.1002/mds.20511.

[19] Arias Vásquez A et al. A deletion in DJ-1 and the risk of dementia—A population-based survey. Neuroscience Letters. 2004;**372**(3):196-199. DOI: 10.1016/j.neulet.2004.09.040.

[20] Aarsland D, Kurz MW. The epidemiology of dementia associated with Parkinson disease. Journal of the Neurological Sciences. 2010;**289**(1-2):18-22. DOI: 10.1016/j.jns.2009.08.034

[21] Belarbi S et al. LRRK2 G2019S mutation in Parkinson's disease: A neuropsychological and neuropsychiatric study in a large Algerian cohort. Parkinsonism & Related Disorders. 2010;**16**(10):676-679. DOI: 10.1016/j.parkreldis.2010.09.003.

[22] Romo-Gutierrez D, Yescas P, López-López M, Boll M. Genetic factors associated with dementia in Parkinson's disease (PD). Gaceta medica de Mexico. 2015;**151**(1):110-118

[23] Williams-Gray CH et al. Apolipoprotein E genotype as a risk factor for susceptibility to and dementia in Parkinson's disease. Journal of Neurology. 2009;**256**(3):493-498. DOI: 10.1007/s00415-009-0119-8

[24] Riboldi GM, Di Fonzo AB. GBA, Gaucher disease, and Parkinson's disease: From genetic to clinic to new therapeutic approaches. Cell. 2019;**8**(4):364. DOI: 10.3390/cells8040364

[25] Crosiers D et al. Mutations in glucocerebrosidase are a major genetic risk factor for Parkinson's disease and increase susceptibility to dementia in a Flanders-Belgian cohort. Neuroscience Letters;**629**:160, 2016-164. DOI: 10.1016/j.neulet.2016.07.008

[26] Halliday GM, Leverenz JB, Schneider JS, Adler CH. The neurobiological basis of cognitive impairment in Parkinson's disease: Neurobiology of Parkinson's disease dementia. Movement Disorders. 2014;**29**(5):634-650. DOI: 10.1002/mds.25857

[27] Dickson DW et al. Neuropathological assessment of Parkinson's disease: Refining the diagnostic criteria. The Lancet Neurology. 2009;**8**(12):1150-1157. DOI: 10.1016/S1474-4422(09)70238-8

[28] de Laat KF et al. Cortical thickness is associated with gait disturbances in cerebral small vessel disease. NeuroImage. 2012;**59**(2):1478-1484. DOI: 10.1016/j.neuroimage.2011.08.005

[29] Waxman EA, Giasson BI. Induction of intracellular tau aggregation is promoted by -synuclein seeds and provides novel insights into the hyperphosphorylation of tau. Journal of Neuroscience. 2011;**31**(21):7604-7618. DOI: 10.1523/JNEUROSCI.0297-11.2011

[30] Kazmierczak A, Strosznajder JB, Adamczyk A. α-Synuclein enhances secretion and toxicity of amyloid beta

peptides in PC12 cells. Neurochemistry International. 2008;**53**(6-8):263-269. DOI: 10.1016/j.neuint.2008.08.004

[31] Parnetti L et al. CSF and blood biomarkers for Parkinson's disease. The Lancet Neurology. Jun. 2019;**18**(6):573-586. DOI: 10.1016/S1474-4422(19)30024-9.

[32] He R, Yan X, Guo J, Xu Q, Tang B, Sun Q. Recent advances in biomarkers for Parkinson's disease. Frontiers in Aging Neuroscience. 2018;**10**. DOI: 10.3389/fnagi.2018.00305

[33] Fairfoul G et al. Alpha-synuclein RT-Qu IC in the CSF of patients with alpha-synucleinopathies. Annals of Clinical Translational Neurology. 2016;**3**(10):812-818. DOI: 10.1002/acn3.338.

[34] Paciotti S, Bellomo G, Gatticchi L, Parnetti L. Are we ready for detecting α-synuclein prone to aggregation in patients? The case of 'protein-misfolding cyclic amplification' and 'real-time quaking-induced conversion' as diagnostic tools. Frontiers in Neurology. 2018;**9**:1-9. DOI: 10.3389/fneur.2018.00415

[35] Shahnawaz M et al. Development of a biochemical diagnosis of parkinson disease by detection of α-synuclein misfolded aggregates in cerebrospinal fluid. JAMA Neurology. 2017;**74**(2):163. DOI: 10.1001/jamaneurol.2016.4547.

[36] Hall S, Surova Y, Öhrfelt A, Zetterberg H, Lindqvist D, Hansson O. CSF biomarkers and clinical progression of Parkinson disease. Neurology. 2015;**84**(1):57-63. DOI: 10.1212/WNL.0000000000001098

[37] Compta Y et al. Combined dementia-risk biomarkers in Parkinson's disease: A prospective longitudinal study. Parkinsonism & Related Disorders. 2013;**19**(8):717-724. DOI: 10.1016/j.parkreldis.2013.03.009.

[38] Bäckström DC et al. Cerebrospinal fluid patterns and the risk of future dementia in early, incident Parkinson disease. JAMA Neurology. 2015;**72**(10):1175. DOI: 10.1001/jamaneurol.2015.1449.

[39] Schrag A, Siddiqui UF, Anastasiou Z, Weintraub D, Schott JM. Clinical variables and biomarkers in prediction of cognitive impairment in patients with newly diagnosed Parkinson's disease: A cohort study. The Lancet Neurology. 2017;**16**(1):66-75. DOI: 10.1016/S1474-4422(16)30328-3

[40] Ffytche DH, Pereira JB, Ballard C, Chaudhuri KR, Weintraub D, Aarsland D. Risk factors for early psychosis in PD: Insights from the Parkinson's progression markers initiative. Journal of Neurology, Neurosurgery & Psychiatry. 2017;**88**(4):325-331. DOI: 10.1136/jnnp-2016-314832.

[41] Irizarry MC et al. Association of homocysteine with plasma amyloid β protein in aging and neurodegenerative disease. Neurology. 2005;**65**(9):1402-1408. DOI: 10.1212/01.wnl.0000183063.99107.5c.

[42] García-Moreno J-M et al. May serum levels of advanced oxidized protein products serve as a prognostic marker of disease duration in patients with idiopathic Parkinson's disease? Antioxidants & Redox Signaling. 2013;**18**(11):1296-1302. DOI: 10.1089/ars.2012.5026.

[43] Yu S et al. Potential biomarkers relating pathological proteins, neuroinflammatory factors and free radicals in PD patients with cognitive impairment: A cross-sectional study. BMC Neurology. 2014;**14**(1):1-7. DOI: 10.1186/1471-2377-14-113.

[44] Liu Z et al. Lack of association between IL-10 and IL-18 gene promoter polymorphisms and Parkinson's disease

with cognitive impairment in a Chinese population. Scientific Reports. 2016;**6**(1):1-6. DOI: 10.1038/srep19021.

[45] Lindqvist D et al. Cerebrospinal fluid inflammatory markers in Parkinson's disease—Associations with depression, fatigue, and cognitive impairment. Brain, Behavior, and Immunity. 2013;**33**:183-189. DOI: 10.1016/j.bbi.2013.07.007.

[46] Lin C-H et al., "Blood NfL: A biomarker for disease severity and progression in Parkinson disease," Neurology, vol. 93, no. 11, pp. e1104–e1111, Sep. 2019, doi: 10.1212/WNL.0000000000008088.

[47] The Parkinson Study Group DATATOP Investigators et al. Longitudinal assessment of tau and amyloid beta in cerebrospinal fluid of Parkinson disease. Acta Neuropathologica. 2013;**126**(5):671-682. DOI: 10.1007/s00401-013-1121-x.

[48] Waragai M et al. Plasma levels of DJ-1 as a possible marker for progression of sporadic Parkinson's disease. Neuroscience Letters. 2007;**425**(1):18-22. DOI: 10.1016/j.neulet.2007.08.010.

[49] Hirayama M et al. Urinary 8-hydroxydeoxyguanosine correlate with hallucinations rather than motor symptoms in Parkinson's disease. Parkinsonism & Related Disorders. 2011;**17**(1):46-49. DOI: 10.1016/j.parkreldis.2010.11.004.

[50] Lin X et al. DJ-1 isoforms in whole blood as potential biomarkers of Parkinson disease. Scientific Reports. 2012;**2**(1):1-10. DOI: 10.1038/srep00954.

[51] Lorio S, Sambataro F, Bertolino A, Draganski B, Dukart J. The combination of DAT-SPECT, structural and diffusion MRI predicts clinical progression in Parkinson's disease. Frontiers in Aging Neuroscience. 2019;**11**:1-13. DOI: 10.3389/fnagi.2019.00057

[52] Kraemmer J, Kovacs GG, Perju-Dumbrava L, Pirker S, Traub-Weidinger T, Pirker W. Correlation of striatal dopamine transporter imaging with post mortem substantia nigra cell counts: Correlation of DAT Imaging with SN cell counts. Movement Disorders. 2014;**29**(14):1767-1773. DOI: 10.1002/mds.25975

[53] Le Bihan D et al. Diffusion tensor imaging: Concepts and applications. Journal of Magnetic Resonance Imaging. 2001;**13**(4):534-546. DOI: 10.1002/jmri.1076.

[54] Ashburner J, Csernansk JG, Davatzikos C, Fox NC, Frisoni GB, Thompson PM. Computer-assisted imaging to assess brain structure in healthy and diseased brains. The Lancet Neurology. 2003;**2**(2):79-88. DOI: 10.1016/S1474-4422(03)00304-1

[55] Burton EJ. Cerebral atrophy in Parkinson's disease with and without dementia: A comparison with Alzheimer's disease, dementia with Lewy bodies and controls. Brain. 2004;**127**(4):791-800. DOI: 10.1093/brain/awh088

[56] Pyatigorskaya N, Gallea C, Garcia-Lorenzo D, Vidailhet M, Lehericy S. A review of the use of magnetic resonance imaging in Parkinson's disease. Therapeutic Advances in Neurological Disorders. 2014;**7**(4):206-220. DOI: 10.1177/1756285613511507

[57] Szewczyk-Krolikowski K et al. Functional connectivity in the basal ganglia network differentiates PD patients from controls. Neurology. 2014;**83**(3):208-214. DOI: 10.1212/WNL.0000000000000592.

[58] Tang Y et al. Identifying the presence of Parkinson's disease using low-frequency fluctuations in BOLD signals. Neuroscience Letters. 2017;**645**:1-6. DOI: 10.1016/j.neulet.2017.02.056.

[59] Mangesius S et al. Novel decision algorithm to discriminate parkinsonism with combined blood and imaging biomarkers. Parkinsonism & Related Disorders. Aug. 2020;**77**:57-63. DOI: 10.1016/j.parkreldis.2020.05.033.

[60] Evers LJ et al. Real-life gait performance as a digital biomarker for motor fluctuations: The Parkinson@ Home validation study. Journal of Medical Internet Research. 2020;**22**(10):e19068. DOI: 10.2196/19068

[61] Mc Ardle R, Del Din S, Galna B, Thomas A, Rochester L. Differentiating dementia disease subtypes with gait analysis: Feasibility of wearable sensors? Gait & Posture. 2020;**76**:372-376. DOI: 10.1016/j.gaitpost.2019.12.028.

[62] Muslimovic D, Post B, Speelman JD, Schmand B. Cognitive profile of patients with newly diagnosed Parkinson disease. Neurology. 2005;**65**(8):1239-1245. DOI: 10.1212/01.wnl.0000180516.69442.95

[63] Hoogland J et al. Risk of Parkinson's disease dementia related to level I MDS PD-MCI. Movement Disorders. 2019;**34**(3):430-435. DOI: 10.1002/mds.27617.

[64] Galtier I, Nieto A, Lorenzo JN, Barroso J. Mild cognitive impairment in Parkinson's disease: Diagnosis and progression to dementia. Journal of Clinical and Experimental Neuropsychology. 2016;**38**(1):40-50. DOI: 10.1080/13803395.2015.1087465

[65] Pagonabarraga J, Kulisevsky J. Cognitive impairment and dementia in Parkinson's disease. Neurobiology of Disease. 2012;**46**(3):590-596. DOI: 10.1016/j.nbd.2012.03.029

[66] Fengler S, Liepelt-Scarfone I, Brockmann K, Schäffer E, Berg D, Kalbe E. Cognitive changes in prodromal Parkinson's disease: A review: Cognitive changes in prodromal PD. Movement Disorders. 2017;**32**(12):1655-1666. DOI: 10.1002/mds.27135

[67] Gratwicke J, Jahanshahi M, Foltynie T. Parkinson's disease dementia: A neural networks perspective. Brain. 2015;**138**(6):1454-1476. DOI: 10.1093/brain/awv104

[68] Kehagia AA, Barker RA, Robbins TW. Cognitive impairment in Parkinson's disease: The dual syndrome hypothesis. Neurodegenerative Diseases. 2013;**11**:79-92. DOI: 10.1159/000341998

[69] Aarsland D et al. Cognitive decline in Parkinson disease. Nature Reviews. Neurology. 2017;**13**(4):217-231. DOI: 10.1038/nrneurol.2017.27.

[70] H. Hall et al., "Hippocampal Lewy pathology and cholinergic dysfunction are associated with dementia in Parkinson's disease," Brain, vol. 137, no. Pt 9, pp. 2493-2508, Sep. 2014, doi: 10.1093/brain/awu193.

[71] Halliday GM, Leverenz JB, Schneider JS, Adler CH. The neurobiological basis of cognitive impairment in Parkinson's disease. Movement Disorders. 2014;**29**(5):634-650. DOI: 10.1002/mds.25857

[72] O'Callaghan C, Lewis SJG. Cognition in Parkinson's disease. In: International Review of Neurobiology. Vol. 133. Elsevier; 2017. pp. 557-583

[73] Olde Dubbelink KTE et al. Predicting dementia in Parkinson disease by combining neurophysiologic and cognitive markers. Neurology. 2014;**82**(3):263-270. DOI: 10.1212/WNL.0000000000000034.

[74] Hoogland J et al. Detecting mild cognitive deficits in Parkinson's disease: Comparison of neuropsychological tests: Detecting mild cognitive deficits

in PD. Movement Disorders. 2018;**33**(11):1750-1759. DOI: 10.1002/mds.110.

[75] Litvan I et al. Diagnostic criteria for mild cognitive impairment in Parkinson's disease: Movement Disorder Society Task Force guidelines. Movement Disorders. 2012;**27**(3):349-356. DOI: 10.1002/mds.24893.

[76] Skorvanek M et al. Global scales for cognitive screening in Parkinson's disease: Critique and recommendations. Movement Disorders. 2018;**33**(2):208-218. DOI: 10.1002/mds.27233.

[77] Dubois B et al. Diagnostic procedures for Parkinson's disease dementia: Recommendations from the movement disorder society task force. Movement Disorders. 2007;**22**(16):2314-2324. DOI: 10.1002/mds.21844.

[78] Campbell MC et al. Parkinson disease clinical subtypes: Key features & clinical milestones. Annals of Clinical Translational Neurology. 2020;**7**(8):1272-1283. DOI: 10.1002/acn3.51102.

[79] Ba F, Obaid M, Wieler M, Camicioli R, Martin WRW. Parkinson disease: The relationship between non-motor symptoms and motor phenotype. Canadian Journal of Neurological Sciences/Journal Canadien des Sciences Neurologiques. 2016;**43**(2):261-267. DOI: 10.1017/cjn.2015.328

[80] Burn DJ et al. Parkinson's disease motor subtypes and mood. Movement Disorders. 2012;**27**(3):379-386. DOI: 10.1002/mds.24041.

[81] Lichter DG, Benedict RHB, Hershey LA. Importance of balance-gait disorder as a risk factor for cognitive impairment, dementia and related non-motor symptoms in Parkinson's disease. Journal of Parkinson's Disease. 2018;**8**(4):539-552. DOI: 10.3233/JPD-181375

[82] Domellöf ME, Elgh E, Forsgren L. The relation between cognition and motor dysfunction in drug-naive newly diagnosed patients with Parkinson's disease. Movement Disorders. 2011;**26**(12):2183-2189. DOI: 10.1002/mds.23814

[83] Martínez-Horta S, Kulisevsky J. Is all cognitive impairment in Parkinson's disease 'mild cognitive impairment'? Journal of Neural Transmission. 2011;**118**(8):1185-1190. DOI: 10.1007/s00702-011-0675-9.

[84] Tessitore A et al. Resting-state brain connectivity in patients with Parkinson's disease and freezing of gait. Parkinsonism & Related Disorders. 2012;**18**(6):781-787. DOI: 10.1016/j.parkreldis.2012.03.018.

[85] Amboni M et al. Gait patterns in parkinsonian patients with or without mild cognitive impairment. Movement Disorders. 2012;**27**(12):1536-1543. DOI: 10.1002/mds.25165.

[86] Bohnen NI et al. Gait speed in Parkinson disease correlates with cholinergic degeneration. Neurology. 2013;**81**(18):1611-1616. DOI: 10.1212/WNL.0b013e3182a9f558.

[87] Seppi K et al. Update on treatments for nonmotor symptoms of Parkinson's disease—An evidence-based medicine review. Movement Disorders. 2019;**34**(2):180-198. DOI: 10.1002/mds.27602.

[88] Kulisevsky J et al. Measuring functional impact of cognitive impairment: Validation of the Parkinson's disease cognitive functional rating scale. Parkinsonism & Related Disorders. 2013;**19**(9):812-817. DOI: 10.1016/j.parkreldis.2013.05.007.

[89] Martinez-Martin P, Rodriguez-Blazquez C, Forjaz MJ, Kurtis MM, Skorvanek M. Measurement of nonmotor symptoms in clinical

practice. International Review of Neurobiology. 2017;**133**:291-345. DOI: 10.1016/bs.irn.2017.04.001.

[90] Mu J, Chaudhuri KR, Bielza C, de Pedro-Cuesta J, Larrañaga P, Martinez-Martin P. Parkinson's disease subtypes identified from cluster analysis of motor and non-motor symptoms. Frontiers in Aging Neuroscience. 2017;**9**:1-10. DOI: 10.3389/fnagi.2017.00301

[91] Kulisevsky J et al. Subclinical affective and cognitive fluctuations in Parkinson's disease: A randomized double-blind double-dummy study of oral vs. intrajejunal levodopa. Journal of Neurology. 2020;**267**(11):3400-3410. DOI: 10.1007/s00415-020-10018-y.

[92] Emre M et al. Rivastigmine for dementia associated with Parkinson's disease. The New England Journal of Medicine. 2004;**351**(24):2509-2518. DOI: 10.1056/NEJMoa041470.

[93] Henderson EJ et al. Rivastigmine for gait stability in patients with Parkinson's disease (ReSPonD): A randomised, double-blind, placebo-controlled, phase 2 trial. The Lancet Neurology. 2016;**15**(3):249-258. DOI: 10.1016/S1474-4422(15)00389-0.

[94] Emre M et al. Memantine for patients with Parkinson's disease dementia or dementia with Lewy bodies: A randomised, double-blind, placebo-controlled trial. Lancet Neurology. 2010;**9**(10):969-977. DOI: 10.1016/S1474-4422(10)70194-0

[95] Weintraub D et al. Atomoxetine for depression and other neuropsychiatric symptoms in Parkinson disease. Neurology. 2010;**75**(5):448-455. DOI: 10.1212/WNL.0b013e3181ebdd79.

[96] Wagle Shukla A et al. Repetitive transcranial magnetic stimulation (rTMS) therapy in Parkinson disease: A meta-analysis. PM & R: The Journal of Injury, Function, and Rehabilitation. 2016;**8**(4):356-366. DOI: 10.1016/j.pmrj.2015.08.009.

[97] Coupland CAC, Hill T, Dening T, Morriss R, Moore M, Hippisley-Cox J. Anticholinergic drug exposure and the risk of dementia: A nested case-control study. JAMA Internal Medicine. 2019;**179**(8):1084. DOI: 10.1001/jamainternmed.2019.0677.

[98] Kalbe E, Aarsland D, Folkerts A-K. Cognitive interventions in Parkinson's disease: Where we want to go within 20 years. Journal of Parkinson's Disease. 2018;**8**(s1):S107-S113. DOI: 10.3233/JPD-181473

[99] Biundo R, Weis L, Fiorenzato E, Antonini A. Cognitive rehabilitation in Parkinson's disease: Is it feasible? Archives of Clinical Neuropsychology. 2017;**32**(7):840-860. DOI: 10.1093/arclin/acx092

Chapter 6

The Role of the Primary Care Physician in the Management of Parkinson's Disease Dementia

Xin-Nong Li and Dawei Zheng

Abstract

Dementia is a frequent complication of Parkinson's disease with an annual incidence of around 10% of patients with Parkinson's disease. If dementia occurs in patients with Parkinson's disease, it is typically many years or decades after the onset of Parkinson's disease. It is devastating for both patient and family or caretaker when a patient with Parkinson's disease develops dementia. Primary care physician is at the center of the care team for the patient. This chapter discusses the pivotal role of the primary care physicians in the management of patients with Parkinson's disease dementia. A guide is provided to emphasize the art of practice for Primary care physicians which consists of knowing when and how to introduce a comprehensive ongoing care plan for individual patient with Parkinson's disease dementia. Recommendations for maintaining some patients with Parkinson's disease dementia in a status of relative independence are discussed. Indications for initiation of palliative care are also discussed.

Keywords: Primary care physicians, Parkinson's disease dementia, management, palliative care

1. Introduction

Parkinson's disease dementia (PDD) is a well-known complication of Parkinson's disease (PD), with an annual incidence of around 10% of patients with PD and a cumulative prevalence of 75–90% of those with a disease duration of 10 years or more [1–3]. Dementia is an overall term that describes a wide range of symptoms associated with a decline in memory or other thinking skills severe enough to reduce a person's ability to perform independent activities of daily living (IADLs) [4]. Symptoms of dementia can be seen in most of the neurodegenerative diseases, such as Alzheimer's disease (AD), vascular dementia (VD), dementia with Lewy bodies (DLB), Creutzfeldt-Jakob disease (CJD), frontotemporal dementia, Huntington's disease, normal pressure hydrocephalus [5, 6]. The general risk factors for dementia include lower education, hypertension, hearing impairment, smoking, obesity, depression, physical inactivity, diabetes, low social contact, excessive alcohol consumption, traumatic brain injury, and air pollution [7]. It is devastating for both patient and family or caretaker when a patient with PD develops dementia because both PD and dementia have a protracted course, with progressive but insidious development of disability [8]. Primary care physicians (PCPs) stand in a unique position for caring for patients from early to terminal stage of their life and play an important role in the management of PDD patients, including in screening, diagnosis, and treatment. It is important to provide individual, realistic, and affordable options of care to every unique patient and his/her family [9, 10].

2. Screening for the early symptoms and signs of PDD

PD impacts people in different ways. Not everyone will experience all the symptoms of PD at the same time or follow the same pattern. But PCPs should be familiar with the common symptoms or typical patterns of progression in PD that are defined in stages [11–13]. PCPs should also know the risk factors that make PD patients more likely to experience dementia because the clinical symptoms of both syndromes can overlap to a high degree. PCPs should always consider seeking reversible medical conditions that can affect mental function in PD patients. A flowsheet (**Table 1**) for screening generated here should help PCPs and their team to achieve this goal during a patient's routine annual wellness visit (AWV) or general visit.

In addition to above mentioned risk factors [7], genetic risk factors are concerning too. One gene, identified to be a risk factor, is the apolipoprotein E gene which presents in three allelic forms (ε2, ε3, and ε4), of which the ε4 allele is a risk factor for AD [23, 24]. Recognizing some other factors in PD patients is also important for early diagnosis of PDD [25, 26]. Those other factors include advanced age at time of diagnosis of PD, experiencing excessive daytime sleepiness, hallucinations before the onset of other dementia symptoms, a history of mild cognitive impairment, more severe motor impairment symptoms than most people with PD, having a specific PD symptom that causes a person to have difficulty starting to take a step or to halt mid-step while walking.

Items	Purpose
Age	recognize this is a risk factor
Stage of PD	severity of motor impairment from PD, another risk factor for PDD
cognitive functions	search cognitive function stage including attention, executive, and visuospatial functions
Dementia Screen Indicator [14]	screening possible high-risk patients. If it is negative, follow up periodically. If it is positive, further investigation is needed.
Geriatric Depression Scale [15, 16]	search for mood disorders
PHQ-9 screen for depression [17, 18]	further evaluation of depression
MoCA [19]	early detection of cognitive impairment
Qmci [20]	differentiating MCI and NC
MMSE + CDT [21, 22]	to stage mental dysfunction, better specificity and sensitivity

AWV: annual wellness visit; PHQ-9: patient health questionnaire-9; MCI: mild cognitive impairment; NC: normal cognitive. MoCA: Montreal cognitive assessment; Qmci: quick mild cognitive impairment; MMSE: mini-mental state examination. CDT: clock drawing test.
The information needed to arrive at the diagnosis requires the clear demonstration that cognitive impairment negatively impacts daily living. This issue is determined by the patient and caregiver interview, and generally focuses on the patient's autonomy, the ability to manage finances, to cope in social situations, and to utilize equipment that is part of daily living.

Table 1.
For routine AWV in PD patient in addition to routine questionnaire.

It is important to search for reversible medical conditions affecting mental dysfunction that may mimic dementia. Electrolyte imbalance, such as hyponatremia or hypernatremia, may cause neuropsychiatric manifestations [27–29]. A personality change such as increasing irritability may be a symptom of hypernatremia, hypercalcemia, hypocalcemia, hypophosphatemia, or hypomagnesemia. In most instances, correction of such underlying electrolyte imbalance will alleviate the psychiatric symptoms. PCPs should pay close attention to age-related limitations of fluid homeostasis, especially in PD patients because that can change the mental function in PD patients gradually and insidiously. Vitamin D deficiency has been associated with neuropsychiatric conditions such as PD, schizophreniform disorder, multiple sclerosis (MS), AD and autism spectrum disorder [30]. PCPs should always be alerted that the side effects of medications can also cause various symptoms and signs of mental disorders that can mimic dementia [31]. Those common drugs include anxiolytics (Benzodiazepines), antiseizure medications (e.g. carbamazepine), antidepressants (e.g. tricyclics), narcotics (e.g. hydrocodone), certain medications for PD (e.g. pramipexole, ropinirole), some hypertension medications (e.g. beta-blockers), sleeping medications (non-benzodiazepine, zolpidem.), medications for incontinence (anticholinergics, oxybutynin.), and some antihistamines (first generation, e.g. hydroxyzine and diphenhydramine).

It is unclear whether early detected cognitive impairment and interventions for dementia patients have a significant effect on their long-term outcomes [32, 33]. But early detection of cognitive impairment can allow for identification and treatment of reversible causes. It also may help patients understand and adhere to medical treatment plans and provide a basis for advance planning for patients and their families [34]. Unfortunately, underdiagnosis of Alzheimer's and other dementias in the primary care setting is not uncommon [35].

Many screening tools have been developed for medical providers to identify dementia patients earlier. These can be used for screening in PD patients. These tools are summarized in **Table 2**. A dementia screening indicator is generated to help PCPs plan the next steps of management [14]. First, it starts with three simple questions if you think your patient may have cognitive impairment based on (1) your observations, (2) concerns of the patient or (3) concerns of family or others. If the answer is yes for one of these three questions, the patient should be screened for cognitive impairment. Second, is the patient 80 or older? If yes, the patient should be screened for cognitive impairment. If not 80 or older, the dementia screening indicator should be administered. The dementia screening indicator consists of 7 items that include (1) age, (2) years of education, (3) body mass index (BMI), (4) history of type 2 diabetes, (5) history of stroke, (6) function of management of

Screening tool	Characteristic	Usage
Screen Indicator [35]	simple, easily administered in PCP settings.	identify high risk patients for MCI and dementia
MoCA [14]	early detection of cognitive impairment	High specificity and sensitivity for screening MCI
Qmci [19]	needs more administrate effort	more sensitive in differentiating MCI and NC
MMSE [20]	comprehensive evaluation	Able to stage dementia, but less sensitive to screen MCI

MCI: mild cognitive impairment; NC: normal cognitive. MoCA: Montreal cognitive assessment; Qmci: quick mild cognitive impairment; MMSE: mini-mental state examination.

Table 2.
Comparison of different screening tools for mental status.

money or medication and (7) depression. If the total point score is more than 22, the patient should be screened for cognitive impairment, with an instrument such as those described below [14].

One commonly used screening tool is the Montreal Cognitive Assessment (MoCA; range 0–30; follow-up evaluation to screening recommended if score is <26). MoCA requires about 10–15 minutes to administer and is useful in early detection of cognitive impairment, including MCI with executive dysfunction [19].

The quick mild cognitive impairment (Qmci) has six domains with total score 100; five orientation items (country, year, month, day, and date with a maximum score of 10), five registration items (score ≤ 5) and a clock drawing test (score ≤ 15), each scored within 1 min. It also has a delay recall (DR) section (timed at 20 seconds with score ≤ 20), a verbal fluency (VF) test (in 60 seconds with score ≤ 20) and a logical memory (LM) test with 30 seconds for administration and 30 seconds for response (score ≤ 30). It can be administered and scored in ~5 minutes. The Qmci is more sensitive than the Standard Mini-Mental State Examination (SMMSE) in differentiating MCI and normal cognition (NC), making it a useful test, for MCI in clinical practice, especially for older adults [20].

The Mini-Mental State Examination (MMSE) that was developed more than 4 decades ago is still a gold standard exam for comparison. It is a brief test, taking ~7 to 10 minutes to complete. The pooled estimate across 15 studies resulted in 89 percent sensitivity (95% CI, 0.85 to 0.92) and 89 percent specificity (95% CI, 0.85 to 0.93) to detect dementia at a cutoff of ≤23 or ≤ 24 [21]. It is less sensitive to the presence of MCI and less thoroughly evaluated in the domains of executive function, higher-level language skills, and complex visuospatial processing. The most sensitive combination of screening tools is the MMSE and Pfeffer Functional Activities Questionnaire (PFAQ) (94.1%). The best specificity is the combination of the MMSE and Clock Drawing test (CDT) [22, 36].

3. Diagnosis of PDD

After the clinical bedside screening test with suspicious PDD as shown in **Table 1**, orchestrating further investigations as outlined in **Table 3** should be the next step to obtain more evidence to make the diagnosis of PDD. Laboratory studies and imagining studies should be carried out before making the diagnosis. Obtaining basic laboratory data on complete blood count (CBC), comprehensive

Items needed to be done	Purpose
Review list of medications that patient is taking	search for side effects of medications.
Laboratory investigation: CMP, CBC, lipid, TSH, B12, CRP	search for reversible causes of mental function change.
Imaging study (MRI of head)	rule out other pathology, identify atrophy of the brain.
Referral for neurological consultation	confirm diagnosis
nonpharmacological intervention	improve symptoms
Pharmacological treatment	prevent or delay the progression of dementia
Health maintenance care	preserve the ability for daily activities
Palliative care/hospice	improve quality of life

Table 3.
Steps for management of suspected PDD patient.

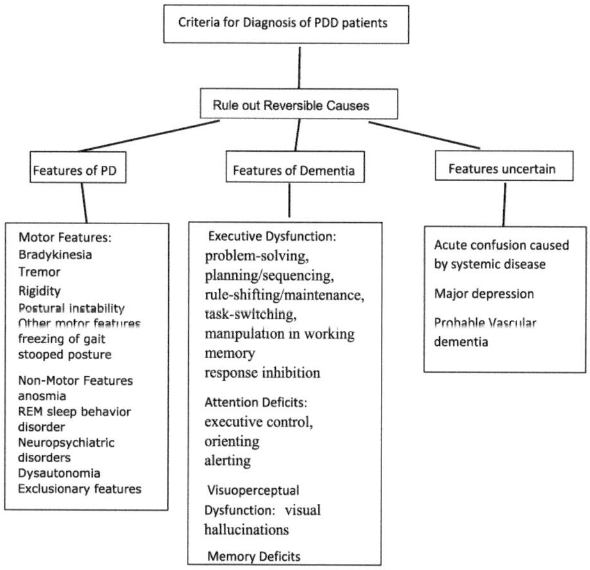

Figure 1.
Criteria for diagnosis of PDD patient.

metabolic panel (CMP), thyroid stimulating hormone (TSH) should be done to understand the basic homeostatic condition of the patients. Checking the levels of vitamin B12, B1, and B6 is proper to search for a reversible pathological cause of mental function change. Brain imaging studies, MRI or CT, will help to distinguish common pathological conditions, including hydrocephalus, atrophy of the brain, vascular disease, or tumor [37, 38].

Criteria to establish the diagnosis of PDD are depicted in **Figure 1**. There are feature domains in these criteria, including features of PD and dementia as well as uncertain features. In the end, a collaborative neurological consultation should be considered to make the diagnosis of PDD [39–43].

4. Treatment guidelines for PDD

The fundamental goals of treatment for PPD patients are to reduce suffering caused by the cognitive and accompanying symptoms, while delaying progressive cognitive and physical decline. How to reach these goals is a challenge to medical providers, patients, and families because the severity of PD, mood disorders, hearing defects, and mental function declining can overlap and affect each other. That needs comprehensive evaluation, planning, and cooperation/coordination with neurologists. An algorithm shown in **Figure 2** will help PCPs to orchestrate the treatment plan with patients and their families.

4.1 Non-pharmacological intervention for PDD

The non-pharmacological interventions that combine diet, exercise, cognitive training, and vascular risk monitoring improve cognition in people at risk for cognitive decline [44–46]. Physical exercise, both aerobic (walking, swimming) and anaerobic/conditioning (resistance training, Tai chi), improves cardiovascular health through benefits on blood pressure and stroke risk [47]. Some trials suggest these interventions may positively affect cognitive and physical function and promote patients' functional independence, improve their well-being and that of their

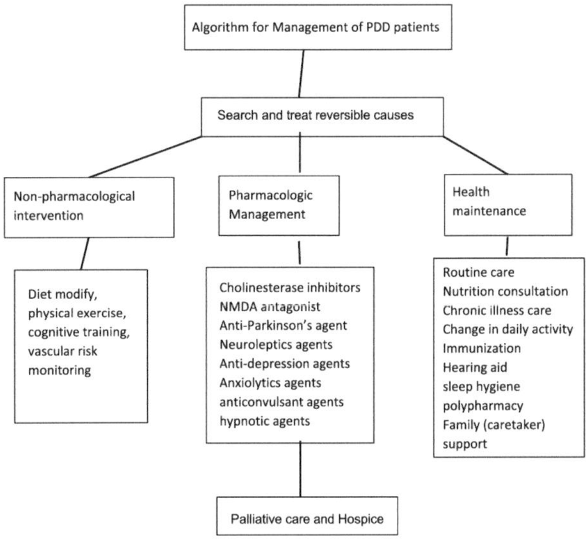

Figure 2.
Algorithm workflow for management of PDD patient.

caregivers. Cognitive training and activities such as reading and playing cognitively engaging games (e.g., chess, bridge) may help maintain cognition and function, improve processing speed, and reduce daytime sleepiness [48].

Music therapy may help maintain cognition or improve quality of life, as some studies revealed that recovery of verbal memory and focused attention improved significantly in patients who listened to their favorite music daily. Besides the improvement in cognitive functions, there was also a substantial mood improvement in this group of patients [49]. Falls have several psychosocial impacts, including fear of falling and reduced self-efficacy, leading to decreased independence, reduced social participation and diminished health-related quality of life [50]. Prescribing cane, walker, or physical and occupational therapies for prevention of falling is one of the responsibilities of PCPs. Moderate intensity outdoor group activities like Nordic Walking and Walking seem to improve motor and non-motor symptoms in patients with Parkinson's disease [51]. Physical activity may assuage the degeneration of motor skills, lessen depression, and increase the quality of life of PDD patients.

4.2 Pharmacologic management for PDD

As described above, PCPs should oversee all medications that PDD patients take before considering pharmacologic treatment for dementia symptoms in PDD patients, because PDD patients usually take medications for PD and other comorbidities. PCP should be familiar with the most common pharmacologic therapies for PD patients, although these are usually initiated by neurologists. These medications include carbidopa-levodopa, monoamine oxidase-B inhibitors, and dopamine agonists. Knowing the effects and side effects of these medications will help PCP to recognize when mental status changes in PD patients are attributable to medication side effects or interactions of medications. It will also help PCPs avoid the interaction of medications when prescribing therapeutic medications either for symptoms of dementia or for other medical conditions. Before any medication is prescribed, potential side effects should be counseled, fully disclosed, and well explained (to the best of your knowledge) to patients and their families or caregivers. This would be critical for those with limited mental capacity to increase compliance and to decrease avoidable incidents. In addition, based on our clinical experience, for lower body mass patients, low-dose initiation of medication and slow titration should be considered. Effective treatment monitoring requires periodic reevaluation of cognition, function, neuropsychiatric and behavioral symptoms, and medication reconciliation. Five drugs, 4 of which are currently available for prescription in the United States, yield modest symptomatic benefit for cognitive symptoms of AD dementia [38]. These drugs may be also beneficial for PDD patients. Their usages are discussed below and summarized in **Tablc 4**.

4.2.1 Acetylcholinesterase inhibitors

This class of medications can exhibit significant clinical impact in mild to moderate dementia patients and can also benefit severe dementia patients. Acetylcholinesterase inhibitors, including Donepezil, Rivastigmine and Galantamine, inhibit the brain enzyme acetylcholinesterase, thereby promoting relative increases in acetylcholine abundance at the synaptic cleft for cholinergic neurotransmission. Donepezil 5 to 10 mg can be taken once a day orally. This is the one most widely used. Side effects of nausea, gastrointestinal (GI) cramps, and dizziness could be minimized by being taken after dinner. Rivastigmine 1.5 to 6 mg twice daily orally, or 4.6 to 9.5 mg transdermal patch once a day is another option. Clinical trials in DLB and PDD have established this agent's clinical efficacy better than other drugs in this class. Another cholinergic drug is Galantamine 4 to 12 mg twice a day orally or extended release 8 to 24 mg once a day orally. This agent has shown less consistent benefit on function and behavior. Tacrine is no longer being used clinically because of liver toxicity, and the above newer agents have better tolerance profiles.

4.2.2 Memantine (Namenda)

Memantine is one of the N-methyl-D-aspartate (NMDA) non-competitive antagonists which might slow down the neurodegenerative process by blocking Glutamate's overstimulation of the NMDA receptors, and thus reduce excitotoxicity. Memantine alone or combined with Donepezil is another option commonly used for moderate to severe Alzheimer's disease. A meta-analysis reported that use of memantine to treat behavioral and psychological symptoms of dementia (BPSD) yielded modest decreases in scores on the Neuropsychiatric Inventory Questionnaire and improvement of symptoms, although sedation was reported to be a major side effect [38]. Memantine can be taken 5 to 10 mg twice a day orally or extended-release form 7 to 28 mg once a day orally. This agent should be considered to initiate at the moderate to severe stages of PDD, because severe dementia in PD most commonly has concomitant AD pathology. In addition to the above 2 categories of drugs, the following other medications that are commonly used in PDD patients are also addressed in below and in **Table 4**.

4.2.3 Anti-Parkinsonian agents

Selegiline 5 mg twice a day orally is also commonly used. Despite lack of confirmatory outcome data, some believe that this anti-Parkinsonian disease medication may have a neuroprotective effect against PDD, based largely on animal models.

Medications commonly used in PCP setting for the pharmacologic management of PDD		
A. Cholinesterase inhibitors.		
1	Donepezil (Aricept)	first line to choose, it should be taken after dinner to lessen the impact of GI side effects.
2	Rivastigmine (Exelon)	Topical patch, Rivastigmine will decrease GI side effects and oral medication burden
B. NMDA antagonist.		
1	Memantine (Namenda)	for moderate to severe dementia, combined with Cholinesterase inhibitor showing better efficacy and less GI side effects
C. Neuroleptics agents		
1	Quetiapine (Seroquel)	commonly first to choose for relative safety profile for sedation and wider dosing range to titrate
2	Olanzapine (Zyprexa)	effective against psychiatric symptoms but less favorable metabolic impacts
3	Risperidone (Risperdal)	usually considered when Quetiapine and Olanzapine failed
D. Anti-depression medications		
a. SSRI		
1	Escitalopram (Lexapro)	low dose initiation, better option towards anxious clinical manifestation
2	Citalopram (Celexa)	good alternative for Escitalopram
3	Sertraline (Zoloft)	long clinical usage and experience for positive psychiatric symptoms
4	Fluoxetine (Prozac)	long clinical usage and experience for negative psychiatric symptoms
b. the Others		
1	Mirtazapine (Remeron)	well adopted in geriatric population for hypnotic and appetite enhancement profiles
2	Trazodone	classical and safe sleep aid in low dose
3	Bupropion (Wellbutrin)	less sexual function disturbance and stamina boosting characters considered
4	Venlafaxine (Effexor)	good feature for general anxiety symptoms
5	Nortriptyline (Pamelor)	well adopted for muscle relaxing, hypnotic and appetite boost but alert on anticholinergic side effect in geriatric population
E. Anxiolytics, anticonvulsant, and hypnotic medications		
1	Buspirone	less clinical effectiveness but very safety profile favored on anxiety background management
2	Valproic acid (Depakote)	mood stabilizer or clinical symptoms complicated with epilepsy
3	Carbamazepine (Tegretol)	mood stabilizer or clinical symptoms complicated with epilepsy
4	Gabapentin (Neurontin)	mood stabilizer or clinical symptoms complicated with neuropathic pain
5	Zolpidem (Ambien)	most widely used hypnotic agent but alert in sleeping walk reported often
6	Zaleplon (Sonata)	short acting for helping waking up in the middle of night

Medications commonly used in PCP setting for the pharmacologic management of PDD		
7	Eszopiclone (Lunesta)	effective hypnotic but dizziness and fainting caution in geriatric population
8	Ramelteon (Rozerem)	quite safe agent but efficacy limited to certain population
9	Suvorexant (Belsomra)	relatively new in market and quite safe agent but efficacy limited in higher dose

Table 4.
Common medications for PDD patients.

4.2.4 Neuroleptics agents

Agitation, aggressive behavior, psychosis, and especially visual hallucinations are often encountered in the early stages, particularly in PDD compared to other types of dementia like AD or VD. For this reason, this class of medicines may be more often required in the early stage PDD compared to other types of dementia, but needs to be dosed and monitored closely. The second-generation antipsychotic agents or atypical antipsychotic agents are currently preferred due to their relatively tolerable side effect profiles with less risk of 'neuroleptic sensitivity', (i.e., motor, and cognitive deterioration) [52]. Also, metabolic abnormalities, especially serum glucose increases, need to be closely monitored during treatment. Over sedation caused by high dose or frequent dosing should be discussed with family members or caregivers for adjusting neuroleptic doses promptly and safely. Institutional abuse of this class of medicine has been reported. These are common second-generation neuroleptics agents: (1) Quetiapine (Seroquel) 12.5 to 100 mg per day orally; (2) Olanzapine (Zyprexa) 2.5 to 10 mg per day orally; (3) Risperidone (Risperdal) 0.25 to 1 mg per day orally; (4) Aripiprazole (Abilify) 10 to 30 mg per day orally; (5) Ziprasidone (Geodon) 20 to 160 mg per orally.

4.2.5 Antidepressant medications

Geriatric depression is a common and treatable comorbidity in patients with dementia. Several tools are validated to screen for depression in older patients. The five-item Geriatric Depression Scale is brief and sensitive. It is as effective as the 15-item Geriatric Depression Scale and does not require clinician administration [52]. In patients with depression and dementia, treatment for depression should usually be initiated first. Pseudodementia, or depression causing cognitive impairment, is diagnosed if the impairment resolves with treatment of the depression. These antidepressant medications have been widely used for mild to moderate uncomplicated depression disorders in the primary care setting [53, 54]. Selective serotonin reuptake inhibitors (SSRIs) are the first line treatment of choice. Patients who do not respond to two or more SSRI agents may choose agents from the other group of antidepressants. These are commonly prescribed SSRI antidepressant medications: (1) Escitalopram 5 to 10 mg per day orally; (2) Citalopram 10 to 20 mg per day orally; (3) Sertraline 25 to 100 mg per day orally; (4) Fluoxetine 10 to 40 mg per day orally. Other antidepressants include: (1) Mirtazapine 7.5 to 30 mg before bedtime orally; (2) Trazodone 50 to 150 mg before bedtime orally; (3) Bupropion 75 to 300 mg per day orally; (4) Venlafaxine 25 to 300 mg per day orally; (5) Nortriptyline 10 to 100 mg before bedtime orally. Three new antidepressants are currently available. One is Vilazodone (Viibryd) that can be started at an initial dose of 10 mg orally once a day for 7 days, followed by 20 mg orally once a day for an additional 7 days, then a maintenance dose of 40 mg orally once a day.

Second one is Levomilnacipran (Fetzima) with initial dose of 20 mg orally once a day for 2 days, then increased to 40 mg orally once a day; Maintenance dose: 40 to 120 mg orally once a day. The third novel antidepressant is Vortioxetine (Trintellix) with dosage of 5 to 10 mg per day orally.

4.2.6 Anxiolytics, anticonvulsants, and hypnotic medications

In advanced disease stages, a significant portion of these patients develop behavioral disorders which are sometimes severe enough to incur a big burden, although not sensed well by patients themselves but mainly by caregivers and family members. Symptoms include anger with exploding tantrums, wandering, suspiciousness or paranoia, wakefulness at nighttime and incontinence, and inappropriate sexual behavior [55, 56].

Benzodiazepines can be carefully prescribed to the patients with agitation and anxiety, using a short acting agent, and on an as needed basis. While prescribing this class of medication, caution must be considered in high priority to balance potential side effects and clinical benefit. Best practices include starting with low dose treatment, while continually monitoring for fall incidence, declines in renal and hepatic function, lethargy, and any other undesirable side effects, especially in elderly patients.

5. Maintaining PDD patients' general health

The most important aspect of the management of PDD is to maintain PDD patients' general health in terms of preventive medicine, and to keep them as independent as possible in activities of daily living (ADL).

Since PDD, like PD itself, is not curable nor reversible, long-term or chronic ongoing care is the highlight of primary care practice. More than 30% of Parkinson's disease patients will eventually develop dementia symptoms [57]. Therefore, early counseling and a scientific based clinical prediction to detect the subtle clinic symptoms of incipient dementia in this group of patients is an advantage that PCPs have over subspecialty physicians during their daily care and more frequent routine encounters. In the last decade, the guidelines for the Annual Wellness Visit (AWV) from Center for Medicare and Medicaid Service (CMS) has provided a good essential structure for PCPs to screen, predict, detect, and manage dementia among PD patients in daily proactive care [58, 59]. During an AWV visit, the companion of family members or caregivers is highly informative and sensitive to obtain information about patients' daily routine life patterns and memory status, and to detect subtle changes in their logical thinking and judgment. Current well-equipped telemedicine setups can provide an even better way of looking into patients' living environment and other real-life situations around them. Periodic proactive monitoring, educational discussions, and prognosis counseling are the cornerstones for taking care of those patients and their family or caregivers. Disease burden, no doubt, is detrimental to the patient. However, family and caregivers' stress and frustration cannot be ignored or underestimated during long-term, chronic stage, ongoing patient management. Especially, advanced PDD patients show hallucinations, wandering, suspiciousness and incontinence, and other behavioral symptoms. The management of these symptoms require tremendous efforts and resources from the caregiver [4, 8]. Early counseling and anticipating this potential development will prepare them psychologically in advance and help alleviate their stresses later. Also, making early arrangements to prepare for catastrophic happenings can lead to better solutions using wider resources and options, and can help avoid caregiver burnout. All these tasks are within the scope of the PCP's practice. The following are the major tasks that PCPs should take care of for PDD patients from the beginning of disease to the end of their lives.

5.1 Annual wellness health maintenance

The mission for PCPs is to promote human beings' wellbeing in aspects of general health and quality of life [60]. According to CMS requirement, recommendations from the United States Preventive Task Force and every professional specialty association practice guideline, all patients including those with PDD must be routinely and properly screened yearly according to their age group. This includes mammograph for breast cancer; fecal occult blood test, Cologuard or colonoscopy accordingly for colon cancer, low dose chest CT for patients at high risk of lung cancer, PSA for high risk of prostate cancer, CBC for leukemia, AFP and liver sonography for liver cancer and so on, even though some clinical benefits are debatable. In most situations, all these cancer screenings are recommended to be held off at age 75 and above [58–60]. However, like anything in life, exceptions should be kept in mind for any individual whose lifespan could be more than 10 years from the day when the PCP performs these screening visits.

5.2 Schedule updating immunization

This group of PDD patients is predominantly within the category of senior citizens. They should follow the recommendation for immunizations per CMS guidelines (summarized in **Table 5**), based on the CDC's Recommended Adult Immunization Schedule for ages 19 years or older, United States, 2021 [61].

5.3 Continuous care of concurrent medical conditions

Maintenance care for chronic illnesses, like hypertension, dyslipidemia, COPD, diabetes mellitus, depression, and chronic pain syndrome, should be routinely monitored. Relevant examination and adjustment of medications should be done as needed on an individual basis. The following should be considered accordingly: RetinaVue and urine microalbumin assay for diabetic retinopathy and nephropathy screening, spirometry for COPD evaluation, office-based tonometry for glaucoma screening, bone density measurement for females aged 65 and above and for males 70 years and above, or for those who have a history of a fracture before the ages specified in the guidelines above [60].

5.4 Counseling patients and their families about PDD

The biggest efforts should be made to communicate thoroughly with patients and their families regarding disease pathophysiology, prognosis, updated treatment guidelines and current options, potential consequences, or complications, and to patiently answer all questions sincerely and honestly in a professional manner [8, 19, 60]. A lengthy and respectful discussion with patients and their family members should be provided. For better results and efficiency, instruction should be given to patients or their families before the appointment, so that they can prepare their questions and do further research if they so choose. During the conference, attention should be paid politely. Use appropriate verbal and body languages and a comfortable office setting. Physicians should try to answer every single question, however, if time is limited or some difficulty arises, it is better to set up another appointment or location for further conversations, and to collect

Vaccine	Starting time	Interval
Influenza vaccine	Starting in autumn, until next spring at any age	1 dose annually
Pneumovax	Starting at age 65 or younger with other comorbidities.	Prevnar 13 and Pneumovax 23; one dose each within one year apart. Boost dose every 5 years
Zoster vaccine, recombinant Shingrix vaccine	Starting at age of 50	2-dose series RZV (Shingrix) 2–6 months apart
Tetanus, diphtheria, and pertussis vaccination (Tdap, Td)	Tdap followed by 1 dose Td or Tdap at least 4 weeks after Tdap and another dose Td	Td or Tdap every 10 years
COVID-19 vaccine	Starting at any age	Pfizer and Moderna mRNA are given two doses with a 3- or 4-week interval. Johnson & Johnson's is given one dose.*

**Boost dose may be needed according to the update information.*

Table 5.
Schedule updating immunization [61].

different perspectives. In this situation, listening is far more important than lecturing. Through this, PCPs might be able to understand a patients' or families' deep concern and real need, to recognize their under-the-table concerns, their inner voice, and agenda. At the end of the meeting, PCPs should make a summary and give a clear detailed picture of the treatment plan. Avoid using academic medical terminology whenever possible. Try to make sure that all medical information is delivered precisely and correctly, using lay language. Patients and their families should be well informed, allowing them to be part of the care team, and given many opportunities to be involved in the treatment, management, and planning. They should be convinced that everyone, including the patient, family, primary care provider, office supporting staff, and specialists are working together towards one goal of providing the best possible care to this individual patient and family.

5.5 General supportive measures

General support is important, not just for PDD patients, but also for their families. Nutritional status should be evaluated, addressed, and emphasized [62]. Nutrition cannot be overemphasized and should be discussed with the caregiver and family. A well-balanced high protein diet, with adequate daily calories, and liquid intake is essential. A handbook with detailed instructions for care planning should be provided for the caregivers. The Mediterranean diet, both alone and in combination with the Dietary Approach to Systolic Hypertension (DASH) diet, may be beneficial for the prevention of cognitive decline. Further research is needed to rule out potential confounds and to better characterize the mechanisms underlying the role of nutrition in cognitive outcomes. Cessation of alcohol and cigarette smoking should be instructed. Supplement of vitamins, especially vitamin D and minerals (calcium, magnesium, zinc) should be discussed and encouraged.

Hearing loss and dementia often occur together, and hearing loss may be an independent but modifiable risk factor for subsequent dementia [63, 64]. PCPs should screen for hearing impairment and manage hearing aids for those who require them to help prevent faster deterioration of cognitive function. Patients should be encouraged to actively take part in socializing activities to maintain cognitive stimulation, such as cooperating with caregivers, family members, support networks, community resources and adult day care facilities. Patients should be arranged to participate in cognitively stimulating activities, e.g., reading, games, etc., and personally meaningful social activities, such as playing music, conversational interactions with others, family events, etc.

Over the past decade, insomnia has variably been associated with deficits in objective cognitive functioning, increased risk of dementia, and reductions in gray matter volume and white matter integrity in networks essential for cognitive functioning [65]. Sleep pattern and sleep hygiene guidance should be discussed in detail. Proper personal hygiene improves quality of life for patients, and also avoids irritation of the oral mucosa, the perineum area, and underneath the breasts, which can also improve the quality of sleep.

Prescribing hypnotic medications may be considered as needed. Benzodiazepines (BZDs) could be an option but should be used with caution. One study showed continuous exposure to BZDs and non-benzodiazepines (non-BZDs) may contribute to the development of cognitive impairment. One should be careful when prescribing BZD or non-BZD hypnotics to patients with long-term insomnia, especially for those that are aged between 50 and 65 years. Additionally, it is best to use short acting sedatives at the lowest dosage for the therapeutic benefit, because greater exposure to these medications leads to a higher risk of developing dementia [65, 66].

The above approaches require cooperation with patients, families, caretakers, or the assisting living facilities. Although there is no concrete data to prove that the above approaches will delay the deterioration of cognitive function, these approaches will assuredly improve the quality of life for PDD patients.

5.6 Polypharmacy

Polypharmacy is another significant and epidemic issue. PCPs are at a critical and unique central position for this matter. In this age group, patients with PD are most likely struggling with multiple medical conditions, such as hypertension, high cholesterol, osteoarthritis, diabetes, malnutrition, depression, etc. Patients often visit different subspecialists such as cardiologists, nephrologists, neurologists, psychiatrists, ophthalmologists, endocrinologists, and dentists. It is a challenge to be vigilant with patients who have impaired cognitive function and are under the care of multiple physicians. It is particularly important to manage their medications to avoid drug interactions, unnecessary pills, conflict among prescriptions from different subspecialties, drug overdose, compliance issues, financial difficulty, monitoring medication refills and reconciliation of medications. Some studies reveal that polypharmacy was associated with cognitive decline in patients with newly diagnosed PD. Those findings suggest that medication reduction might serve as a promising intervention to prevent the development of dementia in patients with early PD [67, 68]. For fixed income senior citizens, financial challenge for medications is an important, but pragmatic issue to discuss. A PCP can help disadvantaged patients get into assistance programs from public or private sources and the pharmaceutical industry.

5.7 Neurology consultation

Neurologists are dependable and reliable allies and consultants in the care of PDD patients, but high-level care should be individualized. Once physician and patient relationships are established long-term, PCPs should be at the center of care planning. PCPs have the advantage of knowing and understanding patients better in terms of their medical and personal history, personality, habits, family members, language, and cultural background. From that point of view, a PCP should be able to coordinate the best fitting specialists to take care of this individual within the guidelines of national and international standards [2, 8, 69].

6. Management of PDD patients in advanced stage

PD and dementia are incurable neurological conditions. PD patients who develop dementia usually progress to the advanced stages of disease. PDD patients often experience specific, complex, and varying needs along their disease trajectory. A palliative approach to PDD should be discussed with patients, their caretakers, and families in advance regarding management of the advanced stages of PDD, especially at the terminal periods. PDD patients may have several needs in the four domains of palliative care (physical, psychological, social, and spiritual) in addition to specific needs for a peaceful, familiar environment, and practical support [70–72]. "Person-centered care, communication and shared decision making" is among the most important domains of palliative care in dementia [73]. An algorithm for the evaluation and management of PDD patients across the disease stages is depicted in **Figure 2**, summarizing much of the above recommendations.

6.1 Counseling and guidance for advance medical directive

Counseling for advance medical directive (AMD) or advance care planning (ACP) should be routine care tasks for PCPs. Medical and advance care directives (e.g., designation of power of attorney) should be discussed as early as possible while the mental functions of patients are still competent, allowing patients and their families to have enough time to discuss and plan. ACP is a special form of ongoing communication about preferred future health care [70]. Long-term health care planning (e.g., living arrangements in the late stage of dementia) and financial planning are other important issues for patients and families to discuss and plan well in advance. In California, the Physician Orders for Life-Sustaining Treatment form or POLST (pink form) is routinely used in the PCP's office for the purpose of making the patients' advanced directives clear and easily obtainable. Physicians should explain the meaning and the consequences of the decision making with patients and family in detail. This process should be highly informative and provide guidance so that patients may come to their informed decision comfortably.

6.2 Management of advanced disease

To optimally promote quality of life and death of a person affected by a complex, incurable, and life-threatening health problem, such as dementia, care teams must address the person's physical, emotional, psychosocial and spiritual needs, as summarized in the WHO definition of palliative care. Dementia usually occurs during the later stages in PD, when clinical symptoms could be progressing quite rapidly, complicated by aging and other comorbidities. Once PD reaches such an advanced stage, the approach towards care should shift towards palliative care, or its consideration. Palliative care can start in the form of ACP if the patient and family caregiver are willing to talk about the future soon after the diagnosis of PDD. The focus of care should be well planned, but simple with straightforward symptom management. Care of the person, not disease per se, is important. This approach includes attention to physical, mental, social, and spiritual aspects, especially since there are no cures available with current interventions. **Figure 3** outlines a model

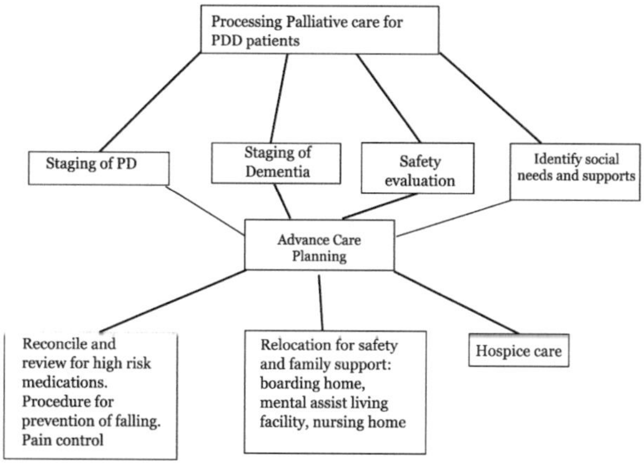

Figure 3.
Model for palliative care of PDD patients.

for palliative care of PDD patients. The palliative care should be carried out by a comprehensive team which includes physicians as leaders, registered nurses, office supportive staff, social workers, religious leaders, family members and/or supporting network, a disease focus group and so forth. An in-home model of palliative care for homebound advanced PD and PDD patients was recently introduced in 2020, which highlights the importance of medication reconciliation, home safety assessments, and appropriate monitoring and treatment of orthostatic hypotension, a leading cause of falls [71]. At this stage not only patients' needs, but also families' needs should be addressed. Options like assisted living homes, boarding care, and skilled nurse facilities should be discussed when those needs arise. The goal at an advanced stage, which may eventually progress to the level of hospice care, is to minimize the suffering and improve the quality of life for both patients and their families or caregivers.

6.3 Pain control

Pain is often difficult to assess in people with advanced dementia due to loss of communicative ability [74]. This can result in patient concerns about pain not being heard or being misinterpreted. Communication difficulties are a challenge to practitioners because there may be several possible causes of distress and possibly no particular localizing behaviors or signs associated with pain in an individual with dementia [72]. Agitation is a frequent symptom in dementia patients and may be associated with untreated pain. Studies show that agitation and aggressive symptoms decrease when pain is effectively treated [75]. Proper and effective pain control and the judicious utilization of opioid and benzodiazepine medications during palliative care is a critical step in successful care. Pain is distressful for both patients and their families and can trigger a cascade of other symptoms. For best results, a specialized pain management team, trained nurse practitioner or physician assistant may be consulted or invited into the care team. Fortunately, in the current healthcare system of the United States of America, well designed palliative care/hospice enterprises are established, and widely available for primary care physicians to adopt and refer their patients and families. This facilitates a well-designed, professional, and individually tailored optimal palliative care plan for the many stresses and discomforts associated with end of life.

6.4 Social needs management

The burden of caring for a dementia patient may be physical/medical (e.g., neglect of caregiver's own health, with potential medical complications), emotional and psychological (stress, burnout, depression), and/or financial. Prevention, early recognition, and treatment of these issues (e.g., referrals to social work for additional support), are integral to an effective management plan [76]. PCPs should engage the office staff, benefit and personnel specialists, and social workers in dealing with disease stage transitioning, personal financial issues, and interfamilial relationships. They, in many cases, need to activate available funding sources at the state and federal levels. Questions regarding the patient's driving safety and privileges should be raised at the appropriate time and stage of the disease. PCPs are the advocates of patients in protecting their loved ones from becoming burned out due to the long term duties of caregiving. In the end, PCPs function as liaisons on behalf of patients and their caregivers in not only coping with but also fighting against this devastating disease.

7. Conclusions

PCPs play an important role in the management of PDD patients. The art of practice for PCPs includes knowing when and how to introduce a comprehensive ongoing care plan for individual PDD patients. A comprehensive ongoing care plan includes (1) screening for changes in mental function regularly, (2) properly diagnosing PDD, (3) applying nonpharmacologic and pharmacologic interventions accordingly, (4) orchestrating multidisciplinary care, special therapies, and auxiliary support accordingly, (5) consulting advance medical directive and palliative care early. The optimal goal is to maintain relative independence for PDD patients, if this is safe. It is reasonable and proper to initiate palliative care and hospice for PDD patients in the advanced stage to provide better qualities of their later life experience.

Acknowledgements

The authors thank Micha Y.Z. Cheng, MPH, MD and Justin Cheng, MD for their assistance. This book chapter is partly supported by the 2021 Mid-Year Innovation Project from Sutter Independent Physician Medical Group.

Conflict of interest

The authors declare no conflict of interest.

Author details

Xin-Nong Li* and Dawei Zheng
Sutter Health/Sutter Independent Physician Medical Group,
Sacramento, California, USA

*Address all correspondence to: drxinnongli@icloud.com

References

[1] Müller J, Wenning GK, Jellinger K, McKee A, Poewe W, Litvan I. Progression of Hoehn and Yahr stages in Parkinsonian disorders: A clinicopathologic study. Neurology 2000;55:888-891.

[2] Garcia-Ptacek S, Kramberger MG. Parkinson Disease and Dementia. J Geriatr Psychiatry Neurol. 2016 Sep;29(5):261-270. doi: 10.1177/0891988716654985. PMID: 27502301.

[3] Gratwicke J, Jahanshahi M, Foltynie T, Parkinson's disease dementia: a neural networks perspective, Brain, Volume 138, Issue 6, June 2015, Pages 1454-1476, https://doi.org/10.1093/brain/awv104

[4] Sancesario GM, Bernardini S. Diagnosis of neurodegenerative dementia: where do we stand, now? Ann Transl Med 2018;6(17):340. doi: 10.21037/atm.2018.08.04

[5] Liu Y, Jin-Hu Fan J-H, Gao X, Ma L, Qiao Y-L, Zhang L. 2015. The Natural Progression of Parkinson's Disease in a Small Cohort with 15 Drug-naïve Patients. Chinese Medical Journal 128 (13): 1761-1764. doi:10.4103/0366-6999.159350. http://dx.doi.org/10.4103/0366-6999.159350.

[6] Armstrong MJ, Okun MS. Diagnosis and Treatment of Parkinson Disease A Review. JAMA. 2020;323(6):548-560. doi:10.1001/jama.2019.22360

[7] Livingston J, Huntley J, Sommerlad A, Ames D, Ballard C, Banerjee S, Brayne C, Burns A, Cohen-Mansfield J, Cooper C, Costafreda SG, Dias A, Fox N, Gitlin LN, Howard R, Kales HC, Kivimäki M, Larson EB, Ogunniyi A, Orgeta V, Ritchie K, Rockwood K, Sampson EL, Samus Q, Schneider LS, Selbæk G, Teri L, Mukadam N. Dementia prevention, intervention, and care: 2020 report of the Lance Commission. The Lancet. 2020 Aug 08:m 413-446.

[8] van der Steen JT, Lennaerts H, Hommel D, Augustijn B, Groot M, Hasselaar J, Bloem BR, Koopmans RTCM. Dementia and Parkinson's Disease: Similar and Divergent Challenges in Providing Palliative Care. Front Neurol. 2019 Mar 11;10:54. doi: 10.3389/fneur.2019.00054.

[9] Goroll AH, Alberta G. Mulley AG, Jr. Primary Care Medicine 6th ed. Wolters Kluwer/Lippincott Williams & Wilkins; 2009. Chapter: 169 Evaluation of Dementia

[10] Davie CA, A review of Parkinson's disease, British Medical Bulletin, Volume 86, Issue 1, June 2008, Pages 109-127, https://doi.org/10.1093/bmb/ldn013

[11] Rating scales | European Parkinson's Disease Association (epda.eu.com)

[12] Hoehn MM, Yahr MD, Parkinson's onset, progression, and mortality. Neurology May 1967, 17 (5) 427; DOI: 10.1212/WNL.17.5.427

[13] Braak H, Ghebremedhin E, Rüb U, Bratzke H, Del Tredici K. Stages in the development of Parkinson's disease-related pathology. Cell Tissue Res. 2004 Oct;318(1):121-134. doi: 10.1007/s00441-004-0956-9. Epub 2004 Aug 24. PMID: 15338272.

[14] Barnes DE, Beiser AS, Lee A, Langa KM, Koyama A, Preis SR, Neuhaus J, McCammon RJ, Yaffe K, Seshadri S, Haan MN, Weir DR. Development and validation of a brief dementia screening indicator for primary care. Alzheimers Dement. 2014 Nov;10(6):656-665.e1. doi: 10.1016/j.jalz.2013.11.006. Epub 2014 Feb 1.

PMID: 24491321; PMCID: PMC4119094. (form https://campuslifeservices.ucsf.edu/clsforms/documentsmedia/dementiarisk/)

[15] Krishnamoorthy Y, Rajaa S, Rehman T. Diagnostic accuracy of various forms of geriatric depression scale for screening of depression among older adults: Systematic review and meta-analysis. Arch Gerontol Geriatr. 2020 Mar-Apr; 87:104002. doi: 10.1016/j.archger.2019.104002. Epub 2019 Dec 19. PMID: 31881393.

[16] https://geriatrictoolkit.missouri.edu/cog/GDS_SHORT_FORM.PDF

[17] Phelan E, Williams B, Meeker K, Bonn K, Frederick J, Logerfo J, Snowden M. A study of the diagnostic accuracy of the PHQ-9 in primary care elderly. BMC Fam Pract. 2010 Sep 1; 11:63. doi: 10.1186/1471-2296-11-63. PMID: 20807445; PMCID: PMC 2940814.

[18] https://integrationacademy.ahrq.gov/sites/default/files/2020-07/PHQ-9.pdf

[19] Nasreddine ZS, Phillips NA, Bédirian V, Charbonneau S, Whitehead V, Collin I, Cummings JL and Chertkow H. (2005), The Montreal Cognitive Assessment, MoCA: A Brief Screening Tool For Mild Cognitive Impairment. Journal of the American Geriatrics Society, 53: 695-699. https://doi.org/10.1111/j.1532-5415.2005.53221.x (form https://www.parkinsons.va.gov/resources/MOCA-Test-English.pdf)

[20] O'Caoimh, R., Y. Gao, C. McGlade, L. Healy, P. Gallagher, S. Timmons and D. Molloy. "Comparison of the quick mild cognitive impairment (Qmci) screen and the SMMSE in screening for mild cognitive impairment." Age and Ageing 41 (2012): 624 - 629.

[21] Aprahamian I, Martinelli JE, Cecato J, Yassuda MS. Screening for Alzheimer's disease among illiterate elderly: accuracy analysis for multiple instruments. J Alzheimers Dis. 2011;26(2):221-229. doi: 10.3233/JAD-2011-110125. PMID: 21593559.

[22] Lessig M, Scanlan J et al. Time that tells: Critical clock-drawing errors for dementia screening. Int Psychogeriatr. 2008 June; 20(3): 459-470.

[23] van der Flier WM, Scheltens P. Epidemiology and risk factors of dementia Journal of Neurology, Neurosurgery & Psychiatry 2005; 76: v2-v7.

[24] Beker N, Ganz A, Hulsman M, et al. Association of Cognitive Function Trajectories in Centenarians with Postmortem Neuropathology, Physical Health, and Other Risk Factors for Cognitive Decline. JAMA Netw Open. 2021;4(1):e2031654. doi:10.1001/jamanetworkopen.2020.31654

[25] Vasconcellos LF, Pereira JS. Parkinson's disease dementia: Diagnostic criteria and risk factor review. J Clin Exp Neuropsychol. 2015;37(9):988-993. doi: 10.1080/13803395.2015.1073227. PMID: 26332178.

[26] Glatt S, L, Hubble J, P, Lyons K, Paolo A, Tröster A, I, Hassanein R, E, S, Koller W, C: Risk Factors for Dementia in Parkinson's Disease: Effect of Education. Neuroepidemiology 1996;15:20-25. doi: 10.1159/000109885

[27] William L. Webb, Mohan Gehi. Electrolyte and fluid imbalance: Neuropsychiatric manifestations. Psychosomatics, Volume 22, Issue 3, 1981, Pages 199-203, ISSN 0033-3182. https://doi.org/10.1016/S0033-3182(81)73532-1.

[28] Luckey AE, Parsa CJ. Fluid and Electrolytes in the Aged. Arch Surg. 2003;138(10):1055-1060. doi:10.1001/archsurg.138.10.1055

[29] Adrogué HJ, Madias NE. Hypernatremia.N Engl J Med 2000; 342:1493-1499. DOI: 10.1056/NEJM200005183422006

[30] Cuomo A, Maina G, Bolognesi S, Rosso G, Crescenzi BB, Zanobini F, Goracci A, Facchi E, Favaretto E, Baldini I, Santucci A, Fagiolini A. Prevalence and Correlates of Vitamin D Deficiency in a Sample of 290 Inpatients With Mental Illness. Front. Psychiatry, 29 March 2019 | https://doi.org/10.3389/fpsyt.2019.00167

[31] Armstrong MJ, Okun MS. Diagnosis and Treatment of Parkinson Disease: A Review. JAMA. 2020;323(6):548-560. doi:10.1001/jama.2019.22360

[32] Lin JS, O'Connor E, Rossom RC, Perdue LA, Eckstrom E. Screening for cognitive impairment in older adults: a systematic review for the U.S. Preventive Services Task Force. Ann Intern Med. 2013;159(9):601-612. doi:10.7326/0003-4819-159-9-201311050-00730

[33] Patnode CD, Perdue LA, Rossom RC, Rushkin MC, Redmond N, Thomas RG, Lin JS. Screening for Cognitive Impairment in Older Adults: An Evidence Update for the U.S. Preventive Services Task Force [Internet]. Rockville (MD): Agency for Healthcare Research and Quality (US); 2020 Feb. Report No.: 19-05257-EF-1. PMID: 32129963.

[34] US Preventive Services Task Force, Owens DK, Davidson KW, Krist AH, Barry MJ, Cabana M, Caughey AB, Doubeni CA, Epling JW Jr, Kubik M, Landefeld CS, Mangione CM, Pbert L, Silverstein M, Simon MA, Tseng CW, Wong JB. Screening for Cognitive Impairment in Older Adults: US Preventive Services Task Force Recommendation Statement. JAMA. 2020 Feb 25;323(8):757-763. doi: 10.1001/jama.2020.0435. PMID: 32096858.

[35] (2020), 2020 Alzheimer's disease facts and figures. Alzheimer's Dement., 16: 391-460. https://doi.org/10.1002/alz.12068

[36] Gomperts SN, Marquie M, Locascio JJ, Bayer S, Johnson KA, Growdon JH. PET Radioligands Reveal the Basis of Dementia in Parkinson's Disease and Dementia with Lewy Bodies. Neurodegener Dis. 2016;16 (1-2):118-124. doi:10.1159/000441421

[37] Arvanitakis Z, Shah RC, Bennett DA. Diagnosis and Management of Dementia: Review. JAMA October 22/29, 2019 Volume 322, Number 16: 1589-1599.

[38] Tarakad A, Jankovic J. Diagnosis and Management of Parkinson's Disease. Semin Neurol. 2017 Apr;37(2):118-126. doi: 10.1055/s-0037-1601888. Epub 2017 May 16. PMID: 28511252.

[39] Dubois B, Burn D, Goetz C, Aarsland D, Brown RG, Broe GA, Dickson D, Duyckaerts C, Cummings J, Gauthier S, Korczyn A, Lees A, Levy R, Litvan I, Mizuno Y, McKeith IG, Olanow CW, Poewe W, Sampaio C, Tolosa E, Emre M. Diagnostic procedures for Parkinson's disease dementia: recommendations from the movement disorder society task force. Mov Disord. 2007 Dec;22(16):2314-2324. doi: 10.1002/mds.21844. PMID: 18098298.

[40] Goetz CG, Emre M, Dubois B. Parkinson's disease dementia: definitions, guidelines, and research perspectives in diagnosis. Ann Neurol. 2008 Dec;64 Suppl 2:S81-S92. doi: 10.1002/ana.21455. PMID: 19127578.

[41] Brooks DJ. Parkinson's disease: diagnosis. Parkinsonism Relat Disord. 2012 Jan;18 Suppl 1:S31-S33. doi: 10.1016/S1353-8020(11)70012-8. PMID: 22166447.

[42] Gomperts SN. Lewy Body Dementias: Dementia With Lewy Bodies

and Parkinson Disease Dementia. Continuum (Minneap Minn). 2016 Apr;22(2 Dementia):435-63. doi: 10.1212/CON.0000000000000309. PMID: 27042903; PMCID: PMC5390937.

[43] Galvin JE. The Quick Dementia Rating System (QDRS): A Rapid Dementia Staging Tool. Alzheimers Dement (Amst). 2015 Jun 1;1(2):249-259. doi: 10.1016/j.dadm.2015.03.003. PMID: 26140284; PMCID: PMC44 84882.

[44] Adan RAH, van der Beek EM, Buitelaar JK, Cryan JF, Hebebrand J, Higgs S, Schellekens H, Dickson SL. Nutritional psychiatry: Towards improving mental health by what you eat. Eur Neuropsychopharmacol. 2019 Dec;29(12):1321-1332. doi: 10.1016/j.euroneuro.2019.10.011. Epub 2019 Nov 14. PMID: 31735529.

[45] Silva MVF, Loures CMG, Alves LCV, de Souza LC, Borges KBG, Carvalho MDG. Alzheimer's disease: risk factors and potentially protective measures. J Biomed Sci. 2019 May 9;26(1):33. doi: 10.1186/s12929-019-0524-y. PMID: 31072403; PMCID: PMC6507104.

[46] Walton CC, Mowszowski L, Gilat M, et al. Cognitive training for freezing of gait in Parkinson's disease: a randomized controlled trial. npj Parkinson's Disease 4, 15 (2018). https://doi.org/10.1038/s41531-018-0052-6

[47] Bloem BR, de Vries NM, Ebersbach G. Nonpharmacological treatments for patients with Parkinson's disease. Mov Disord. 2015 Sep 15;30(11):1504-1520. doi: 10.1002/mds.26363. Epub 2015 Aug 14. PMID: 26274930.

[48] Hindle JV, Watermeyer TJ, Roberts J, Martyr A, Lloyd-Williams H, Brand A, Gutting P, Hoare Z, Edwards RT, Clare L. Cognitive rehabilitation for Parkinson's disease dementia: a study protocol for a pilot randomised controlled trial. Trials. 2016 Mar 22;17:152. doi: 10.1186/s13063-016-1253-0. Erratum in: Trials. 2017 Mar 23;18(1):138. PMID: 27000036; PMCID: PMC4802850.

[49] Jäncke L. Music, memory and emotion. J Biol. 2008 Aug 8;7(6):21. doi: 10.1186/jbiol82. PMID: 18710596; PMCID: PMC2776393.

[50] O'Malley N, Clifford AM, Comber L, Coote S. Effectiveness of non-pharmacological falls prevention interventions for people with Multiple Sclerosis, Parkinson's Disease and stroke: protocol for an umbrella review. HRB Open Res. 2020 Dec 1;3:17. doi: 10.12688/hrbopenres.13023.2. PMID: 33392439; PMCID: PMC7745191.

[51] Granziera, S., Alessandri, A., Lazzaro, A. et al. Nordic Walking and Walking in Parkinson's disease: a randomized single-blind controlled trial. Aging Clin Exp Res (2020). https://doi.org/10.1007/s40520-020-01617-w

[52] Rinaldi P, Mecocci P, Benedetti C, Ercolani S, Bregnocchi M, Menculini G, Catani M, Senin U, Cherubini A. Validation of the five-item geriatric depression scale in elderly subjects in three different settings. J Am Geriatr Soc. 2003 May;51(5):694-698. doi: 10.1034/j.1600-0579.2003.00216.x. PMID: 12752847.

[53] Samudra N, Patel N, Womack KB, Khemani P, Chitnis S. Psychosis in Parkinson Disease: A Review of Etiology, Phenomenology, and Management. Drugs Aging. 2016 Dec;33(12):855-863. doi: 10.1007/s40266-016-0416-8. PMID: 27830568; PMCID: PMC6760850.

[54] Tible OP, Riese F, Savaskan E, von Gunten A. Best practice in the management of behavioural and psychological symptoms of dementia. Therapeutic Advances in Neurological

Disorders. August 2017:297-309. doi:10.1177/1756285617712979

[55] Yuan M, Sperry L, Malhado-Chang N, Duffy A, Wheelock V, Farias S, O'Connor K, Olichney J, Shahlaie K, Zhang L Atypical antipsychotic therapy in Parkinson's disease psychosis: A retrospective study. Brain Behav. 2017 Jun; 7(6): e00639. doi: 10.1002/brb3.639

[56] Connolly BS, Lang AE. Pharmacological treatment of Parkinson disease: a review. JAMA. 2014 Apr 23-30;311(16):1670-83. doi: 10.1001/jama.2014.3654. PMID: 24756517.

[57] Jeannette E. South-Paul, Samuel C. Matheny & Evelyn L. Lewis Current Diagnosis & Treatment: Family Medicine 4th ed; 2016. Chapter 44: Movement Disorders; Chapter 67: Hospice & Palliative Medicine

[58] Beckman AL, Becerra AZ, Marcus A, DuBard CA, Lynch K, Maxson E, Mostashari F, King J. Medicare Annual Wellness Visit association with healthcare quality and costs. Am J Manag Care. 2019 Mar 1;25(3):e76-e82. PMID: 30875175.

[59] Pfoh E, Mojtabai R, Bailey J, Weiner JP, Dy SM. Impact of Medicare Annual Wellness Visits on Uptake of Depression Screening. Psychiatr Serv. 2015 Nov;66(11):1207-1212. doi: 10.1176/appi.ps.201400524. Epub 2015 Jul 15. PMID: 26174947.

[60] Robert E. Racquel and David P. Raquel Textbook of The Family Medicine 9th ed. Elsevier Sanders; 2016. Chapter: 1 Family Physician.

[61] https://www.cdc.gov/vaccines/schedules/hcp/imz/adult.html

[62] Szeto, J.Y.Y., Walton, C.C., Rizos, A. *et al.* Dementia in long-term Parkinson's disease patients: a multicentre retrospective study. *npj Parkinsons Dis.* 6, 2 (2020). https://doi.org/10.1038/s41531-019-0106-4

[63] Ray M, Dening T, Crosbie B. Dementia and hearing loss: A narrative review. Maturitas. 2019 Oct;128:64-69. doi: 10.1016/j.maturitas.2019.08.001. Epub 2019 Aug 5. PMID: 31561826.

[64] Hubbard HI, Mamo SK, Hopper T. Dementia and Hearing Loss: Interrelationships and Treatment Considerations. Semin Speech Lang. 2018 Jul;39(3):197-210. doi: 10.1055/s-0038-1660779. Epub 2018 Jun 22. PMID: 29933487.

[65] Sexton CE, Sykara K, Karageorgiou E, Zitser J, Rosa T, Yaffe K, Leng Y. Connections Between Insomnia and Cognitive Aging. Neurosci Bull. 2020 Jan;36(1):77-84. doi: 10.1007/s12264-019-00401-9. Epub 2019 Jun 20. PMID: 31222500; PMCID: PMC694 0406.

[66] Chen PL, Lee WJ, Sun WZ, Oyang YJ, Fuh JL. Risk of dementia in patients with insomnia and long-term use of hypnotics: a population-based retrospective cohort study. PLoS One. 2012;7(11):e49113. doi: 10.1371/journal.pone.0049113. Epub 2012 Nov 7. PMID: 23145088; PMCID: PMC3492301.

[67] Csoti I, Herbst H, Urban P, Woitalla D, Wüllner U. Polypharmacy in Parkinson's disease: risks and benefits with little evidence. J Neural Transm (Vienna). 2019 Jul;126(7):871-878. doi: 10.1007/s00702-019-02026-8. Epub 2019 Jun 20. PMID: 31222606.

[68] Ishii N, Mochizuki H, Sakai K, Ogawa G, Shiomi K, Nakazato M. Polypharmacy Associated with Cognitive Decline in Newly Diagnosed Parkinson's Disease: A Cross-Sectional Study. Dement Geriatr Cogn Dis Extra. 2019 Sep 10;9(3):338-343. doi: 10.1159/000502351. PMID: 31608098;

[69] Robert E. Raquel Essentials of Family Practice 2nd ed. WB Sanders

company; 1998. Chapter 5: Disease Prevention.

[70] van der Steen JT, Lennaerts H, Hommel D, Augustijn B, Groot M, Hasselaar J, Bloem BR, Koopmans RTCM. Dementia and Parkinson's Disease: Similar and Divergent Challenges in Providing Palliative Care. Front Neurol. 2019 Mar 11;10:54. doi: 10.3389/fneur.2019.00054. PMID: 30915012; PMCID: PMC6421983.

[71] Fleisher JE, Klostermann EC, Hess SP, Lee J, Myrick E, Chodosh J. Interdisciplinary palliative care for people with advanced Parkinson's disease: a view from the home. Ann Palliat Med. 2020 Feb;9(Suppl 1):S80-S89. doi: 10.21037/apm.2019.09.12. Epub 2019 Oct 14. PMID: 31735037; PMCID: PMC7341729.

[72] Raymond M, Warner A, Davies N, Nicholas N, Manthorpe J, Iliffe S. Palliative and end of life care for people with dementia: lessons for clinical commissioners. Prim Health Care Res Dev. 2014 Oct;15(4):406-417. doi: 10.1017/S146342361300039X. Epub 2013 Nov 26. PMID: 24280024.

[73] van der Steen JT, Lennaerts H, Hommel D, et al. Dementia and Parkinson's Disease: Similar and Divergent Challenges in Providing Palliative Care. Frontiers in Neurology. 2019 ;10:54. DOI: 10.3389/fneur.2019.00054. PMID: 30915012; PMCID: PMC6421983.

[74] Achterberg WP, Pieper MJ, van Dalen-Kok AH, de Waal MW, Husebo BS, Lautenbacher S, Kunz M, Scherder EJ, Corbett A. Pain management in patients with dementia. Clin Interv Aging. 2013;8:1471-82. doi: 10.2147/CIA.S36739. Epub 2013 Nov 1. PMID: 24204133; PMCID: PMC3817007.

[75] Pergolizzi JV, Raffa RB, Paladini A, Varrasi G, LeQuang JA. Treating pain in patients with dementia and the possible concomitant relief of symptoms of agitation. Pain Manag. 2019 Nov;9(6):569-582. doi: 10.2217/pmt-2019-0024. Epub 2019 Nov 22. PMID: 31755371.

[76] Arvanitakis Z, Shah RC, Bennett DA. Diagnosis and Management of Dementia: Review. JAMA. 2019 Oct 22;322(16):1589-1599. doi: 10.1001/jama.2019.4782. PMID: 31638686; PMCID: PMC7462122.

Section 3

Management and Comprehensive Care

Chapter 7

Dementia and Physical Therapy

Constanza I. San Martín Valenzuela

Abstract

Cognitive functions allow us to perform complex tasks on a day-to-day basis. When we move or want to perform a functional task, not only the integrity of the motor systems is needed, but also those cognitive functions that help plan and execute movement in challenging environments. Currently, the physical therapy of people with Parkinson's disease, little by little, integrates the cognitive abilities of patients to the motor rehabilitation of the disease. Most studies to date have proven the effectiveness of this dual-task integration in mild or moderate stages of the disease. However, in more serious stages, we do not fully know the effectiveness of physical rehabilitation in patients who already have dementia or cognitive impairment. This chapter aims to review the latest findings in this regard, to know what are the implications of dementia in Parkinson's disease on the motor performance, and to unravel the new lines of study that researchers and clinicians should follow in the area of physical rehabilitation in advanced stages of Parkinson's disease.

Keywords: cognitive impairment, functional movement, physical therapy, Parkinson's dementia, executive functions

1. Introduction

The cognitive abilities of people who start a physical rehabilitation program are essential to ensure the effectiveness of therapeutic exercise. The ability to understand and follow instructions, the ability to perform exercise with the indicated frequency, as well as the ability to integrate physical improvements into activities of daily living are factors that influence the success of physical treatment in the short and long term. In people with Parkinson's disease (PD), the effects of physical rehabilitation are widely documented in the scientific literature, establishing the possibility of motor learning in people with PD during early stages of the disease. However, patients could experience cognitive impairment over the evolution of PD whose clinical expression, severity, and progression can be variable. These cognitive changes can range from subtle impairment to mild cognitive impairment (PD-MCI) or to more severe deficits such as dementia due to Parkinson's disease (PDD), and they can appear from early to more advanced stages of the disease [1]. In people with PD-MCI or PDD, the implementation of a rehabilitation program acquires additional challenges that can hinder its effectiveness. This may be one of the reasons why in the scientific literature on the effects of physical treatments, we constantly see that having a normal cognitive state is included as a criterion for participation of people with PD, frequently evaluated by a quick cognitive screening with the mini-mental Parkinson's examination [2] or the Montreal Cognitive Assessment [3].

 IntechOpen

Comparing with age-matched healthy groups, people with PD exhibit a faster decline in certain cognitive domains like executive, attentional, visuospatial, and memory functions [4]. Even though these cognitive alterations of people with PD are greater than typical for normal aging, they are measurable through standardized cognitive scales, and they are consistent with PD-MCI, they do not critically interfere with daily functioning. Conversely, PDD involve more severe cognitive deficits, and these have a significant impact on day-to-day and functional activities [1, 5]. In addition, PDD is often accompanied by behavioral features such as apathy, mood disorders, excessive daytime sleepiness, and psychosis [6]. Despite these differences, it should be noted that PD-MCI increases the risk of conversion to dementia 6-fold [1].

2. How does cognitive impairment influence functional movement?

A person's functional capability is the result of the interaction of three factors: the individual, the objective task, and the environment where the task takes place [7]. This means that the movements respond to a specific demand that involve what we going to do and where we going to do it. From the individual, not only is the indemnity of the motor system necessary to exercise functional movement, but an interaction with the sensory and cognitive systems is also required. We can say with total certainty that movement is a cognitive-sensory-motor phenomenon. More specifically, when we exercise a voluntary movement, the cognitive system acquires special relevance in the motor control.

Action planning and selection, action initiation, online adaptation during actual execution, and inhibition of an ongoing action are among the main cognitive tasks directly involved in the execution of the voluntary movement, although not the only ones involved [8]. These components related to the action control belong to higher cognitive processes to modulate and produce behavior: the executive functions. Associated with the prefrontal cortex, the impairment in one or more of the components of executive functions has been related to motor abilities such as walking efficiently and safely. Seen from an example, poor self-awareness of limitations, an aspect of volition, might result in an increased risk of falling, or the impaired planning skills could result in getting lost or choices that produce inefficient pathways or unnecessary effort to arrive at a destination [9]. Other executive functions related to functional movement under multiple stimuli are dual execution and multitasking, considered as the ability to organize and perform tasks optimally simultaneously, intercalating them. This ability to perform more than one task at the same time is the basis of the functional environment, where people are exposed to several cognitive demands.

On the other hand, attention has been also determined as essential in goal-directed movement. Attention can be classified into separate functions, including focused or selective, sustained, divided, and alternating. This cognitive function is defined as the state of observation and alert that allows awareness of what happens in the environment. It is a capacity or process by which specific mental resources are generated and directed on the most relevant aspects of the environment or the most appropriate actions, maintaining the appropriate state of activation to achieve a goal or purpose. To carry out this process, it is necessary to focus on specific stimuli, ignoring other minor ones. The attention is necessary to initiate and adapt a movement that is developed voluntarily. For example, when we want to start walking in unfamiliar terrain or modify the gait pattern to change direction or avoid an obstacle, the first thing we do is direct our attention to this requirement, controlling the gait from the motor cortex.

In addition to attention and executive functions, other authors have mentioned that cognitive processes such as emotion (motivation) or memory are also crucial to develop motor tasks with a certain objective within a certain environment [7]. Anyway, either by the connections of the basal ganglia with the primary motor cortex, supplementary motor area, premotor cortex, and cingulate motor area (motor circuit) or, on the other hand, with the dorsolateral prefrontal cortex and lateral orbitofrontal cortex (executive circuit), movement in Parkinson's disease is threatened from mild to moderate stages long before dementia appears.

3. Can physical therapy improve the cognitive performance?

In the previous section we have seen the relationship that cognitive functions have to generate voluntary movement. But what happens the other way around? Can motor practice influence cognitive performance? The truth is that non-pharmacological interventions are an essential part of the treatment in PD. Physiotherapy, speech therapy, psychology, and occupational therapy are the most common nondrug health strategies to alleviation the symptoms directly related with a poor development a functional live. Even when pharmacological and surgical treatment improved immediate parkinsonian symptoms and, in consequence, quality of life, there has been a limited effect on axial symptoms, i.e. gait, posture, balance, speech, and swallowing [10] and also on cognitive deficiencies [11]. These disabilities not only have a powerful impact on the activities of daily living for people with PD but are also strongly related to dependency and mortality [12].

In this regard, physical rehabilitation, physiotherapy, or physical therapy has shown an effect beyond the physical characteristics itself that it pretends to rehabilitate, and in addition, it will also depend on the type of physical therapy that is implemented. This has been demonstrated in aging people without associated pathologies, as well as in people with PD. In healthy aged people it has been shown that resistance exercises and resistance training are powerful physical intervention strategies to induce meaningful functional brain changes, especially in the frontal lobe, which are accompanied by improvements in executive functions [13]. In the same way, aerobic and coordination exercises seem to be more beneficial to cognitive processes than other exercises such as stretching or balancing to improve cognitive functions like memory, processing and perceptual speed, and attention [14]. On other hand, in recent years, the effectiveness of multi-domain physical therapy in different population has gained much prominence. This kind of therapy involves both motor and cognitive practice, and it has been studied through dual-task or multi-task training, where the persons performs a primary task, such as gait, while performing other secondary cognitive (or motor) task. In this type of exercise, the patients have to shift attention from one task to another in order to achieve the objective of both, e.g. walking and saying aloud a shopping list [15]. In this way, the dual-task in physical rehabilitation imitates a habitual functional context within the therapy itself, where people practice a motor exercise subjected to the usual demands of the environments in activities of daily living. That is why studies generally report greater cognitive improvements with multi-domain training in older age [16]. Specifically, clinical trials using dual motor-cognitive tasks led to improvements of domains related to global cognitive functions and inhibitory control in older people [17].

In people with PD this also has been widely studied. Besides the poor pharmacological effect on cognition, the importance of finding noninvasive therapies that improve cognitive deficiencies is crucial for two main reasons. The first is that cognitive impairment in people with PD can appear in the early stages of the disease, and on the other hand, mild cognitive impairment represents a significant risk factor for early dementia [10]. Recently published systematic reviews have been summarized that physical therapy has a positive effect on global cognitive function, processing speed, sustained attention, mental flexibility, visuospatial, and executive functions in people with Parkinson's disease [10, 18–21], besides motor function. However, the main function benefiting from the different physical training is the executive and global cognitive function measured through different cognitive screening (**Figure 1**). This may be due to the described relationship of the executive functions in the planning and initiation of the voluntary movement. Although it has been described that several physical therapy programs can have an impact on cognitive performance, it is worth asking what type of strategy achieves the best effects. Aerobic [22–25], multimodal [26–28], and multi-domain [29] are the most referenced techniques in the literature that measures the effects of cognitive functions through a standardized test for it. While multi-domain refers to interventions targeting two or more domains, as physical exercise and cognitive training, in this section we use multi-modal as different components of the same domain, e.g., the combination of strength and balance training in the same program. However, in some publications, both terms may refer to intervention programs with components from different domains.

Studies with multi-domain intervention have shown that the ability to transfer the performance improvements depended largely on the demands, particularly cognitive, of the specific task involved [30]. One of the most repeated examples in the literature is the use of virtual-reality-based training; however, this requires that patients have individual sessions and the availability of the respective equipment. A more feasible multi-domain training option is dual-task training, which can be applied individually or in groups. The studies so far that analyze the effectiveness of dual-cognitive task training assess the performance of the secondary cognitive task itself, but not the cognitive function through a standardized test. Even so, studies have been published indicating that dual motor and cognitive tasks improve executive functions measured through the Trail Making Test [15].

Finally, the revised systems reviews indicate that trials that used longer interventions were associated with improved attention and processing speeds, whereas

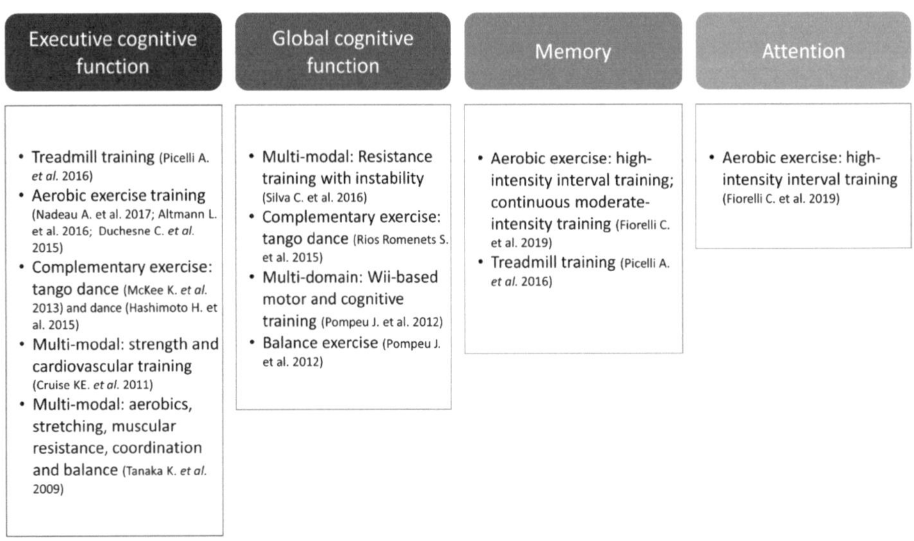

Figure 1.
Physical training applied to people with Parkinson's disease has shown a significantly positive effect on one or more cognitive functions, measured through standardized tests for cognitive performance.

trials conducted among individuals with mild cognitive impairment tended to show more memory improvement compared to non-dementia samples [19, 21].

4. Physical performance in people with and without dementia

We have reviewed that physical rehabilitation can have effects on cognitive functions even when these are not the objective of the intervention. But what happens to the physical performance when people with PD have dementia, have mild cognitive impairment, or do not have any cognitive disability? Regardless of the range of signs and motor dysfunctions that we can find in PD, we will analyze this issue from the functionality of the hand and gait.

4.1 Hand functionality

Impairment in voluntary hand movements results from deficits characteristics of PD such as slowness of movements and difficulty in executing sequential movements. Also, the performance of hand fine motor skills is not the same for people with PD without cognitive impairment and people with PD as well as cognitive impairment and dementia. Although the scientific evidence of these differences in samples exclusively with PD is limited, a few authors specifically indicate in which domains of hand functionality we can observe these differences (**Table 1**). Dahdal et al. determined that people with PD and mild cognitive impairment exhibited a significant worse motor performance in precision (to guide a stylus through a narrow curved track without touching the sides), dexterity (to insert 25 long and short pins into holes in a platform), and velocity of arm-hand movement (time spent to precisely hit 20 subsequent points lined in a row) tasks [31]. Likewise, Tan et al. found that people with PD and dementia have poorer hand function in pen-holding, buttoning, and knotting actions than do the patients without dementia [32].

Authors	Task/test	PD MCI	PD non-MCI
Dahdal et al. [31]	*Precision*: number of errors made by touching the sides while patients guide a stylus through a narrow curved track	−0.36 (1.04)	0.25 (0.74)
	Dexterity: duration needed to complete the task of inserting 25 long and short pins into holes in a platform	−0.28 (0.8)	0.14 (0.7)
	Velocity of arm-hand: velocity required to precisely hit 20 subsequent points lined in a row	−0.28 (0.9)	0.16 (0.6)
		PDD	**Non-PDD**
Tan et al. [32]	Pen-holding	1.2 (1.5)	0.8 (1.3)
	Buttoning	2.0 (1.6)	1.7 (1.5)
	Knotting	2.0 (1.6)	1.6 (1.5)

Means and standard deviations of the hand function outcomes. MCI, mild cognitive impairment; PDD, Parkinson's disease dementia. Differences founded by Dahdal et al. show p values <0.05. Differences founded by Tan et al. show p values <0.001. Tan et al. assessed the domains 8.1 (pen holding), 8.2 (buttoning), and 8.3 (knotting) of the Functioning Disability Evaluation Scale Adult Version with a 4-point scale that designate if there was total independence or a need for assistance when accomplishing tasks (0 = total independence, 1 = need for supervision or mild assistance, 2 = need for moderate assistance, 3 = need for maximal assistance, 4 = need for total assistance).

Table 1.
Significant differences found between people with PD, with and without cognitive impairment/dementia in hand functionality performance.

In addition to these differences, the authors demonstrated the significant correlation of precision task with age of participants and the MiniMental State Examination results [31]. Also, pen-holding and knotting performance was significantly associated with dementia in patients with moderate-to-advanced PD, which allowed the researchers to establish there is a 13% higher probability of dementia for PD patients if they had any level of disability in pen holding [32].

4.2 Gait

Gait performance has been become in an indicator of health in many pathologies. In fact, gait speed in older adults has been accepted as a reliable and sensitive measure for assessment of physiologic performance and prediction of clinical outcomes, and indeed has been regarded as the "sixth vital sign" [33]. Added to this, people with PD report that gait impairments are the most disabling motor symptoms of the disease [34]. Most of the studies when analyzing the effects of gait rehabilitation programs exclude patients with dementia or cognitive disorders in their samples, even though this group of patients suffers a worse deterioration of the walking pattern than do people with PD without cognitive disorders (**Table 2**). PD patients with cognitive impairment walked slower and had shorter step length and stride length than those without cognitive impairment [35, 36]. In those studies that only analyzed a sample of patients with dementia or cognitive impairment without a control group [37, 38], the values recorded are below normal gait pattern.

As with the parameters of hand functionality, correlations between gait variables and other parameters related to dementia have also been demonstrated in gait. Mini Mental State Examination is significantly associated with step length [35] and stride length [35]. Also, cognitive domains such as attention and visuospatial have been positively correlated with step and stride length [35].

In addition to the classic correlations between gait performance and cognitive performance, studies that search to predict cognitive decline in PD people demonstrate that gait variability is associated with lower cognitive performance [39, 40]. The variability is usually calculated through the coefficient of variation (CV = [standard deviation/mean] × 100) and indicates how stable or repeatable the analyzed

	Authors	PD MCI/PDD	PD non-MCI/PDD
Velocity (m/s)	Kim et al. [35]	0.55 ± 0.29	0.66 ± 0.30
	Chen et al. [36]	1.07 ± 1.51*	1.21 ± 1.69
	Chen et al. [37]	0.88	—
	Mc Ardle et al. [38]	0.89 ± 0.25	—
Step length (m)	Kim et al. [35]	0.30 ± 0.16*	0.38 ± 0.14
	Mc Ardle et al. [38]	0.51 ± 0.12	—
Stride length (m)	Kim et al. [35]	0.62 ± 0.30*	0.74 ± 0.28
	Chen et al. [36]	0.62 ± 0.21*	0.64 ± 0.16
	Chen et al. [37]	0.66	
Cadence (steps/min)	Chen et al. [36]	98.13 ± 16.81*	97.61 ± 11.11

*Means and standard deviations of the gait outcomes. MCI, mild cognitive impairment; PDD, Parkinson's disease dementia. *Comparison with PD non-MCI/PDD is statistically significant. Authors who assess participants with mild cognitive impairment: Kim et al.; Chen, Cheng et al.; Chen, Lien et al. Authors who assess participants with dementia: Mc Ardle et al.*

Table 2.
Gait performance in people with PD and mild cognitive impairment or Parkinson's dementia.

sample is when walking. It answers the question whether the participants with PD always walked in all repetitions at the same speed or with the same stride length. These studies indicate that gait variability is an indicator or biomarker of specific cognitive domains (fluctuating attention and visual memory) in early PD, and even that it is a stronger predictor than baseline cognition [39].

5. Future of research in physical rehabilitation focused on people with PD and dementia

While dementia caused by traumatic brain injury is usually static, dementia caused by neurodegenerative diseases is usually progressive and can eventually be fatal [41]. Although motor rehabilitation impact on people with PD is widely referenced in the scientific literature, the physical effects that can be achieved with physiotherapy in people with PD and dementia are hardly documented. That is why the steps of the new research that seek to clarify the relationship between motor performance and the cognitive impairment and dementia in PD should be as follows:

Randomized control trials about the effectiveness of physical rehabilitation should be include as secondary outcomes the assessment of cognitive functions which performed may be impaired in PD: executive function, attention, speech and language, visuospatial, memory and psychological and behavioral functioning [1].

Although usually in randomized controlled trials on physical rehabilitation, the sample is subdivided by the severity of the disease, according to either the Hoehn and Yahr scale or the Unified Parkinson's Disease Rating Scale, researchers must take into account the analysis of the scope of the effectiveness of physical rehabilitation in patients with different degrees of cognitive impairment or dementia, which implies not excluding their participation in research.

Likewise, studies that introduce cognitive training in people with PD should study the effects of the intervention on motor functions such as gait, balance, and hand functionality.

Scientific publications suggest that physical interventions that include multidomain interventions have better results than physical programs that focus on a single physical aspect.

Moreover, cognitive disorder and dementia are not the only mental disorders that PD patients suffer during the course of the disease. While cognitive decline is one of the most frequent and important nonmotor symptoms in PD [4], mental disorders such as depression, anxiety, insomnia, apathy, and psychosis are other aspects that people with PD deal throughout the disease [42]. Although the alteration of executive functions is part of mild cognitive impairment, dysexecutive syndrome is a clinical picture that requires a specialized study in people with PD. Dysexecutive behavioral disorders may include distractibility, perseverative behavior, poor flexibility, and impulse control, strongly affecting the social functioning of patients. However, these symptoms are not included in the regular executive functions assessment, which is frequently focused on the initiation, inhibition, flexibility, generation, deduction, planning, and coordination of a motor task with some cognitive requirement. Roussel et al. evaluated both cognitive and behavioral domains of the dysexecutive syndrome. These authors determined that dysexecutive syndrome was observed in 80.6% (sample size = 88) of PD patients, and selectively affected either the behavioral domain or the cognitive domain in more than half of the patients [43]. Although there are still aspects to study about the scope of physical therapy for people with dementia in PD, researchers should not ignore the mental disturbances that can appear in the course of the disease.

6. Conclusions

It has been identified that people with PD and cognitive impairment have lower physical functional performance than do people with PD without cognitive impairment. This may be due to alterations in specific cognitive functions that are involved in the planning and execution of voluntary movements, such as executive functions and attention.

Studies that analyze the effects of physical rehabilitation with aerobic exercises, multi-modal or in a multi-domain context, observe cognitive improvements in their participants in addition to physical improvements. Future research should study the effects of physical rehabilitation on the different characteristics of the disease and on people with cognitive impairment and dementia since it constitutes a powerful non-pharmacological treatment tool with benefits in multiple systems.

Conflict of interest

The author declares no conflict of interest.

Abbreviations

PD	Parkinson's disease
PD-MCI	Mild cognitive impairment in Parkinson's disease
PDD	Dementia due to Parkinson's disease (PDD)
CV	Coefficient of variation

Author details

Constanza I. San Martín Valenzuela
Research Unit in Personal Autonomy, Dependence, and Mental Disorder, INCLIVA Health Research Institute, Physiotherapy Department, University of Valencia, Valencia, Spain

*Address all correspondence to: constanza.martin@uv.es

References

[1] Goldman JG, Sieg E. Cognitive impairment and dementia in Parkinson disease. Clinics in Geriatric Medicine 2020;36(2):365-377. DOI: 10.1016/j.cger.2020.01.001.

[2] Mahieux F, Michelet D, Manifacier MJ, Boller F, Fermanian J, Guillard A. Mini-mental Parkinson: First validation study of a new bedside test constructed for Parkinson's disease. Behavioural Neurology 1995;8(1):15-22. DOI: 10.3233/BEN-1995-8102.

[3] Nasreddine ZS, Phillips NA, Bédirian V, Charbonneau S, Whitehead V, Collin I, et al. The Montreal Cognitive Assessment, MoCA: A brief screening tool for mild cognitive impairment. Journal of the American Geriatrics Society 2005;53(4):695-699. DOI: 10.1111/j.1532-5415.2005.53221.x.

[4] Aarsland D, Creese B, Politis M, Chaudhuri KR, ffytche DH, Weintraub D, et al. Cognitive decline in Parkinson disease. Nature Reviews. Neurology 2017;13(4):217-231. DOI: 10.1038/nrneurol.2017.27.

[5] Litvan I, Goldman JG, Tröster AI, Schmand BA, Weintraub D, Petersen RC, et al. Diagnostic criteria for mild cognitive impairment in Parkinson's disease: Movement disorder society task force guidelines. Movement Disorders 2012;27(3):349-356. DOI: 10.1002/mds.24893.

[6] Emre M, Aarsland D, Brown R, Burn DJ, Duyckaerts C, Mizuno Y, et al. Clinical diagnostic criteria for dementia associated with Parkinson's disease. Movement Disorders. 2007;22(12):1689-1707; quiz 1837. DOI: 10.1002/mds.21507.

[7] Anne Shumway-Cook, Marjorie H. Woollacott. Motor Control: Translating Research into Clinical Practice. 5th ed. Philadelphia, PA: Lippincott Williams & Wilkins; 2012. 4-5 p. ISBN: 978-1-4963-0263-2.

[8] Ruitenberg MFL, Koppelmans V. Cognition in motion: Evidence for intact action control with healthy aging. The Journals of Gerontology. Series B, Psychological Sciences and Social Sciences 2021;76(2):252-261. DOI:10.1093/geronb/gbaa184.

[9] Yogev-Seligmann G, Hausdorff JM, Giladi N. The role of executive function and attention in gait. Movement Disorders 2008;23(3):329-342. DOI: 10.1002/mds.21720.

[10] Sharpe G, Macerollo A, Fabbri M, Tripoliti E. Non-pharmacological treatment challenges in early Parkinson's disease for axial and cognitive symptoms: A mini review. Frontiers in Neurology 2020;11:576569. DOI: 10.3389/fneur.2020.576569.

[11] Hely MA, Reid WGJ, Adena MA, Halliday GM, Morris JGL. The Sydney multicenter study of Parkinson's disease: The inevitability of dementia at 20 years. Movement Disorders 2008;23(6):837-844. DOI: 10.1002/mds.21956.

[12] Macleod AD, Counsell CE. Predictors of functional dependency in Parkinson's disease. Movement Disorders 2016;31(10):1482-1488. DOI: 10.1002/mds.26751.

[13] Herold F, Törpel A, Schega L, Müller NG. Functional and/or structural brain changes in response to resistance exercises and resistance training lead to cognitive improvements—A systematic review. European Review of Aging and Physical Activity 2019;16(1):10. DOI: 10.1186/s11556-019-0217-2

[14] Muiños M, Ballesteros S. Does physical exercise improve perceptual skills and visuospatial attention in older adults? A review. European Review of Aging and Physical Activity 2018;15(1):2. DOI: 10.1186/s11556-018-0191-0

[15] San Martín Valenzuela C, Moscardó LD, López-Pascual J, Serra-Añó P, Tomás JM. Effects of dual-task group training on gait, cognitive executive function, and quality of life in people with Parkinson disease: Results of randomized controlled DUALGAIT trial. Archives of Physical Medicine and Rehabilitation 2020;101(11):1849-1856.e1. DOI: 10.1016/j.apmr.2020.07.008.

[16] Levin O, Netz Y, Ziv G. The beneficial effects of different types of exercise interventions on motor and cognitive functions in older age: A systematic review. European Review of Aging and Physical Activity 2017;14(1):20. DOI: 10.1186/s11556-017-0189-z.

[17] Wollesen B, Wildbredt A, van Schooten KS, Lim ML, Delbaere K. The effects of cognitive-motor training interventions on executive functions in older people: A systematic review and meta-analysis. European Review of Aging and Physical Activity 2020;17(1):9. DOI: 10.1186/s11556-020-00240-y.

[18] Cheng Y-C, Su C-H. Evidence supports PA prescription for Parkinson's disease: Motor symptoms and non-motor features: A scoping review. International Journal of Environmental Research and Public Health 2020;17(8):2894. DOI: 10.3390/ijerph17082894

[19] da Silva FC, Iop R da R, de Oliveira LC, Boll AM, de Alvarenga JGS, Gutierres Filho PJB, et al. Effects of physical exercise programs on cognitive function in Parkinson's disease patients: A systematic review of randomized controlled trials of the last 10 years. PLoS ONE 2018;13(2):e0193113. DOI: 10.1371/journal.pone.0193113.

[20] Feng Y-S, Yang S-D, Tan Z-X, Wang M-M, Xing Y, Dong F, et al. The benefits and mechanisms of exercise training for Parkinson's disease. Life Sciences 2020;245:117345. DOI: 10.1016/j.lfs.2020.117345.

[21] Stuckenschneider T, Askew CD, Menêses AL, Baake R, Weber J, Schneider S. The effect of different exercise modes on domain-specific cognitive function in patients suffering from Parkinson's disease: A systematic review of randomized controlled trials. Journal of Parkinson's Disease 2019;9(1):73-95. DOI: 10.3233/JPD-181484.

[22] Altmann LJP, Stegemöller E, Hazamy AA, Wilson JP, Bowers D, Okun MS, et al. Aerobic exercise improves mood, cognition, and language function in Parkinson's disease: Results of a controlled study. Journal of the International Neuropsychological Society 2016;22(9):878-889. DOI: 10.1017/S135561771600076X.

[23] Duchesne C, Lungu O, Nadeau A, Robillard ME, Boré A, Bobeuf F, et al. Enhancing both motor and cognitive functioning in Parkinson's disease: Aerobic exercise as a rehabilitative intervention. Brain and Cognition 2015;99:68-77. DOI: 10.1016/j.bandc.2015.07.005.

[24] Fiorelli CM, Ciolac EG, Simieli L, Silva FA, Fernandes B, Christofoletti G, et al. Differential acute effect of high-intensity interval or continuous moderate exercise on cognition in individuals with Parkinson's disease. Journal of Physical Activity & Health 2019;16(2):157-164. DOI: 10.1123/jpah.2018-0189.

[25] Nadeau A, Lungu O, Duchesne C, Robillard M-È, Bore A, Bobeuf F, et al. A 12-week cycling training regimen improves gait and executive functions concomitantly in people with Parkinson's disease. Frontiers in Human Neuroscience 2017; 10:690. DOI: 10.3389/fnhum.2016.00690.

[26] Cruise KE, Bucks RS, Loftus AM, Newton RU, Pegoraro R, Thomas MG. Exercise and Parkinson's: Benefits for cognition and quality of life. Acta Neurologica Scandinavica 2011;123(1):13-19. DOI: 10.1111/j.1600-0404.2010.01338.x.

[27] Silva-Batista C, Corcos DM, Roschel H, Kanegusuku H, Gobbi LTB, Piemonte MEP, et al. Resistance training with instability for patients with Parkinson's disease. Medicine and Science in Sports and Exercise 2016;48(9):1678-1687. DOI: 10.1249/MSS.0000000000000945.

[28] Tanaka K, Quadros AC de, Santos RF, Stella F, Gobbi LTB, Gobbi S. Benefits of physical exercise on executive functions in older people with Parkinson's disease. Brain and Cognition 2009;69(2):435-441. DOI: 10.1016/j.bandc.2008.09.008.

[29] Pompeu JE, Mendes FA dos S, Silva KG da, Lobo AM, Oliveira T de P, Zomignani AP, et al. Effect of Nintendo WiiTM-based motor and cognitive training on activities of daily living in patients with Parkinson's disease: A randomised clinical trial. Physiotherapy 2012;98(3):196-204. DOI: 10.1016/j.physio.2012.06.004.

[30] dos Santos Mendes FA, Pompeu JE, Modenesi Lobo A, Guedes da Silva K, Oliveira T de P, Peterson Zomignani A, et al. Motor learning, retention and transfer after virtual-reality-based training in Parkinson's disease—Effect of motor and cognitive demands of games: A longitudinal, controlled clinical study. Physiotherapy. 2012;**98**(3):217-223. DOI: 10.1016/j.physio.2012.06.001.

[31] Dahdal P, Meyer A, Chaturvedi M, Nowak K, Roesch AD, Fuhr P, et al. Fine motor function skills in patients with Parkinson disease with and without mild cognitive impairment. Dementia and Geriatric Cognitive Disorders 2016;42(3-4):127-134. DOI: 10.1159/000448751.

[32] Tan S, Hong CT, Chen J-H, Chan L, Chi W-C, Yen C-F, et al. Hand fine motor skill disability correlates with cognition in patients with moderate-to-advanced Parkinson's disease. Brain Sciences 2020;10 (6):337. DOI: 10.3390/brainsci10060337

[33] Middleton A, Fritz SL, Lusardi M. Walking speed: The functional vital sign. Journal of Aging and Physical Activity 2015;23(2):314-322. DOI: 10.1123/japa.2013-0236.

[34] Tan D, Danoudis M, McGinley J, Morris ME. Relationships between motor aspects of gait impairments and activity limitations in people with Parkinson's disease: A systematic review. Parkinsonism & Related Disorders 2012;18(2):117-124. DOI: 10.1016/j.parkreldis.2011.07.014.

[35] Kim SM, Kim DH, Yang Y, Ha SW, Han JH. Gait patterns in Parkinson's disease with or without cognitive impairment.
Dementia and Neurocognitive Disorders 2018;17(2):57-65. DOI: 10.12779/dnd.2018.17.2.57.

[36] Chen P-H, Lien C-W, Wu W-C, Lee L-S, Shaw J-S. Gait-based machine learning for classifying patients with different types of mild cognitive impairment. Journal of Medical Systems 2020;44(6):107. DOI: 10.1007/s10916-020-01578-7.

[37] Chen P-H, Cheng F-Y, Cheng S-J, Shaw J-S. Predicting cognitive decline in Parkinson's disease with mild cognitive impairment: A one-year observational study. Parkinson's Disease 2020; 2020:8983960. DOI: 10.1155/2020/8983960.

[38] Mc Ardle R, Del Din S, Galna B, Thomas A, Rochester L. Differentiating dementia disease subtypes with gait

analysis: Feasibility of wearable sensors? Gait & Posture 2020;76:372-376. DOI: 10.1016/j.gaitpost.2019.12.028.

[39] Morris R, Lord S, Lawson RA, Coleman S, Galna B, Duncan GW, et al. Gait rather than cognition predicts decline in specific cognitive domains in early Parkinson's disease. The Journals of Gerontology. Series A, Biological Sciences and Medical Sciences 2017;72(12):1656-1662. DOI: 10.1093/gerona/glx071.

[40] Pieruccini-Faria F, Black SE, Masellis M, Smith EE, Almeida QJ, Li KZH, et al. Gait variability across neurodegenerative and cognitive disorders: Results from the Canadian consortium of neurodegeneration in aging (CCNA) and the gait and brain study. Alzheimer's & Dementia 2021;1-12. DOI: 10.1002/alz.12298.

[41] Yinglong Chen, Xinyan Tan, Di Yan, Zengmeng Zhang, Yongjun Gong. A composite fabric-based soft rehabilitation glove with soft joint for dementia in Parkinson's disease. IEEE Journal of Translational Engineering in Health and Medicine 2020; 8:1400110. DOI: 10.1109/JTEHM.2020.2981926.

[42] Grover S, Somaiya M, Kumar S, Avasthi A. Psychiatric aspects of Parkinson's disease. Journal of Neurosciences in Rural Practice 2015;6(1):65-76. DOI: 10.4103/0976-3147.143197.

[43] Roussel M, Lhommée E, Narme P, Czernecki V, Gall DL, Krystkowiak P, et al. Dysexecutive syndrome in Parkinson's disease: the GREFEX study. Neuropsychology, Development, and Cognition. Section B, Aging, Neuropsychology and Cognition 2017;24(5):496-507. DOI: 10.1080/13825585.2016.1226248.

Chapter 8

Role of Social Work as Part of PD Treatment

Lisa Marie Mooney

Abstract

The goals of treatment for PD is to maximize function and attempt to minimize the negative impact symptoms may have on a person's qualify of life. To achieve this physicians, patients and family members may need to explore additional medical professionals to address all the needs, challenges and concerns associated with living with Parkinson's Disease. Social Workers can play a valuable role in the care, coping and overall well being of the patient and family members and play an integral part of the treatment team providing in depth psychosocial assessment and recommendations to improve adherence to the treatment plan for each patient/family. Social Workers can assist with a range of needs from the time of diagnosis to end of life. Social Workers can provide assistance at all stages of disease progression to the patient, family and the entire treatment team, therefore it is important for treatment teams consider integrating social workers into the multidisciplinary team approach and opportunities in effort to best address the entire needs of the Parkinson's patient and their psychosocial needs as the disease progresses.

Keywords: social work, social worker, social care needs, multidisciplinary team, social work role

1. Introduction

"While the medical model has promoted great progress in the scientific understanding of etiology and treatment of distinct and unique diseases, the exclusive focus on illness and disease has left out important contextual influences, such as the subjective understanding and adaptation to illness, environmental and social factors" [1]. In my professional experience in working as part of a interprofessional medical department and working with hundreds of Parkinson's patients or family members, I believe medical providers and patients/family member believe the goals of treatment for Parkinson's Disease (PD) is to maximize function and attempt to minimize the negative impact symptoms may have on qualify of life. To achieve this physicians, patients and family members may need to explore additional medical professionals to address all the needs, challenges and concerns associated with living with Parkinson's. Social Workers can play a valuable role from diagnosis to end of life in the success of the medical treatment, coping and wellbeing of the patient and their family members. Integrating social workers into the multidisciplinary/interdisciplinary/interprofessional integrated approach to Parkinson's care can assist with treatment compliance, identify challenges, problems, and barriers to care all while working with other professionals to ensure proper care and treatment to address the patients complex needs. "Integrative Care represents a promising direction for the future of health services and may be leveraged to improve population health across the life course" [2].

2. Social worker role in health care settings

In many health systems there are social workers providing social care/addressing social needs to patients and families, however it is not widely integrated in all aspects of the health system structure (in my experience social workers are often found in inpatient health settings and less frequently in outpatient settings) therefore some patients are getting social worker support, while others are not. For the sake of this chapter, I will keep the integration of social care to focus on how social workers can be an integral part of the Parkinson's Care Team which ideally would include a multidisciplinary or interprofessional approach with doctors, nurses and other allied medical professionals and providers that can contribute a benefit to the overall health, coping and well being of the patient and family during their Parkinson's disease course.

According to a recent publication, "the United States spends 16.3% on health care and only 9.1% on social services, which doesn't appear to be that telling on its own, but when you compare to other countries that spend more on social services, those countries actually spend less on health care services. This information demonstrates that investing into social service resources and professional's health institutions can reduce the spending for health care" [3]. Currently there is not many evidenced based studies to reference showing that a social work "service or task" reduces cost of "this or that", however several small qualitative studies do demonstrate via survey's and questionnaires that addressing social care needs has demonstrated positive outcomes for the patients in the study. "Integrative models of patient care have been advocated and successfully implemented with positive outcomes for patients with chronic conditions such as cancer, chronic pain and diabetes, leading to higher survival rates as well as significant reductions in pain intensity and disability" [4].

With any recommendations that suggest adding another medical provider to the clinical team comes the question of finances and how do we "pay" for this added service or care. Currently some medical clinics or health systems may recognize the value a social worker can provide to patients and may cover the costs, in other cases specialty clinics will get grants from organizations to help support the costs of a social worker or receive philanthropic support from private individuals. Ultimately the hope is that insurance companies will recognize and be able to quantify the value of social workers time and effort as part of the team to be billed as a provider for reimbursement, but that is not the case in most situations at this time. In 2019, a committee on Integrating Social Needs Care into the Delivery of Health Care to Improve the Nation's Health; Board of Health Care Services; Health and Medicine Division; National Academies of Sciences, Engineering and Medicine published a book that discussed this particular issue and found data to suggest that focusing spending on social care of patients can reduce the overall medical spending of a health system. "Though many other industrialized nations spend less per capita on medical services that the United States does, the spend a larger proportion on social services relative to medical services and their residents have better health and lead longer lives" [3]. Improving the health and quality of life for our patients is the reason most professionals got into the healthcare profession therefore, it would be in the best interest of our patients to consider and offer social care as a part of their medical care and treatment and find opportunities to fund this added cost of a social worker on the team which can and will improve treatment success.

3. What is social care or psychosocial care as it relates to treating PD

Treating patients with PD can be challenging for a variety of reasons some of which can be due to issues or barriers not directly related to PD (depression, anxiety, apathy, stress, housing, finances, lack of motivation, etc). For example, a patient may have difficulty maintaining compliance with medical care if they have financial limitations, insurance challenges, depression, anxiety, limited or no family/community support or if they have unstable housing. These are issues that can be a barrier to medical care and treatment specifically for PD, however they are issues that often can be addressed and resolved with community resources and/or support programs. These barriers or difficulties in adhering to recommended treatment can also negatively impact a person's health and mortality. Thus, identifying these social care needs or psychosocial stressors will take a specific assessment, most thoroughly done by a social worker (in my opinion) to ask the questions about living environment, employment, financial limitations, functional abilities, emotional health etc. All areas that can be asked by other professionals however is challenging for a doctor, medical assistant, nurse or nurse practitioner, etc. to incorporate into the already lengthy PD medical assessment and neurological exam. Therefore, integrating a social worker as part of your PD care team can address these social care needs and barriers in an effort to better identify patient needs and appropriate treatment plan.

As we all know, life does not happen in silos, we cannot just focus on health and not work, or focus on kids and not address financial needs, etc. We must find an effective balance or way to address all that life presents. In my experience and as literature also suggests, "Illnesses or diseases have been treated as separate entities and by separate specialists. This episodic and fragmented treatment approach, prevalent in the medical model, can be effective for individuals who encounter an illness that is discrete, of short duration and has limited consequences to work and family, but it is rarely effective for people with chronic conditions" [1]. This is where a social worker's assessment skills can be used to provide more information to the care team to best address the medical needs and social care needs specifically for Parkinson's disease. The social worker's role will extend beyond the day to day management of symptoms and include a fuller picture to try to meet the multiple medical and social care needs of a person with PD both now and in the future. A social workers role in a health system setting is to be aware of therapeutic strategies for treating and coping with PD as well as community resources that will offer support and benefit the patient and family in their PD journey. It is unrealistic to expect that other medical professionals can stay current and up to date on the community programs, or resources that are outside the scope of their practice or education. Medical doctors, nurses, assistants, etc. are educated and skilled in medical intervention for a particular symptom or disease; physical therapists focus on a person's physical well-being, strength, and safety; genetic counselors will focus on the biology and genetic implications for the person and future generations and researchers and scientists will focus on finding meaningful and effective treatments. All these professionals are needed and required to effectively treat and support a PD patient and family, but also needed is a professional to focus on the emotional and social care needs of the person, which is where social workers can be an integral and valuable part of the treatment care team to address the needs of the whole person.

4. Social worker education

Social workers are educated and skilled in many areas. However, the cornerstone of social work practice and skill is building trust and rapport with patients to gain better understanding of the person to best meet their complex needs as a human being. Social workers attempt to provide a safe and judgment free, culturally sensitive and collaborative environment in which we can work with the patient to address needs or concerns. In addition to offering support to individuals' social workers will advocate and develop plans to better meet individual and community needs. I describe social workers as part detectives, part negotiators and 100% advocates for others. "The core values of social work support the role of social workers on integrated care teams to be advocates for patients [2]. At minimum social workers will have a bachelor's of social work (BSW) degree however many social workers will also pursue higher education and get master's level or even doctoral degrees (MSW or PhD in Social Work). Social workers are not required to be licensed to practice social work, but many will pursue State or Federal licensures which require adherence to a code of ethics, participating in continuing education and annual professional development. There are practice standards and guidelines that social workers are encouraged to follow (unlicensed or licensed) called the Social Work Code of Ethics which guide social work principles and practice in all environments from working with individuals, families, to communities or social systems.

> *"Social work education in the bio-psych-social perspective focuses on the biopsychosocial stressors of chronic illness for the individual and the family. Its person-in-environment approach encourages continuous assessment of the whole person, his/her unique situational context and the social determinants of health. Social work training and skills in relationship building, facilitating communication, counseling, advocacy and community resource access bring unique strengths to interprofessional and integrated chronic care practice settings" [5].*

The interdisciplinary or sometimes called interprofessional team approach can be very beneficial not only to the patient, family but also to the medical care team. Social workers can be available to identify issues and challenges and help the other medical providers in establishing a care plan that will best work for the patient. For example if the patient would benefit from a specialized procedure (i.e. Deep Brain Stimulation, DBS) but does not have transportation to get to surgery or a person to care for them after the surgery or to get to follow up appointments, they are not likely to get that procedure done. In some cases this patient might be labeled, uncompliant or does not seem to care about their health, however if a social worker was able to complete an assessment, identify this social care need, then social worker and team can explore more realistic options or assist in finding resolution to the barrier to treatment. This can reduce the providers frustration with patient, reduce what might be labeled as "non-compliant", and may assist in avoiding crisis or unnecessary hospitalizations or emergency room visits.

5. What does social work involvement look like?

"Social workers frequently support patients and their families as they navigate complex health systems, coordinate multifaceted care plans, provide patient psychoeducation on health and wellness, address behavioral health through a variety of treatment modalities, facilitate connections to needed non-medical resources, and advocate for patients across care teams to improve overall access of care" [6]. Initially when social workers meet patients or family members for this first time we take time to establish rapport and trust with the patient, the biggest focus is to ensure that the patient is the person in charge (if appropriate) and the social worker is there to assist and help as the patient/family needs or requests. The first step is to share what the social worker role is as often times patients may have misunderstanding of what social workers do, and in fairness there are social workers in various aspects of life and thus the roles are different for the setting we are working in. In this case we are referring to social workers in a medical setting working as part of an interdisciplinary team for person's with PD. Once the patient is aware of our role and has opportunity to ask questions, express concerns, and agree or disagree to move forward with the assessment we can start building trust and better understanding of the whole patient. As alluded to above, if a patient does not want to participate at that time, social workers will respect that wish and let them know that if they change their mind or would like assistance at another time they can always reach out then. With patient/family participation, social workers will move forward with psychosocial assessment (assessment of the social aspects of the person—education, employment, family, finances, fun, personal care needs/ability, responsibilities, etc. as well as the psychological—emotional health, coping strategies, life stressors, trauma, safety, etc). The assessment will offer additional insight for the treatment team about the patient's daily life, family life, emotional health, coping skills, motivation, stressors, abilities, needs and limitations. Some of this can and will be gathered from other medical professionals as many medical professionals will assess mood symptoms, however with a Social Worker we can dive deeper into the triggers or cause for increased mood symptoms or changes in behavior, which can free up the doctor, physical therapist, nurse practitioner, etc. from having to explore these nuances and human complexities that maybe even the patient has not fully explored or identified and thus the other treatment team professionals can focus on their area of expertise. The Social worker can then work with the patient or family on how all the recommendations from the other professionals can be implemented into their daily life for better medical management of their PD.

Maybe this sounds too good to be true. And truth be told some patients/families will embrace the social work assistance and others will not, but even having the knowledge of a person not wanting social worker involvement can speak to other issues/concerns that the patient is experiencing. If a patient has had a negative interaction with a social worker, they may be reluctant to utilize that resource again, just as if a patient has a negative experience with a medical professional they may seek care elsewhere or stop seeking care altogether. So, no, social workers cannot solve, identify, and make all patients cooperative and compliant (that is a miracle worker and when you find one, please let me know). However, when the social worker is able to complete the assessment and identify stressors, barriers or areas that may cause interference with compliance or quality of life, he/she can offer information, education as well as resources to address these social care needs. For another example, if finances are a challenge or concern and the patient is having to choose between this or that due to limited money, the social worker can explore with the patient what he/she might be eligible for in regards to government financial programs or explore reduced rate utility programs, or medication assistance programs so the person can make their income cover more needs and maintain the wellbeing of the family.

Equally impactful for the patient is a social workers role to help patients cope with PD. Parkinson's symptoms cannot be stopped or cured and therefore patients and families are forced to adapt to the changes to maintain a quality of life of which they seek. This can be difficult to cognitively and emotionally process and, in most cases, patients will need support and education to effectively process this new "road" they are forced to go down. This is another area in which a social worker can assist patients: supportive counseling, compassion, and education about what to expect, normalizing their experience and connecting them with others in similar situations so they do not feel so isolated and depressed. Helping them process the impact PD will have on future hope, dreams, and abilities is important to maintain their sense of purpose, value and quality of life. Social workers can intervene at that time of diagnosis to lessen the negative emotional impact this may have on a person's life as the disease progresses.

For this they need to have a trusted professional to discuss what they may be feeling and to normalize and offer strategies to help them process their feelings to minimize potential exacerbation of depression, anxiety, irritability, anger or suicidal thoughts. Mood and cognitive changes are common in persons with PD and while medication is effective to treat it, we also want to ensure that the patient and family has effective coping strategies to manage mood, cognitive changes and any stress in an effort to positively impact their overall compliance with treatment plan and quality of life. To address emotional health and improve ability to cope, we have resources such a talk therapy, counseling, exercise programs, education, support groups, community events, social gatherings and events, etc. that can offer emotional support but are also effective strategies to manage mood and quality of life. Some patients may not want to accept support because maybe they feel they are not deserving or others are worse than they are and they deserve the help more, or it may trigger feelings of failure that they cannot "do it all themselves, independently". All these feelings are valid and must also be addressed and explored to help the person process the feelings and changes they are experiencing and to help them find a way through the feelings (which are often related to grief/loss) as a result of the PD diagnosis.

Living with PD can be described as a series of grief/losses that patients and their loved ones will have to go through as the disease progresses that will impact quality of life. Learning how to live with the disease knowing that the symptoms of Parkinson's will change their life in many ways (i.e. impact on interpersonal relationships, ability to work, ability to engage in pleasurable activities, ability to take care of themselves, etc.) takes time and will not be resolved in one clinic appointment. Therefore, the social worker can continue to monitor and assess for any impact grief and loss the patient or family may be experiencing throughout the PD journey and address them as appropriate in hopes to minimize any negative impact on treatment or prevent a crisis situation.

In a clinical environment the medical doctor can only prescribe treatment to the patient, however the patients well-being, compliance and ability to participate is often directly influenced by the family (spouse, adult children, siblings, friend, or other care providers) and without addressing the stressors and social care needs of the family, the Parkinson's Care team is ignoring a large and influential piece of the patient's success with treatment. While other professionals are not able to put the time and effort into the family needs or have the skills to navigate the complex family dynamics that are often involved, the social worker can take the time to address these complexities and social care needs which often does improve cooperation and treatment compliance. Which leads us to another aspect of where social workers can be increasingly valuable and effective on the PD care team is identifying the family or social support system the patient lives within.

Throughout this chapter I have referenced patients meaning the persons diagnosed with PD symptoms AND I have referenced family referring to those that interact, support or provide care to the person with PD. While the patient is the center or direct focus of the treatment and the one receiving direct medical intervention and care for PD they are not the only person that may be impacted by this diagnosis. In most situations patients are a part of a family system which also needs to be included in the assessment of social care or psychosocial needs, because family support is often a significant influence on a successful or unsuccessful treatment plan. The entire family or support system of the patient and needs to be recognized and understood as interrelated to best treat the patient successfully. While the patient and doctor relationship are essential to the management and effective treatment of PD symptoms, the rapport and relationship the PD care team has with the family is also essential to the overall cooperation, compliance and success of the individual's medical care.

In my experience, most people do not recognize their limitations, severity or impact one's health or symptoms can have on others around them. For example, it is rare that a person will acknowledge they are a "bad" driver yet ask their partner or passengers and you may get a different perspective. This is clearly an oversimplified analogy to demonstrate that the family or other persons involved in the PD patient's daily life can offer a different, sometimes more accurate, perspective on what is being experienced outside the medical office. PD patients might report feeling good and doing well, taking medications, getting their exercise, following all the medical recommendations, but then you look at their family sitting next to them and their body language, facial expressions or words tell a different story. Exploring what the family is experiencing is necessary and will positively or negatively influence the patient's medical treatment. If the family is struggling because now they are shouldering the responsibilities the patient used to manage, they may not be able to continue to take the patient to therapies, or manage the medications, or get them to appointments, etc. and this will negatively impact the patients compliance with PD care.

6. WHEN to involve social work and WHAT needs will be addressed

As with most illness early intervention and treatment usually brings the best benefit to the patient and that is certainly the case with involving social workers early on as close to the time of diagnosis as possible. The earlier social workers can build the trust and rapport, the earlier they can have difficult discussions, avoid struggles and help the patient/family avoid possible crisis situations. Early social care intervention can help people with coping, but also with practical life issues that come up with a disease like Parkinson's. For example, social workers can help patients think about workplace accommodations or future in home care needs and discuss what is available now and what they may need to consider in the future. Social workers can help a person prepare for the changes he/she will face as PD progresses. Social Workers can educate and assist the medical team in knowing what to document so that the patient/family can obtain or utilize disability programs, government programs or long term care needs. Having the medical documentation that medically justifies symptom progression and functional decline early on will assist in avoiding delays in the application process and approval for most programs. This will help reduce stress for patient and the team, allowing for a better transition for the patient and family as the personal care or social care needs of the patient as PD progresses.

7. Social work role at each Parkinson's disease stage

7.1 Early stage/initial diagnosis (stage 1 or 2)

In early stages social workers can assist with connecting patients and families to education, information and support specific to Parkinson's so the patient and family can better understand and process what this diagnosis means for both the short term and long term. This can be addressing patient and/or family members feelings about the diagnosis, addressing any questions about disease process as well as assistance with patient and family establishing the support system, they will need to address their social care needs. Areas of focus in early stages often include:

- Coping: emotional health and coping with new diagnosis, mood symptoms,
- Finances: income, financial responsibilities, limitations, or concerns
- Safety: both physical and emotional safety. Suicide assessment
- Employment: workplace accommodations, short term and long-term disability,
- Future planning: Advance Health Care Directives, Wills, Trusts
- Transportation: driving concerns/issues, ability to access and use public transportation
- Education: linking to accurate and reliable education and information about Parkinson's or Parkinson's support.
- Social Support: building their support system, linking to support groups, therapy, or nonprofits to integrate into PD community.
- Case Management: care coordination (where to go for PT, equipment, ongoing documentation of needs and disease progression for the care team) as well as advocacy for community needs/resources.
- Exercise: desire and ability to exercise, how to incorporate despite functional changes, linking to community exercise programs for PD.
- Life essentials: access to food, water, housing, clothing, etc.
- Faith-based needs: linking to faith-based resources

7.2 Social work role in middle stage (stage 3 or 4)

As the disease progresses and symptoms increase, social workers can assist the patient or family in identifying safety concerns, long term plans and desires, as well as assist in addressing any issues/concerns that tend to come up in the process of living. Social workers will often start the hard and difficult conversations early with patients about end of life wishes, advance care planning, safety, etc. so that the patient/family and the team have some idea of what the patient wants, this very much can evolve and change over the course of care and treatment, but opening these conversations early can avoid having them under stressful or when a patient/family is in a crisis. While these are similar areas of focus as was in the early stage, however in middle stage is usually when the family will need to implement certain resources to address the changes and disease progression and a social worker can assist in implementing the ideas or thoughts discussed in early stages. For example, in the middle stage patients may need more supervision for safety, may be increased fall risk, may need more assistance with home and life responsibilities, etc. therefore the social worker can link the family to community resources or agencies that fit within their financial constraints, and/or ways to increase independence and safety in the home, fall prevention strategies and as always will provide emotional support during the disease journey. In some cases, legal issues, capacity, guardianship/conservatorship may have to be discussed and explored, which is something social workers can help explore and link to appropriate government or community agencies.

7.3 Social work role in late stage PD (stage 5)

During this stage the role of the social worker will be mostly directed to supporting the family where the role of the medical provider will be comfort and management of symptoms and medication. This stage the social worker will provide a great deal of emotional support, coping strategies and involvement of outside community agencies (like in home assistance, home health services or hospice services) as appropriate. At all stages, but often in later stages family is emotionally drained and unable to advocate or ask for what is needed and in these situations the social worker familiar with the patient and family can advocate to the care team or other providers or agencies to address any needs.

8. Social work role post-mortem

If the family has been involved and engaged in the medical care and treatment of the PD person, it is likely that they have formed a relationship and bond with the care team and may reach out to the team, because that is what they were used to doing throughout the PD journey. In these cases, the Social Worker is likely to be the point of contact and will continue to offer guidance, supportive counseling and linking family to bereavement resources within their community to address any grief symptoms they may be experiencing. It is common for persons that are grieving to seek support from someone familiar and that really understood the complexities of what the family went through during their loved ones Parkinson's disease.

Social workers can be supportive and validate the feelings of the family because he/she will have historical understanding of how and what the family had to do and sacrificed during the PD journey. Caring for a PD loved one often occurs over a long period of time often 10 or more years and includes many ups and downs and certainly changes the family dynamic, social interactions and purpose to primarily revolve around the PD person. Having this routine and purpose, just end can be confusing and paralyzing for the family in identifying their new normal and moving forward with their lives. In addition, each family member will grieve differently and may require different support or intervention to process and move forward. Aside from processing their feelings and finding ways to emotionally move forward with life, the family may have challenges establishing new routines or priorities, establishing or reestablishing family dynamics and new social interactions. Staying connected to the Social Worker can provide a sense of connectiveness, comfort and normalcy that others not involved in the long term journey PD journey may not recognize or understand and thus assist the family in their grief and moving forward with their lives.

9. Conclusions

Most, if not all, PD patients and families will experience more than just the physical, cognitive or emotional symptoms of PD, but will also experience psychosocial stressors, changes and social care needs for example: altering one's sense of self or purpose, change the family dynamics, how one interacts with others, how one maintains relationships, and their plans and dreams for the future. These changes can have a profound impact on their compliance with medical care and coping at all stages of the disease. Literature suggests" taking social risk factors into account is critical to improving both primary prevention and the treatment of acute and chronic illness because social contexts influence the delivery and outcomes of health care" [3]. The National Academies of Sciences, Engineering and Medication, also recommends that "effectively integrating social care into the delivery of health care requires effective interprofessional teams that include experts in social care" [3] which can be most effectively addressed by a social worker.

Social workers can be an integral and valuable member of a Parkinson's Care Team in providing insight and perspective to the team about the patient's social care needs, limitations and barriers to treatment, but can also support the patient and the family to achieve maximum effectiveness, cooperation and compliance of the medical recommendations. While minimal research and studies have been completed to direct specific interdisciplinary integration, some literature and study results show "an integrative model of treatment, involving a variety of specialties, allows clinicians to interact and treat arising PD symptoms in a more fluid manner than on a strictly referral basis" [4]. Social workers have extensive education, experience, and skills in a variety of areas to address needs, advocate and navigate the complexities of family systems, community systems, health systems, government systems, etc. To provide effective, successful, and comprehensive care to our patients, we must look at all aspects of health and life. Patients are unable to treat Parkinson's on their own, therefore seek out knowledgeable and competent doctors to assist them, and doctors cannot be expected to be able to address all the physical, emotional, and social needs of Parkinson's patients without other providers to support them, guide them and be experts in their area of education. It's the timeless sentiment of "it take a village" and in the case of Parkinson's disease, establishing an interdisciplinary care team of professionals to address the needs of the whole person will provide improved health, quality of life and over all well-being to individuals and families living with PD.

Conflict of interest

The author declares no conflict of interest.

Notes/thanks/other declarations

Thank you to the expert and caring faculty and staff at the UC Davis Health, Department of Neurology for their support, guidance, patience and trust in me to be part of the amazing Department, it is my honor to work alongside such compassionate professionals. Most of all thank you for recognizing the value of social workers and integrating my skills into the care of your patients.

A specific thank you to Dr. Lin Zhang for his validation and gratitude for my work and giving me the opportunity to share my Parkinson's and Social Work knowledge and experience through this book and chapter.

Special thank you to Dr. Vicki Wheelock, Terry Tempkin, NP and the Northern California Huntington's Disease Society of America (HDSA) Chapter for hiring me, teaching me and guiding me, 11 years ago, to work with the Huntington's Community, which led me to expanded my skills, knowledge and understanding that afforded me the opportunity to work with other patients and families living with Neurological illness, specifically Parkinson's disease.

Thank you to the Parkinson's patients and families that trust me with their story to support them in their disease journey. It is an honor and a privilege to work with such courageous and inspiring patients and families.

An extra special thanks to my family and friends that are always loving, supportive and happily listen and participate in local events to support my patients and families because it is important to me and therefore important to them.

Author details

Lisa Marie Mooney
LCSW, Department of Neurology, UC Davis Health, Sacramento, California, United States

*Address all correspondence to: lmooney@ucdavis.edu

References

[1] Stanhope V, Videka L, Thorning H, McKay M. Moving toward integrated health: An opportunity for social work. Social Work in Health Care. 2015;**54**(5):383-407. DOI: 10.1080/00981389.2015.1025122

[2] de Saxe Zerden L, Lombardi BM, Jones A. Social workers in integrated health care: Improving care throughout the life course. Social Work in Health Care. 2019;**58**(1):142-149. DOI: 10.1080/00981389.2019.1553934

[3] National Academies of Sciences, Engineering and Medicine. Integrating Social Care into the Delivery of Health Care: Moving Upstream to Improve the Nation's Health. Washington, DC: The National Academies Press; 2019. DOI: https://doi.org/10.17226/25467

[4] Prizer LP, Browner N. The Integrative Care of Parkinson's Disease: A Systematic Review. Journal of Parkinson's Disease. 2012;**2**:79-86. DOI: 10.3233/JPD-2012-12075

[5] Gonzalez-Ramos G, Cohen EV, Luce V, Gonzalez MJ. Clinical social work in the care of Parkinson's disease: Role, functions, and opportunities in integrated health care. Social Work in Health Care. 2019;**58**(1):108-125. DOI: 10.1080/00981389.2018.1544600

[6] Fraser MW, Lombardi BM, Wu S, de Saxe Zerden L, Richman EL, Fraher EP. Integrated primary care and social work: A systematic review. Journal of the Society for Social Work and Research. 2018;**9**:175-215. DOI: 10.1086/697567

Chapter 9

Sleep in Parkinson's Disease Dementia

Matthew Chow

Abstract

Sleep disruption and daytime somnolence are common in Parkinson's disease dementia (PDD). In this condition, the clinical features of Parkinson's disease (PD) and dementia with Lewy bodies (DLB) converge. Both PD and DLB populations have different sleep disturbances that are amplified when combined. Hence, sleep disruption is often significant and multifactorial in PDD. It is proposed that sleep–wake neural networks are affected early in the neurodegenerative process. The resultant lack of sleep results in impaired clearance of toxic metabolites, hastening disease progress. As the motor and nonmotor symptoms of PDD worsen, sleep becomes more disturbed. Medications used to control these symptoms can be sedating or cause insomnia. Comorbid sleep disorders are also often present. All of these factors contribute to poor sleep in these patients. Management is centered on symptom control, quality of life, and treatment of comorbidities.

Keywords: Parkinson's disease dementia, Lewy body dementia, glymphatic system, REM sleep behavior disorder, circadian rhythm disturbance, insomnia, obstructive sleep apnea, restless legs syndrome, nocturia

1. Introduction

Sleep–wake disturbances play an important role in the clinical presentation of the disease in patients with PDD. Involvement of brainstem and diencephalic structures result in dysfunction of the reticular activating system and other structures related to sleep-wake homeostasis. The resultant sleep disruption may impair the clearance of these abnormal proteins through slow wave sleep-mediated glymphatic drainage. Thus, neurodegeneration and sleep disruption interact in a feedforward loop, increasing the progression of disease. PD is classically recognized for its motor symptoms of tremor, rigidity, bradykinesia, and postural instability. However, sleep disturbances, broadly classified as one of the nonmotor manifestations of the condition, are quite common and associated with significant morbidity. Nocturnal motor symptoms, nocturia, dopaminergic medications, comorbid medical, psychiatric, sleep disorders, and environmental factors can all contribute to poor sleep in these patients. On the other end of the clinical spectrum, disturbance of sleep–wake mechanisms is a core feature of DLB. There are fluctuations of attention and arousal manifesting as variability in the ability to organize thoughts throughout the day and frequent daytime lethargy and napping despite an adequate sleeping period at night. The presence of REM sleep behavior disorder (RBD), a sleep disorder characterized by the enactment of dream activity due to loss of the normal muscle paralysis associated with REM sleep, is highly prevalent in DLB and is often one of

IntechOpen

the first signs of the disease. DLB patients are also notably sensitive to neuroleptic medications, which can present as confusion, inattention, and somnolence upon exposure to this class of medication. Unfortunately, this is often discovered on the road to diagnosis in an attempt to manage the behavioral manifestations of the disease. These clinical features are often present in PD as well; however, they are often identified retrospectively or later in the course of the disease. PDD, on the spectrum of PD and DLB, is characterized by the onset of cognitive decline in patients with an established diagnosis of PD. All of the aforementioned sleep disturbances seen in PD and DLB can coexist in PDD and are often historically difficult to disentangle. While present as a core feature of DLB and a common nonmotor manifestation of PD, sleep disturbances are often underappreciated in these diseases, especially in the prodromal phase. The presence of disturbed sleep and/or daytime sleepiness in a patient with cognitive impairment or subtle signs of Parkinsonism should alert the clinician to the possibility of a neurodegenerative process. Sleep disruption often presents years prior to the motor or cognitive stigmata of these conditions; however, it may be overlooked as nonspecific or regarded as typical of age-related changes in sleeping patterns. A sleep-focused history, review of systems, standardized questionnaires, neurological examination, and polysomnography can aid in identifying sleep–wake disturbances in these patients. Early recognition is important for expectant disease management, counseling, and research into neuroprotective agents with the aim of halting or altering the trajectory of illness in these diseases.

2. Neurodegeneration of sleep–wake systems

Primary neurodegeneration in PDD causes excessive daytime sleepiness and disruption of sleep–wake architecture. Sleepiness and daytime napping are common in the older general population and not specific for the presence of a neurodegenerative condition. Clinical tools used to assess daytime sleepiness include quantitative questionnaires of subjective sleepiness like the Epworth Sleepiness Scale (ESS) as well as nocturnal polysomnography in combination with daytime nap testing, such as the multiple sleep latency test (MSLT). Patients with alpha-synuclein disease present with increased sleepiness by both subjective and objective measures compared to age-matched controls [1]. Within this population, daytime sleepiness also tends to increase with the presence of dementia with patients with PDD exhibiting increased sleepiness compared to patients with PD alone [2]. This daytime somnolence is in large part due to sleep disruption at night with associated alterations in underlying sleep architecture seen with polysomnography. Studies in patients with PD have shown poorer sleep quality with a delay in sleep onset, reduced N3 sleep, REM sleep, total sleep time, and sleep efficiency. This is similar to studies in patients with DLB that have also shown increased wake after sleep onset and N2 sleep [3]. These patients are also more frequently afflicted with EMG augmentation during REM sleep and confusional arousals from NREM sleep. These polysomnographic findings suggest that disruption of sleep–wake neural networks is common to both clinical conditions with overlap in their neuropathological spread. Posterior dominant slowing of background rhythms in REM sleep and wakefulness, temporal slowing with wakefulness, and impairment in spindle generation appear to be electrographic biomarkers for the development of PDD [4, 5]. This mirrors neurohistopathological findings that show increased Lewy body deposition in brainstem and limbic structures, which colocalize with the wake-promoting reticular activating system (RAS) and thalamocortical circuitry involved with spindle generation, respectively. The Unified Staging System for Lewy Body Disorders suggests that the involvement of these structures occurs early on in the disease course with brainstem involvement

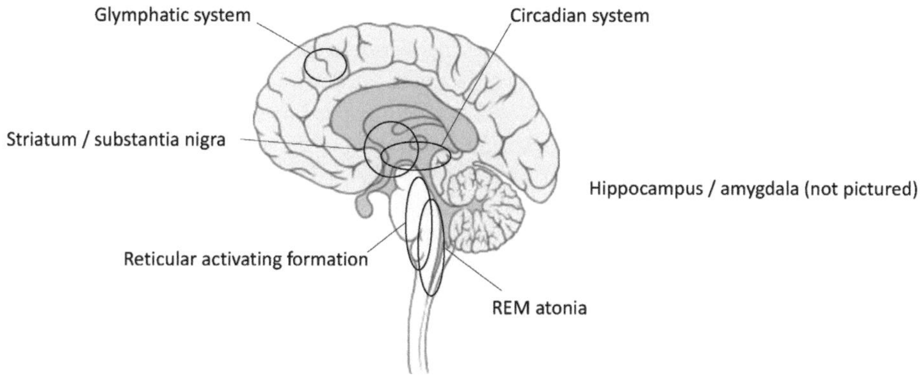

Figure 1.
Relevant neuroanatomical regions implicated in the pathogenesis of PDD.

(IIa) characteristic of more parkinsonian-type features and limbic involvement (IIb) characteristic of a more dementing-type illness. It is at these stages of disease that sleep disturbances likely become apparent. PDD would be identified in the transition from mostly brainstem involvement (IIa) to both brainstem and limbic involvement (III). After both neuroanatomical regions become involved, there is subsequent spread to the neocortex (IV) (**Figure 1**) [6].

Of course, it is important to note that the clinical picture is not always this clear. PD patients can also have Alzheimer's and cerebrovascular disease. These patient populations also suffer from daytime sleepiness and sleep disturbances. Amyloid plaques, neurofibrillary tangles, and ischemic changes can be seen on pathological examination. Often, a detailed neurologic history can aid in distinguishing these entities. In summary, PDD patients have increased sleepiness compared to healthy elderly subjects and PD patients without dementia. This is in large part due to degradation of sleep architecture from Lewy body disease in the brainstem and limbic structures.

3. Impaired clearance and disease progression

Impaired clearance of abnormal proteins in the central nervous system has been hypothesized as a mechanism for disease progression in alpha-synuclein disease as well as other neurodegenerative conditions. Recent discovery of the glymphatic system, a perivascular pathway that promotes the clearance of waste products facilitated by aquaporin-4 (AQ4) astrocytic water channels, has shown to be associated with amyloid-beta clearance. The glymphatic system is most active during sleep, notably slow wave sleep, due to reduced cellular swelling, expansion of the extracellular space with flow driven by cardiac pulsations [7]. These findings have implications in the pathogenesis of Alzheimer's disease and the role of sleep in general. While amyloid-beta levels have been shown to oscillate in CSF analysis of human subjects with the sleep–wake cycle, no such data exist with regard to alpha-synuclein. In a mouse model of PD, reduced glymphatic flow via ligation of deep cervical lymph nodes, yielded worsening of motor deficits and perivascular aggregation of alpha-synuclein [8]. Given sleep disturbances often occur early in alpha-synuclein disease and associated with more cognitive dysfunction, a feed forward mechanism for disease progression has been proposed. Primary neurodegeneration of sleep–wake structures in the brainstem leads to increased sleep disruption, which then impairs glymphatic clearance of abnormal proteins accumulated during wakefulness. This then causes worsening of the underlying neurodegenerative disease further disrupting sleep. Even if alpha-synuclein is not cleared by the glymphatic system, PD patients are not immune from developing Alzheimer's disease (AD) pathology, which likely contributes to a subset of the PDD phenotype as mentioned previously. Reduction of comorbid amyloid-beta pathology could reduce central nervous system disease burden. Aging itself may be a risk factor for impaired glymphatic drainage as mouse models have demonstrated reduced beta-amyloid clearance with advancing age [9]. The importance of screening for comorbid sleep disorders in patients suspected of alpha-synuclein disease cannot be understated, as many of these disorders have established and effective therapies. Treatment of sleep disorders represents one of the significant modifiable risk factors in disease progression in patients who go on to develop PDD. In summary, the glymphatic system is hypothesized to play a role in alpha-synuclein accumulation through feed forward mechanisms. Comorbid AD pathology, advancing age, and sleep disorders can be contributory.

4. REM sleep behavior disorder as a biomarker

REM sleep behavior disorder is often prodromal in PDD and may represent a unique subtype of PD patients. The early and often initially isolated presence of RBD provides a window into the prodromal stages of Lewy body disease. The perilocus coeruleus in the pontine tegmentum projects to medullary magnocellularis neurons via the lateral tegmental-reticular tract. These neurons then project to motor neurons in the anterior horn cells of the spinal cord to produce paralysis during REM sleep. Disruption of this pathway can lead to REM sleep without atonia (RSWA) and manifest clinically as RBD. Consistent with the hypothesis that Lewy body disease presents early in brainstem structures, the presence of RBD can predate the onset of parkinsonism or cognitive decline by years (**Figure 2**).

PD patients with RBD appear to have increased cognitive impairment than PD patients without RBD [10]. They also share a number of clinical features more characteristic of patients with DLB than classic tremor-predominant idiopathic Parkinson's disease patients. An akinetic-rigid motor phenotype, hallucinations, and autonomic dysfunction have been more frequently described in PD patients with RBD than in those without. They also have more dense and diffuse pathology

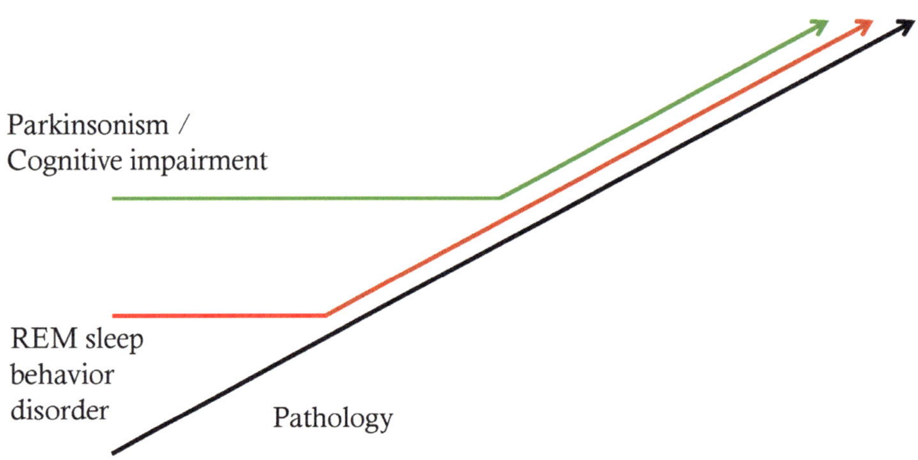

Figure 2.
Relative symptom onset with disease progression in Lewy body disease.

on autopsy [11]. These clinical findings are supportive of a specific pathological subtype among patients with PD. Prospective studies in patients with idiopathic RBD who have yet to develop symptoms of parkinsonism or dementia have yielded similar conclusions. A study in a cohort of presumably idiopathic RBD (iRBD) patients has uncovered a number of interesting findings. (1) The large majority of iRBD patients actually have prodromal alpha-synucleinopathy. (2) Quantitative motor evaluation was both predictive of phenoconversion to parkinsonism AND dementia. (3) The diagnoses of DLB and PDD may mostly be a clinical distinction in that phenoconversion to parkinsonism first versus dementia first was similarly predictive of DLB [12]. These findings suggest a predictable pattern of disease in patients with iRBD with a common endpoint, which can be assessed in the clinic. A patient with iRBD who develops motor features consistent with parkinsonism is at risk for PDD. Similarly, opposed to the notion that dementia precedes parkinsonian features in DLB, this did not seem to matter in patients with RBD with patients presenting with parkinsonism first having a similar risk for developing DLB. Of note, most of these studies focused on the prodromal or early stages of PD and dementia. Less is known about patients with longstanding PD who develop RBD later in the disease course. In summary, the mere presence of RBD may portend the development of PDD and DLB, which likely have the same pathological underpinnings with a more aggressive disease progress and poor prognosis.

5. Case study

History of present illness:

A 57-year-old left-handed retired salesman with a past medical history significant for restless legs syndrome (RLS), transient ischemic attack (TIA) with word-finding difficulties at the time, and concussion in his youth presents with a 10-year history of episodes of violent dream reenactment with sleep. Episodes occur monthly to a couple of times per week. They usually occur a couple of hours upon falling asleep. He will often kick off his covers, talk, yell, and curse. This is accompanied by dreams of trying to run away from an attacker or kick himself free. He may wake up in the midst of one of these episodes and realize they have occurred. It has also been witnessed by others. Alcohol and sweets prior to bedtime may precede an episode. Ropinirole and imipramine prescribed by a neurologist in the past seemed to be beneficial. Clonazepam was ineffective. He denies any associated symptoms, specifically, no difficulties with memory, complex tasks or judgment, visuospatial ability, language, or behavior. He also denies a loss of taste or smell, constipation, muscle stiffness, slowness of movement, tremor, or falls. He feels his mood is good and denies any hallucinations. He denies any loss or near loss of consciousness.

The patient presents with isolated violent dream enactment behavior suspicious for RBD. His age of onset is consistent with the usual initial presentation for Lewy body disease (>50 years old). Violent content, usually in the act of defense, is common. Time of onset in the night is usually in the latter half of the night due to more prolonged REM periods with successive sleep cycles; however, episodes can occur anytime the patient enters REM sleep. Waking in the midst of episodes and dream recall is common as REM sleep is a "lighter" stage of sleep with an EEG profile similar to wakefulness (low amplitude mixed frequency EEG). Some studies have reported an association with RBD and alcohol, however, only in the context of chronic and heavy consumption. Clonazepam is usually first line in the treatment of RBD; however, the patient felt this was subjectively ineffective. There is little data to support the use of dopamine agonists or tricyclic antidepressants in the treatment of RBD, with some concern that this may exacerbate the condition; however, the patient found these medications subjectively beneficial.

Medications: Aspirin, atorvastatin, vitamin D, and a multivitamin.

Allergies: No known drug allergies.

Past medical history: RLS, TIA, concussion, hypertension, hyperlipidemia, Gilbert's syndrome, and vitamin D deficiency.

Past surgical history: Tonsillectomy.

Social history: No history of learning difficulties. Earned his bachelor's degree. Recently retired due to work-related stress (not due to disability or job performance). Lives with his wife. Independent with his activities of daily living. Good social support. Rare alcohol. No smoking or recreational drug use.

Family history: Mother diagnosed with DLB, stroke in her 60s, and colon cancer. Died at 80 years old. Sister with breast cancer. Alive.

Of note, the patient is not on antidepressant or anticholinergic medications, which can mimic or "unmask" RBD. The patient has a family history of DLB in his mother. Having a family member with DLB may increase one's risk of developing DLB; however, DLB is generally not considered a genetic disease with most mutations being sporadic. Genes implicated in DLB include APOE, GBA, SNCA, BIN1, and TMEM175 [13].

Exam: The patient is obese with stage 1 hypertension. All other vital signs were stable. General physical exam was normal. On neurological exam, he scored a 26/30 on the MOCA with points missed for copying the image of the cube (visuospatial), identifying the association between a train and bicycle (abstraction), and 3/5 on word recall (delayed recall). He also had difficulty with identification with the alcohol sniff test. Otherwise, his neurological exam was unremarkable.

The patient was within the lower end of the normal range on his MOCA with deficits in visuospatial, abstraction, and delayed recall. Cognitive deficits in Lewy body disease have attention, executive function, and visuospatial perception disproportionately involved. Nonspecific but possibly the most clinically relevant finding on exam was his impaired sense of smell with olfactory bulb involvement common in prodromal Lewy body disease and consistent with his largely isolated RBD presentation.

Neuropsychological testing: Evaluation revealed normal cognition with testing in the average to superior range in attention, processing speed, language abilities, memory, and executive functioning. His performance in visuospatial tasks was overall normal; however, this may possibly reflect area of very subtle weakness in comparison to other areas.

MRI of the brain: Mild generalized brain parenchymal volume loss without lobal predilection.

Diagnostic polysomnogram revealed the following (**Figure 3**):

Phasic EMG activity in the bilateral arms and leg leads throughout as well as increased chin tone in the latter half of this 30-second epoch is observed. The background EEG is of low amplitude and mixed frequency with phasic "sail wave" eye movements observed in the EOG. The sleep technologist noted a behavioral manifestation in the corresponding video recording (not pictured here). These polysomnographic findings are consistent with RSWA and confirmatory of a diagnosis of RBD in the appropriate clinical setting.

6. Sources of sleep disturbance

There are a number of clinical symptoms associated with PDD that contribute to sleep disruption. Nocturnal motor and cognitive symptoms, pharmacologic

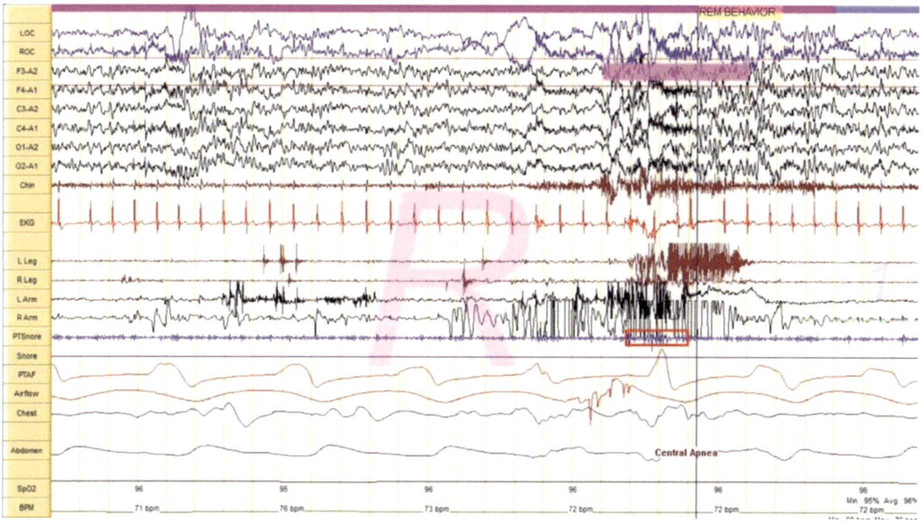

Figure 3.
A 30-second epoch from a polysomnogram showing RSWA.

(dopaminergic, acetylcholinesterase, antidepressant, and neuroleptic) therapy, circadian rhythm disturbances, mood disorder, nocturia, insomnia, obstructive sleep apnea (OSA), and RLS can all play a role.

6.1 Nocturnal motor symptoms

While the motor manifestations of parkinsonism classically abate with sleep, sleep is often disturbed by the presence of akinesia, rigidity, cramping, tremor, and dystonia. These motor manifestations of PD are caused by the loss of dopaminergic neurons in the substantia nigra. The degree to which these motor symptoms cause sleep disruption trends with the progression of the disease. The obvious challenge with assessing nocturnal motor symptoms is that treatment decisions are largely based on retrospective patient report and daytime motor assessment, which can be challenging in patients with PDD. There are a couple of tools that have been developed to address this need. The Parkinson's disease sleep scale (PDSS) is a validated, short, 15-item inventory covering some of the most common sleep-related complaints in patients with PD with items 9–13 particularly focused on motor-related symptoms. However, this too relies on accurate patient or caregiver report [14]. More recently, and perhaps more objectively, actigraphy has emerged as an effective means of assessing nocturnal motor symptoms [15]. Patients in the early phase of the disease tend to show more frequent turning, similar to controls, however, with reduced speed and amplitude. More advanced PD patients show less turning, overall, with more time spent upright. This can be used to not only track disease progression but also response to therapy. Polysomnography would represent the "gold standard" assessment for these motor symptoms; however, it is not used clinically for this purpose outside of drug trials. It is mostly helpful in the identification of comorbid sleep disorders, such as RBD, OSA, and periodic limb movement disorder (PLMD). It would be impractical in monitoring the response to dopaminergic therapy. Long-acting preparations of levodopa, pramipexole, ropinirole, and a transdermal rotigotine patch have been developed. These medications have shown to be effective in treating nocturnal motor symptoms and reducing PDSS scores. Such preparations reduce the need for nocturnal medication administration. They also increase the amount of time the patient spends in the therapeutic range, without having to augment the dose, which can cause toxicity. In summary, motor symptoms of PDD can cause sleep disruption. Accurate assessment of these symptoms can be challenging in patients with cognitive impairment. Actigraphy offers an objective measure of motor symptoms that can be tracked over time and assessed in response to therapy. Long-acting dopaminergic preparations are helpful in alleviating motor symptoms causing sleep disruption.

6.2 Dopaminergic therapy

Proper timing and titration of dopaminergic therapy to address nocturnal motor symptoms specifically, as opposed to simply sleep disturbance in general, are critical. Bradykinesia, rigidity, and tremor can give way to dyskinesias in a hyperdopaminergic state. Dopamine also has direct wake-promoting properties and can cause insomnia. Most stimulant medications exert their wake-promoting effects through dopamine pathways. Rebound "sleep attacks" are also a well-known phenomenon, mostly related to dopamine agonists. While this may be less of a concern at night, it can be problematic for PDD patients who already exhibit fluctuations in attention and arousal. Dopamine-promoting medications have also been implicated in circadian rhythm disruption, causing increased melatonin production and an "uncoupling" of circadian phase and behavioral sleep onset (delayed relative to dim light melatonin onset [DLMO]) in PD patients on versus off therapy [16]. Lastly, PDD patients are also prone to complex visual hallucinations, which can be exacerbated by these drugs. In summary, while dopaminergic medications can treat motor symptoms causing sleep disruption, they can also disturb sleep through dyskinesias, insomnia, fluctuations in arousal, circadian uncoupling, and hallucinations. Caution is advised. Long-acting and levodopa-based medications are preferred. Short-acting dopamine agonists should be avoided.

6.3 Cognition

"Sundowning" or nocturnal delirium, hallucinations, and fluctuations in cognition, attention, and arousal can disturb sleep in patients with PDD. These symptoms can cause difficulty with sleep onset, long periods of wakefulness in the middle of the night, and disturb the homeostatic drive for sleep at night due to daytime somnolence (**Figure 4**).

Such symptoms can be seen across the spectrum of dementia. Nocturnal agitation can be one of the most disturbing and disabling symptoms for patients and their caregivers. This can lead to injury, particularly falls at night, in patients already prone to these issues. The mechanism for "sundowning" is unknown; however, it is felt to be multifactorial with circadian rhythm dysfunction and absence of environmental sensory cues hypothesized to play a driving role. Management can be challenging. Alternative causes should be excluded, such as toxic/metabolic encephalopathies, infection, and subdural hematoma. Nonpharmacologic interventions are considered first line despite the lack of randomized controlled trials in the PDD population due to their relative safety. Bright light therapy (on the order of 10,000 s of lux) in the morning for delayed sleep phase chronotype and in the evening for advanced sleep phase chronotype can be helpful. Daytime physical exercise can help entrain daytime wakefulness while consolidating sleep at night. It has also shown to improve multiple metrics in PD including: cognition [17], motor symptoms, and falls. Behavioral multicomponent interventions (cognitive behavioral therapy for insomnia) have shown to be effective in elderly adults with mixed results in patients with dementia. This can take the form of stimulus control, sleep restriction, relaxation exercises, paradoxical intention, psychotherapy, and

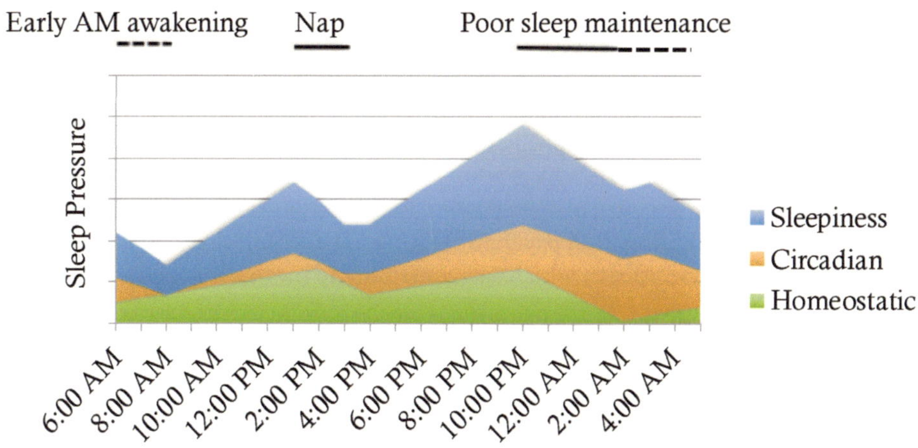

Figure 4.
Sleep–wake disturbance with circadian and homeostatic sleep drive dyssynchrony.

sleep hygiene. However, such interventions may be challenging in PDD patients due to the degree of understanding and participation required. This is most useful early in the disease course and with caregiver support. Melatonin has shown to be helpful with "sundowning" in patients with Alzheimer's dementia [18]. This agent has a dual benefit in PDD as melatonin is effective in suppressing the behavioral manifestations of RBD as well. In summary, nocturnal delirium, hallucinations, and fluctuations in arousal seen in PDD can cause sleep disturbance. Secondary causes should be considered. Nonpharmacologic strategies in the form of bright light and physical exercise are preferred as they carry little risk and show some benefit. Melatonin may help with delirium and improve RBD symptoms.

6.4 Medical management of behavioral symptoms

Pharmacological interventions in PDD are largely centered on improving cognitive symptoms and psychosis with improvements in sleep being of secondary benefit. Donepezil, rivastigmine, and memantine have been studied in PDD and DLB and have been shown to be effective in mitigating cognitive symptoms and hallucinations. Cognitive benefits seen in PDD and DLB may even exceed the benefits seen in AD [19] as patients with Lewy body disease have more relative cholinergic deficiency. However, similar to dopaminergic therapy, finding the minimum effective dose is important as acetylcholinesterase inhibitors (AChEIs) can cause nightmares due to their REM sleep-enhancing and consolidating effects. If hallucinations and delusions are distressing and dopaminergic therapy has been optimized, an atypical antipsychotic can be considered to facilitate sleep in psychotic patients. These typically have less D2 receptor blockade than typical antipsychotics to which PDD and DLB patients are particularly sensitive owing to the deficiency in striatal D2 receptors in these patients [20]. The lowest effective dose of quetiapine, clozapine, or aripiprazole dosed at night due to their sedating effects, is preferred. Pimavanserin, a selective serotonin 2A receptor inverse agonist, is a newer dopamine-sparing antipsychotic used in the treatment of PD psychosis. Its effects appear more robust in patients with greater cognitive impairment with concomitant AChEI use [21]. Of note, neuroleptic sensitivity and increased morbidity and mortality with antipsychotics are of concern in this particularly vulnerable population. Antipsychotics should be used sparingly for distressing hallucinations and delusions impacting the patient's quality of life. As previously mentioned, excessive daytime sleepiness, daytime napping, and fluctuations in arousal are common in PDD. If behavioral interventions are insufficient, stimulants can be considered. These largely exert their effects through dopaminergic and adrenergic mechanisms. Modafinil, armodafinil, methylphenidate-based derivatives, and amphetamine salts can all help to promote wakefulness. Monitoring of cardiovascular parameters and symptoms of sympathetic hyperactivation is required. In summary, AChEIs, NMDAR antagonists, atypical antipsychotics, and stimulants are effective in managing cognitive fluctuations and psychotic features disturbing sleep in PDD with monitoring for adverse effects, which can contribute to morbidity and mortality.

6.5 Mood disorders

Depression and anxiety are common comorbidities in PDD and DLB that can impact sleep and neurocognitive outcomes. Despite evidence showing higher rates of depression in patients with Lewy body disease (~20%) compared to AD (~9%) [22], guidelines regarding treatment in this patient population are lacking. Depression can cause a delay in sleep onset, earlier REM sleep onset, poorer sleep efficiency, earlier waking, and increased time in bed. Medications in the selective serotonin reuptake inhibitor (SSRI) and serotonin norepinephrine reuptake inhibitor (SNRI) classes seem to be similarly effective. Tricyclic antidepressants (TCAs) are generally avoided owing to their anticholinergic properties. At least in the general population, treatment of depression appears to improve sleep quality, regardless of whether the medication used is activating or sedating. In PDD, caution must be given to worsening of RBD and RLS/PLMD with antidepressant medication initiation as these are known sleep-related side effects of these medications. In such cases, a reduction in dose or retiming of the medication is effective. If not, bupropion can be used as an alternative agent as it is the only antidepressant that has not been associated with these conditions. In summary, mood disorders are common in PDD and can disturb sleep. SSRIs and SNRIs are recommended if depression/anxiety is present. These can potentially worsen RBD and RLS/PLMD. Bupropion is a viable alternative.

6.6 Nocturia

Nocturia, or the need to urinate at night, significantly disrupts sleep in patients with Lewy body disease. Urinary urgency and frequency are well-known nonmotor symptoms in patients with PD and DLB with the highest prevalence in DLB [23]. Lewy body disease causes disinhibition of the micturition reflex causing an overactive bladder [24]. Obstructive uropathy in men and pelvic insufficiency in women are often contributory. While frequent trips to the bathroom may be tolerated during the day, these trips cause sleep fragmentation and can be dangerous at night. The combination of akinesia, postural instability, dementia, and autonomic instability in PDD patients is a recipe for falls. Additionally, patients may restrict fluid intake to mitigate symptoms that can cause dehydration and exacerbate orthostatic hypotension. Historically, neurologists have been limited in their interventions with nonpharmacologic therapies being the mainstay. Scheduled toileting (before bed), pelvic floor exercises, and adaptive techniques (bedside commode) have been used. Medications have generally been avoided due to the anticholinergic mechanism action of these drugs, which can worsen confusion. Mirabegron, a beta 3-adrenoreceptor agonist, can be used in those seeking to avoid this medication class. If an anticholinergic medication is to be chosen, trospium and darifenacin have shown to have less blood–brain barrier penetrance. Botulinum toxin injection into the detrusor muscle and percutaneous stimulation of the tibial nerve (PTNS) represent third-line therapies, which have been found to be effective in small studies of PD patients. In summary, nocturia in PDD can cause sleep disruption and precipitate falls. Behavioral modification, beta-adrenoreceptor agonists, quaternary amine antispasmodics, botulinum toxin, and PTNS can help treat symptoms.

6.7 Insomnia

Insomnia is common in PDD as well as the general population, affecting up to 30% of the industrialized world. It also increases with age, cognitive impairment, and medical and psychiatric illness. Given its prevalence in the general population, it is not unsurprising that insomnia and daytime sleepiness do not appear to be biomarkers for the development of neurodegenerative disease in RBD patients [25]. The quandary in PDD lies in identifying the contributions of insomnia to sleep disruption from secondary causes and underlying neurodegeneration. Insomnia is conventionally a state of hyperarousal characterized by difficulty with sleep onset, maintenance, and early waking. Excessive daytime sleepiness and sleep maintenance out of proportion to sleep onset difficulties should alert the clinician to secondary causes for the patient's insomnia suggestive of sleep deprivation due to sleep fragmentation. However, in PDD, especially as the disease progresses, daytime hypersomnolence and disruption of sleep–wake architecture usually occur. Comorbid sleep disorders like OSA, RLS, RBD, and circadian rhythm disturbances are common. It is for these reasons that primary insomnia should be considered a diagnosis of exclusion in PDD patients with disturbed sleep. Behavioral measures (see recommendations for "sundowning" above), such as bright light, physical exercise, and cognitive behavioral therapy for insomnia are recommended. Patients with objectively shorter sleeping periods (<6 hours) may be less responsive to behavioral therapy [26]. Pharmacotherapy should be reserved for patients whose insomnia is refractory to these measures and cause distress and impairment in daytime functioning. PDD patients are particularly vulnerable to the side effects of sedative/hypnotic medications as these can cause morning after sedation, cognitive and motor slowing, amnesia, and parasomnias. Clinical practice guidelines for the pharmacologic treatment of chronic insomnia for elderly and cognitively impaired patients do not exist. Choice of therapy should take into account a number of factors: (1) type of problem (sleep onset, maintenance, or both), (2) duration of therapy, (3) adverse effects, (4) medical/psychiatric comorbidities, (5) medication interactions, (6) secondary indication, (7) patient preference, and (8) cost. For isolated sleep onset difficulties, dual orexin receptor antagonists (suvorexant and lemborexant), a melatonin agonist (ramelteon), and a short-acting benzodiazepine receptor agonist (zaleplon) could be considered. Suvorexant, lemborexant, and ramelteon have been studied in patients with dementia [27]. Benzodiazepines should generally be avoided due to their amnestic effects. Some nonbenzodiazepine receptor agonists (BzRAs) have been associated with an increase in parasomnias. For sleep onset and maintenance difficulties, a dual orexin receptor antagonist (DORA) is recommended. For patients with comorbid depression, low-dose trazodone or mirtazapine can be effective. TCAs are generally avoided due to their increased anticholinergic effects. For patients with comorbid RBD, high-dose melatonin or low-dose clonazepam (with caution and if RBD refractory to melatonin) is used. For patients with comorbid, disabling, and refractory psychosis, quetiapine can be considered. In summary, insomnia is common in PDD as well as the general population. Secondary causes for insomnia should be investigated. Behavioral interventions are first line in the treatment of insomnia in PDD. If refractory, there are a number of medication options available based on insomnia subtype and safety profile.

6.8 Obstructive sleep apnea

High rates of OSA have been observed in polysomnographic studies in patients with PD and DLB, affecting up to one-third of these patients [28]. Bulbar symptoms related to parkinsonism are presumed to contribute to airway collapse. This is partially offset by weight loss, often observed as the disease progresses. Patients with loud snoring, witnessed apneas, excessive daytime sleepiness, hypertension, obesity, large neck circumference, older age, and male gender are at increased risk for OSA. Sleep disruption and hypoxia from this condition contribute to neurocognitive decline, affecting attention, concentration, and mood. Additionally, OSA is associated with increased cerebrovascular disease, which can lead to vascular dementia. Motor outcomes in PD patients with OSA are also poorer compared to PD patients without OSA [29]. OSA can also be associated with REM sleep fragmentation with arousal-related motor manifestations out of REM sleep simulating RBD, or so-called pseudo-RBD. Due to REM atonia, the upper airway becomes more relaxed and accessory muscles of respiration become paralyzed, worsening OSA during this stage of sleep. Due to the effects OSA has on these aforementioned PDD-related symptoms, it is important to screen all patients for this condition. There are a number of OSA screening questionnaires that have been developed; however, it is important to note that these have not been validated in the PDD population. Polysomnography and increasingly, home-based sleep apnea testing, are used to diagnose this condition. In-lab testing is preferred in PDD patients as it is monitored by a sleep technologist who can assist with the setup and maintain the quality of the recording. Patients with PDD also often have other sleep disorders, such as RBD and PLMD, which home testing is usually not powered to detect. Continuous positive airway pressure (CPAP) remains the gold standard therapy for OSA. While studies have showed mixed results, CPAP appears to improve cognitive, motor, mood, and sleep quality outcomes in PD [30]. It also improves excessive daytime sleepiness. The cardiometabolic benefits of CPAP remain controversial. As with any behavioral therapy, but especially in PDD patients, adherence and tolerance to CPAP therapy are challenges. The cognitive impairment, trips to the restroom due to nocturia, dryness, and lack of dexterity to apply and adjust the mask are frequently reported issues. Patient education, frequent follow-up, and heated humidification have shown to improve compliance. In mild–moderate cases of OSA, a mandibular advancement device (MAD), a dental appliance that protrudes the jaw and increases the anterior to posterior upper airway diameter at the level of the tongue base, can be used as an alternative therapy. Upper airway surgery can be considered in patients with moderate–severe OSA in which CPAP is not tolerated; however, the risks of surgery and likely more prolonged postoperative course outweigh the benefits in the PDD population. Neuromodulation with a hypoglossal nerve stimulator (HGNS) that promotes tongue protrusion and airway patency represents an interesting less invasive option with minimal postoperative discomfort. Lifestyle measures including weight loss (if obese), positional therapy (side sleeping or head of bed elevation), and myofunctional therapy (mouth and throat exercises) are supplemental and recommend for all patients. It is worth noting that PDD patients spend more time in the supine sleeping position in which OSA is shown to be worse. In summary, OSA contributes to the symptomatology of PDD through different mechanisms. CPAP can improve the impact of OSA on these symptoms; however, adherence and tolerance are issues in this population. MAD, HGNS, and lifestyle measures are alternative and complementary options.

6.9 Restless legs syndrome/periodic limb movement disorder

RLS and PDD pathogenesis, clinical presentation, and therapy significantly overlap. In PD, there is a loss of dopaminergic neurons in the substantia nigra resulting in reduced striatal dopamine. In RLS, there is dopaminergic dysregulation and reduced iron in the basal ganglia with increased striatal dopamine, suggesting reduced sensitivity as opposed to deficiency. Interestingly, as opposed to RLS that shows reduced brain iron transport, PD patients show brain iron accumulation. It is unclear whether iron has a toxic effect in PD or whether this is a by-product of neurodegeneration. RLS is characterized by an urge to move the legs, sometimes associated with an unpleasant sensation, worse with rest, better with movement, and predominant in the evening. Akinesia, tremor, and dystonia may be misinterpreted as restless legs symptoms leading to overdiagnosis. It is important to make sure patients meet all clinical criteria before making the diagnosis of RLS. Periodic limb movements of sleep (PLMS) are common in RLS and PD, which may or may not be of clinical significance. PLMS must cause significant sleep fragmentation with resultant daytime symptoms to make a diagnosis of PLMD. This phenomenology can overlap with the nocturnal motor manifestations of PD and are often difficult to distinguish. Ultimately, RLS is a clinical diagnosis based on patient or caregiver history, which can be challenging in patients with dementia. The symptoms of RLS and motor manifestations of PD are treated similarly, making the diagnostic distinction between the two entities less critical. Oftentimes, PD patients are already on dopaminergic therapy, which can be adjusted to address evening and nighttime RLS symptoms. While generally not first line in RLS-only patients due to high rates of augmentation, levodopa is the preferred choice in PDD due to its dual benefit and lower rates of augmentation [31] in this population. This difference may best be explained by the dopamine deficiency seen in PD. Long-acting oral dopamine agonists and transdermal preparations can also be used. Alpha-2-delta ligand medications, such as gabapentin encarbil and pregabalin, are also considered first line in RLS. These can help with neuropathic pain and sleep induction but do not have activity on the motor manifestations of PD. Serum ferritin is checked systematically and iron supplemented if <50 ng/ml. A trial of oral iron supplementation is reasonable; however, due to constipation, which is already an issue in PD, an iron infusion may be required. Lifestyle measures include light exercise, stretching, avoidance of alcohol and sleep deprivation, and various forms of counter stimulation (vibrating pad, compression stockings, etc.). If medically refractory, a low-potency opioid could be considered with precautions. In summary, RLS and PDD both involve dysfunction in basal ganglia dopaminergic pathways, have overlapping symptoms that can make them difficult to distinguish, and benefit from dopaminergic therapy. Iron, alpha-2-delta ligand medications, behavioral interventions, and opioids are additionally used in RLS.

7. Conclusions

PDD is a clinical subtype on the spectrum of Lewy body disease. It is characterized by multidimensional and multifactorial sleep disturbances, which occur early and contribute significantly to the overall disease burden. Daytime sleepiness and disturbed sleep at night are merely symptomatic endpoints. Predictable brainstem, limbic, and subsequent neocortical spread of Lewy body pathology is responsible for early sleep disruption, followed by motor and then cognitive symptoms. This prodromal sleep disruption is hypothesized to perpetuate disease progression through a feed forward mechanism involving impaired glymphatic clearance. RBD is an example of sleep's role as a biomarker for the alpha-synucleinopathies. The convergence of PD and DLB symptoms in PDD causes further deterioration in sleep. Treatment of these symptoms is a double-edged sword. Medications can ameliorate but also exacerbate sleeping difficulties. Trial data on therapeutics in PDD are lacking with most recommendations being inferred from studies in PD and AD. Sleep disorders, such as circadian rhythm disturbances, insomnia, OSA, and RLS, are common. These often go unrecognized due to attribution to the underlying neurodegenerative process. Most of these conditions have established treatment protocols that can be adapted to the PDD population.

Acknowledgements

I would like to thank Drs. Lin Zhang and John Olichney for inviting me to be a part of this book. I would also like to thank the Department of Neurology at the University of California, Davis, for its support.

Conflict of interest

The authors declare no conflict of interest.

Thanks

I would also like to thank my family for their love and support.

Author details

Matthew Chow
University of California, Davis Medical Center, Sacramento, California, USA

*Address all correspondence to: mtchow@ucdavis.edu

References

[1] Monaca C, Duhamel A, Jacquesson JM, Ozsancak C, Destée A, Guieu JD, et al. Vigilance troubles in Parkinson's disease: A subjective and objective polysomnographic study. Sleep Medicine. 2006;**7**(5):448-453. DOI: 10.1016/j.sleep.2005.12.002

[2] Compta Y, Santamaria J, Ratti L, Tolosa E, Iranzo A, Muñoz E, et al. Cerebrospinal hypocretin, daytime sleepiness and sleep architecture in Parkinson's disease dementia. Brain. 2009;**132**(12):3308-3317. DOI: https://doi.org/10.1093/brain/awp263

[3] Bugalho P, Salavisa M, Marto JP, Borbinha C, Alves L. Polysomnographic data in dementia with Lewy bodies: Correlation with clinical symptoms and comparison with other α-synucleino pathies. Sleep Medicine. 2019;**55**:62-68. DOI: 10.1016/j.sleep.2018.12.006

[4] Latreille V, Carrier J, Gaudet-Fex B, Rodrigues-Brazète J, Panisset M, Chouinard S, et al. Electroencephalographic prodromal markers of dementia across conscious states in Parkinson's disease. Brain. 2016;**139**(Pt 4):1189-1199. DOI: 10.1093/brain/aww018

[5] Latreille V, Carrier J, Lafortune M, Postuma RB, Bertrand JA, Panisset M, et al. Sleep spindles in Parkinson's disease may predict the development of dementia. Neurobiology of Aging. 2015;**36**(2):1083-1090. DOI: 10.1016/j.neurobiolaging.2014.09.009

[6] Beach TG, Adler CH, Lue L, et al. Unified staging system for Lewy body disorders: Correlation with nigrostriatal degeneration, cognitive impairment and motor dysfunction. Acta Neuropathologica. 2009;**117**(6):613-634. DOI: 10.1007/s00401-009-0538-8

[7] Xie L, Kang H, Xu Q, et al. Sleep drives metabolite clearance from the adult brain. Science. 2013;**342**(6156):373-377. DOI: 10.1126/science.1241224

[8] Zou W, Pu T, Feng W, Lu M, Zheng Y, Du R, et al. Blocking meningeal lymphatic drainage aggravates Parkinson's disease-like pathology in mice overexpressing mutated α-synuclein. Translational Neurodegeneration. 2019;**8**(1):7. DOI: 10.1186/s40035-019-0147-y

[9] Kress BT, Iliff JJ, Xia M, et al. Impairment of paravascular clearance pathways in the aging brain. Annals of Neurology. 2014;**76**(6):845-861. DOI: 10.1002/ana.24271

[10] Vendette M, Gagnon JF, Décary A, Massicotte-Marquez J, Postuma RB, Doyon J, et al. REM sleep behavior disorder predicts cognitive impairment in Parkinson disease without dementia. Neurology. 2007;**69**(19):1843-1849. DOI: 10.1212/01.wnl.0000278114.14096.74

[11] Kim Y, Kim YE, Park EO, Shin CW, Kim HJ, Jeon B. REM sleep behavior disorder portends poor prognosis in Parkinson's disease: A systematic review. Journal of Clinical Neuroscience. 2018;**47**:6-13. DOI: 10.1016/j.jocn.2017.09.019

[12] Postuma RB, Lang AE, Gagnon JF, Pelletier A, Montplaisir JY. How does parkinsonism start? Prodromal parkinsonism motor changes in idiopathic REM sleep behaviour disorder. Brain. 2012;**135**(Pt 6):1860-1870. DOI: 10.1093/brain/aws093

[13] Chia R, Sabir MS, Bandres-Ciga S, et al. Genome sequencing analysis identifies new loci associated with Lewy body dementia and provides insights into its genetic architecture. Nature Genetics. 2021;**53**(3):294-303. DOI: 10.1038/s41588-021-00785-3

[14] Chaudhuri KR, Pal S, DiMarco A, et al. The Parkinson's disease sleep scale: A new instrument for assessing sleep and nocturnal disability in Parkinson's disease. Journal of Neurology, Neurosurgery, and Psychiatry. 2002;**73**(6):629-635. DOI: 10.1136/jnnp.73.6.629

[15] Mirelman A, Hillel I, Rochester L, Del Din S, Bloem BR, Avanzino L, et al. Tossing and turning in bed: Nocturnal movements in Parkinson's disease. Movement Disorders. 2020;**35**(6):959-968. DOI: 10.1002/mds.28006.

[16] Bolitho SJ, Naismith SL, Rajaratnam SM, Grunstein RR, Hodges JR, Terpening Z, et al. Disturbances in melatonin secretion and circadian sleep-wake regulation in Parkinson disease. Sleep Medicine. 2014;**15**(3):342-347. DOI: 10.1016/j.sleep.2013.10.016

[17] da Silva FC, Iop RDR, de Oliveira LC, et al. Effects of physical exercise programs on cognitive function in Parkinson's disease patients: A systematic review of randomized controlled trials of the last 10 years. PLoS One. 2018;**13**(2):e0193113. DOI: 10.1371/journal.pone.0193113

[18] Cardinali DP, Brusco LI, Liberczuk C, Furio AM. The use of melatonin in Alzheimer's disease. Neuro Endocrinology Letters. 2002;**23** (Suppl 1):20-23

[19] Samuel W, Caligiuri M, Galasko D, Lacro J, Marini M, McClure FS, et al. Better cognitive and psychopathologic response to donepezil in patients prospectively diagnosed as dementia with Lewy bodies: A preliminary study. International Journal of Geriatric Psychiatry. 2000;**15**:794-802. DOI: https://doi.org/10.1002/1099-1166(200009)15:9<794::AID-GPS178>3.0.CO;2-1

[20] Piggott MA, Marshall EF, Thomas N, Lloyd S, Court JA, Jaros E, et al. Striatal dopaminergic markers in dementia with Lewy bodies, Alzheimer's and Parkinson's diseases: Rostrocaudal distribution. Brain. 1999;**122**(8):1449-1468. DOI: https://doi.org/10.1093/brain/122.8.1449

[21] Espay AJ, Guskey MT, Norton JC, Coate B, Vizcarra JA, Ballard C, et al. Pimavanserin for Parkinson's disease psychosis: Effects stratified by baseline cognition and use of cognitive-enhancing medications. Movement Disorders. 2018;**33**(11):1769-1776. DOI: 10.1002/mds.27488

[22] Chiu PY, Wang CW, Tsai CT, Li SH, Lin CL, Lai TJ. Depression in dementia with Lewy bodies: A comparison with Alzheimer's disease. PLoS One. 2017;**12**(6):e0179399. DOI: 10.1371/journal.pone.0179399

[23] Ransmayr GN, Holliger S, Schletterer K, et al. Lower urinary tract symptoms in dementia with Lewy bodies, Parkinson disease, and Alzheimer disease. Neurology. 2008;**70**(4):299-303. DOI: 10.1212/01.wnl.0000296826.61499.26

[24] Sakakibara R, Tateno F, Kishi M, Tsuyuzaki Y, Uchiyama T, Yamamoto T. Pathophysiology of bladder dysfunction in Parkinson's disease. Neurobiology of Disease. 2012;**46**(3):565-571. DOI: 10.1016/j.nbd.2011.10.002

[25] Postuma RB, Gagnon JF, Pelletier A, Montplaisir JY. Insomnia and somnolence in idiopathic RBD: A prospective cohort study. npj Parkinson's Disease. 2017;**3**:9. DOI: 10.1038/s41531-017-0011-7

[26] Bathgate CJ, Edinger JD, Krystal AD. Insomnia patients with objective short sleep duration have a blunted response to cognitive behavioral therapy for insomnia. Sleep. 2017;**40**(1):zsw012. DOI: 10.1093/sleep/zsw012

[27] McCleery J, Sharpley AL. harmacotherapies for sleep disturbances

in dementia. Cochrane Database of Systematic Reviews. 2020;**11**:CD009178. DOI: 10.1002/14651858.CD009178.pub4

[28] Terzaghi M, Arnaldi D, Rizzetti MC, et al. Analysis of video-polysomnographic sleep findings in dementia with Lewy bodies. Movement Disorders. 2013;**28**(10):1416-1423. DOI: 10.1002/mds.25523

[29] Elfil M, Bahbah EI, Attia MM, Eldokmak M, Koo BB. Impact of obstructive sleep apnea on cognitive and motor functions in Parkinson's disease. Movement Disorders. 2021;**36**(3):570-580. DOI: 10.1002/mds.28412

[30] Kaminska M, Mery VP, Lafontaine AL, et al. Change in cognition and other non-motor symptoms with obstructive sleep apnea treatment in Parkinson disease. Journal of Clinical Sleep Medicine. 2018;**14**(5):819-828. DOI: 10.5664/jcsm.7114

[31] Stefani A, Högl B. Sleep in Parkinson's disease. Neuro psychopharmacology. 2020;**45**(1):121-128. DOI: 10.1038/s41386-019-0448-y

Chapter 10

Current Research on Deep Brain Stimulation and Cognitive Impairment in Parkinson's Disease

Kiarash Shahlaie, Laura Sperry, Luhua Wei and Lin Zhang

Abstract

Cognitive impairment is one of the common non-motor complications in Parkinson's disease. The underlying mechanism remains elusive due to multiple reasons. As a result, treatment options for cognitive decline in Parkinson's disease are limited and not as effective as those for motor symptoms. Recent advances in neuroscience have developed new models for the pathophysiology of Parkinson's disease dementia, based on which clinical research have showed promising results. The role of multiple neurotransmitter systems in cognitive impairment have been emphasized. The change in different functional neural networks (including microscale, mesoscale, and macroscale) resulting from abnormal neurobiochemical environment partly explains the clinical picture. Accordingly, neuromodulation methods can be good candidates for symptomatic management. Several preliminary studies on deep brain stimulation have demonstrated positive results. The nucleus basalis of Meynert, a hub in the cognitive network, is chosen by most studies as the stimulation target. Deep brain stimulation for motor symptoms, on the other hand, may also cause or aggravate patients' cognitive dysfunction. Their influence on cognition is multifaceted and should be taken into account during patient selection, target design, and programming.

Keywords: parkinson's disease, cognitive impairment, dementia, deep brain stimulation

1. Introduction

Cognitive impairment in Parkinson's disease (PD) is a common non-motor symptom (NMS) frequently encountered by patients and practitioners. The cumulative prevalence of PD dementia (PDD) is about 75–90% in patients with a disease course of more than 10 years [1, 2]. It increases the mortality rate and severely impacts the quality of life in patients with PD. With the development of effective pharmacologic and non-pharmacologic interventions, motor symptoms are being better controlled than before, leaving NMSs more frustrating due to a lack of effective treatment. There are several possible reasons. First, it was not until recent years that researchers started to focus on the NMSs of PD. Although cognitive decline in PD is common, our understanding in PD with mild cognitive impairment and PDD is far from adequate. Second, compared with motor symptoms, the underlying mechanism in cognitive impairment seems to be more complicated and involves multiple neurotransmitters and neural circuits. It is not easy to define a single biochemical system or functional hub as a treatment target from the perspective of neural network. Despite the slow progress in the development of treatment for cognitive decline, efforts have been made in this trending field.

Deep brain stimulation (DBS), a well-established treatment for PD as well as other neurological disorders, has been tested in patients with cognitive impairment. New targets such as the nucleus basalis of Meynert (NBM) were chosen based on the underlying pathophysiology of cognitive impairment in PD [3]. Recent advances in DBS have shown some promising results and will enlighten future development of more robust treatment strategies. On the other hand, traditional DBS targets and programming schemes for PD per se may cause cognitive impairment in the long run [4]. Evidence on this topic has been updated and new strategies have been proposed in target selection and programming in patients with signs of cognitive dysfunction. Here, we review the current research on DBS and the cognitive impairment in PD.

2. Mechanisms underlying the use of DBS in patients with cognitive impairment

The mechanism of PDD is multifaceted. Proposed mechanisms that contribute to cognitive decline include protein misfolding, neurotransmitter activities, synaptic dynamics, neuroinflammation, mitochondrial dysfunction, change in glial cells, genetics, epigenetics, adenosine receptor activation, and abnormal brain connectivity [5]. From the neurotransmitter point of view, evidence has shown that not only the dopaminergic system, but also non-dopaminergic activity is associated with cognitive functioning [6]. Cholinergic system is one of the most important transmitter systems involved in cognitive dysfunction in PD. Cholinesterase inhibitors are supported by robust evidence to treat PDD [7, 8]. The effectiveness of cholinesterase inhibitors further proves the essential role of cholinergic system in PDD.

The NBM is a structure of gray matter located in the substantia innominate of the basal forebrain. It harbors 90% of the cholinergic neurons and is considered as a hub in the cholinergic network [9]. The NBM has an important role in cognition including attention, arousal/sleep cycles, memory, praxis, perception, drive and spontaneity. This vast complicated array of connections results in variability in its effect from stimulation [10]. For stimulation of the NMB to be effective, identifying the appropriate targeting to activate a specific network will be essential [10]. The significance of NBM has been proposed in dementia of various etiologies, including PD (**Figure 1**).

Increasing evidence has shown that both the structural and functional networks related to NBM are compromised in PD patients with cognitive impairment. Smaller volumes in the region of NBM are associated with greater change in global cognitive functioning, higher risk of mild cognitive impairment, and more severe and rapid decline in some certain cognitive domains [11]. Increased mean diffusivity in the NBM is also predictive for the development of cognitive dysfunction [12]. Reduced density of the gray matter in the cholinergic basal forebrain correlates with impaired global cognition, attention, and visuospatial function [13]. A recent longitudinal study reported more severe cognitive impairment and significant decline in parietal and occipital metabolism in patients with NBM atrophy, further supporting that structural change in the NBM is associated with cognitive dysfunction in PD [14].

In addition to structural abnormalities, the functional network involved in the development of cognitive impairment is also remarkably disrupted. An EEG-based study showed a significantly greater reduction in alpha reactivity in Lewy body dementia than Alzheimer's disease and healthy controls. This impairment of alpha reactivity might be associated with volume loss of the NBM [15]. One study

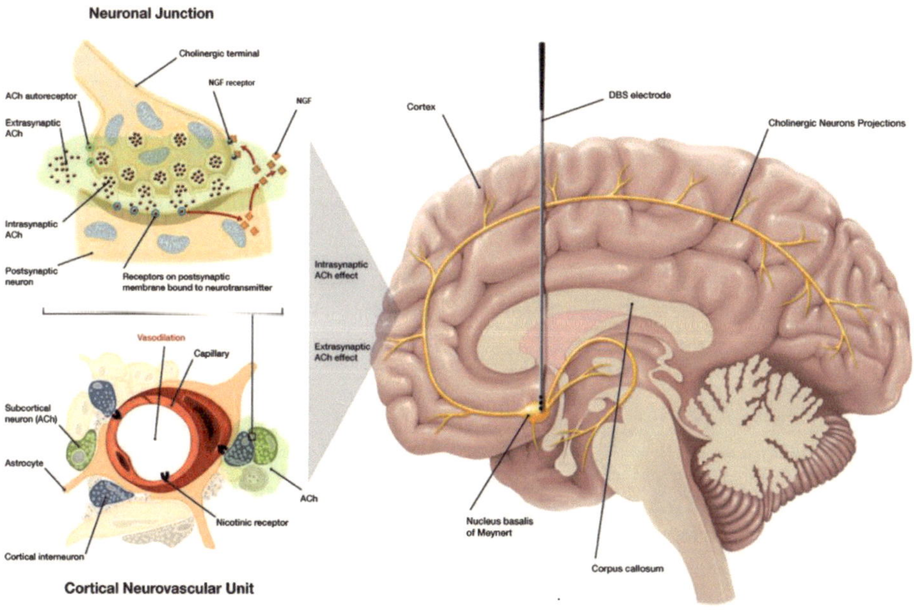

Figure 1.
"Schematic representation of the putative effect of deep brain stimulation (DBS) of the nucleus basalis of Meynert. Intra- and extra-synaptic effects of acetylcholine (ACh) are shown. Top left shows potential effect of DBS by altering cholinergic neurotransmission. Bottom left shows vasodilative effects of DBS via cholinergic activation. Right side shows NBM projection sites after DBS. NGF, nerve growth factor." ["Reprinted from the Journal of Alzheimer's Disease, volume 69 (4), Koulousakis, P, Andrade, P, Visser-Vandewalle, V, Sesia, T, The Nucleus Basalis of Meynert and Its Role in Deep Brain Stimulation for Cognitive Disorders: A Historical Perspective, Pages 905–919, 2019 with permission from IOS Press. The publication is available at IOS Press through http://dx.doi.org/10.3233/JAD-180133"].

calculated the functional connectivity via resting state functional magnetic resonance imaging (fMRI). Compared with PD without cognitive impairment, PD with mild cognitive impairment showed alterations in dynamic functional connectivity in multiple brain networks [16]. This is supported by another study with fMRI which found that the resting state functional connectivity of NBM is reduced in the right superior parietal lobe and the right postcentral gyrus in PD-MCI [17].

Abnormalities in brain networks other than those related to NBM have also been demonstrated. The cerebellar vermis consists of a rich population of cholinergic neurons and is involved in cognitive function. Compared with PD patients with normal cognitive function, those with cognitive impairment show a reduction in the functional connectivity between the vermis and dorsolateral prefrontal cortex, which is associated with deficits in attention, executive functioning, and global cognition [18].

The use of DBS to cause a functional blockade at specific target sites, replacing abnormal neural activity with a more tolerable pattern of activity, is considered standard therapy for several disease processes. It is currently hypothesized that the chronic high frequency electrical stimulation of the target nucleus acts as a brain pacemaker, entraining irregular neuronal firing patterns and desynchronizing pathological hypersynchronization within sensorimotor circuits. DBS is "local" therapy and affects only local circuits and brain regions within the target region [19, 20].

3. Deep brain stimulation surgery

DBS currently has FDA approval to be used in the treatment of motor symptoms for PD, essential tremor and epilepsy and FDA approval under a Humanitarian

Indications	Target
FDA-approved targets	
Parkinson's disease	Subthalamic nucleus (STN), Globus pallidus internis (GPi) Ventral intermedius nucleus (VIM) (tremor)
Essential tremor	Ventral intermedius nucleus (VIM)
Dystonia (HDE approval)	GPi
Medically resistant obsessive-compulsive disorder (OCD) (HDE approval)	Anterior limb of the internal capsule
Epilepsy	Anterior nucleus of the thalamus
Emerging/investigational targets	
Epilepsy (alternative target)	Hippocampus
Medically resistant OCD	Medial thalamus
Medically resistant depression	Nucleus accumbens
Obesity	Nucleus accumbens, Ventromedial nucleus of the hypothalamus
Anorexia nervosa	Nucleus accumbens, Ventromedial nucleus of the hypothalamus
Posture/gait in movement disorders	Pedunculopontine nucleus (PPN)
Medically refractory cluster headache	Posterior hypothalamus (PHypTh)
Medically refractory depression	Subgenual cortex (Brodmann area 25)
Dementia	Nucleus basalis of Meynert (NBM)

Table 1.
Current and emerging deep brain stimulation targets [25].

Device Exemption (HDE) application for dystonia and obsessive-compulsive disorder [21]. DBS of the subthalamic nucleus (STN) or of the internal segment of globus pallidus (GPi) has been shown to significantly improve motor symptoms in PD (such as rigidity, tremor, bradykinesia and, occasionally, disturbances of gait) [22, 23], while DBS of the ventral intermediate thalamic nucleus (Vim) has been shown to reduce tremors in PD and ET [24] (**Table 1**).

Potential candidates are those whose symptoms are refractory to standard medical interventions. As a part of this extensive workup for movement disorder indications, the neurological examination is often videotaped on and off medications to help assess potential treatment response post-surgery and to get a clear understanding of a patient's underlying symptoms. For patients with PD, a 30% improvement on the Unified Parkinson Disease Rating Scale (UPDRS) on and off medications is recommended [26]. In addition, patients will undergo an extensive neuropsychological evaluation to rule out untreated mood disorders and to get a baseline for cognitive status. Patients will complete a screening MRI of the brain to evaluate for atrophy and any structural issues that may complicate implantation of brain leads.

Once the evaluation is completed, a multidisciplinary case conference is held to review the patient's medical history, motor testing scores, neurocognitive and psychiatric data, neuroimaging results and clinical assessment. This process provides a thorough determination of patient eligibility prior to scheduling DBS surgery.

During this meeting, the team will determine the appropriate target nucleus as well as which DBS system will be implanted. These decisions vary depending upon the therapeutic goals, patient symptoms, cognitive and behavioral issues, and surgeon's expertise [27].

To accurately implant a DBS lead into a deep brain structure, an operative plan is developed using a special high-resolution MRI scan. Targets are first identified using a 3-dimensional coordinate system, and further refined for each patient's specific neuroanatomical characteristics. A safe entry point and trajectory are determined, and the surgical plan is stored in a neuronavigation station (**Figure 2A**). Under local anesthesia, a ring is secured to the patient's skull and an additional study is obtained using a localizer box that allows the software program to guide the surgeon along the previously developed plan (**Figure 2B**).

This procedure can be done with the patient asleep or awake during the placement of the electrode(s). Traditionally, the patient is awake during microelectrode recording above and below the surgical target, which results in a physiological map that determines if the intended surgical target represents the dysfunctional area of the brain that is involved in movement (**Figure 2C** and **D**). Once the final DBS electrode is implanted, test stimulation is performed to confirm that the patient experiences therapeutic benefit without significant clinical side effects (**Figure 2E**). A final head CT is obtained to confirm that the actual lead placement is consistent with the clinical evaluation. If needed, adjustments to lead placement can be made at that time. Patients are typically discharged from the hospital 1 day after surgery.

Many patients may experience a temporary microlesion effect following surgery where their PD symptoms briefly improve. To allow sufficient time for this brief effect to subside, providers often wait approximately four weeks following lead implantation before the patient returns to the clinic to have the stimulator turned on and programmed. With lead placements targeting motor symptoms, tremor and rigidity are typically the primary focus although motor speed and gait are also

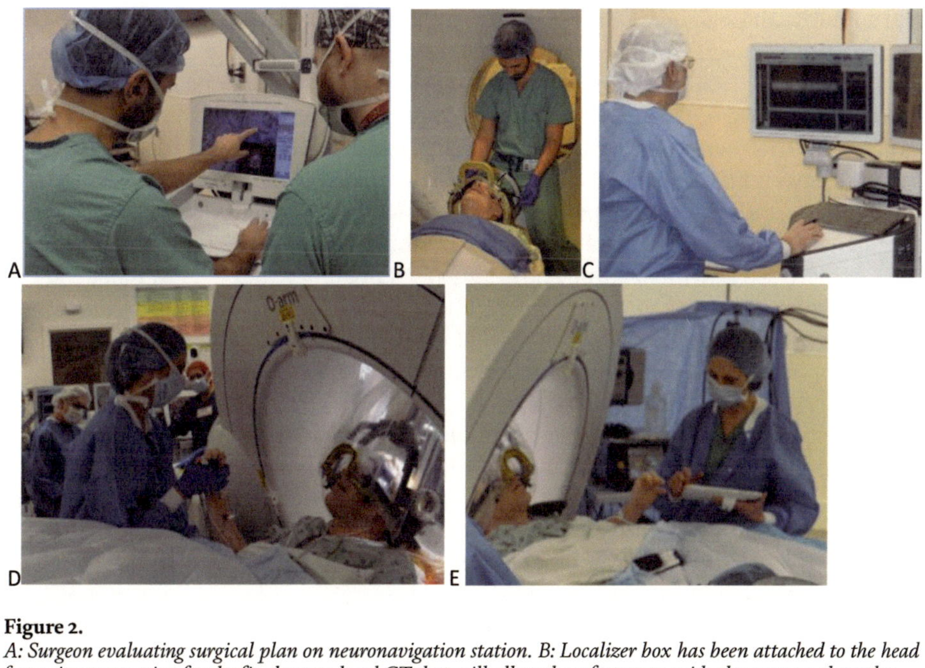

Figure 2.
A: Surgeon evaluating surgical plan on neuronavigation station. B: Localizer box has been attached to the head frame in preparation for the final preop head CT that will allow the software to guide the surgeon along the previously developed plan. C: Microelectrode recording during electrode placement. D: Motor testing during microelectrode testing. E: Intraop test stimulation after electrode placement.

assessed [28]. Adjustments in the stimulation field, amplitude, frequency, and pulse-width control the stimulation response [29]. DBS suppresses symptoms; it does not alter disease progression [20].

The patient will then return for subsequent visits to adjust the stimulator and medications, as needed. Once therapy is optimized, often within 3–6 months, patients will return to their neurologist for ongoing management [28]. It is common to conduct a 6–12-month postoperative neuropsychological evaluation to evaluate the impact of DBS surgery on cognition, psychological, emotional, and behavioral symptoms [27]. The implanted pulse generator (IPG) typically requires surgical replacement every 3–5 years, which is done on an outpatient basis under general or local anesthesia. Current rechargeable IPGs are approved for 15 years. DBS requires life-long monitoring and follow-up [30].

4. Patient selection

Proper patient selection is critical in order to maximize the post-operative benefits and minimize the surgical risks for the patient, especially for those with cognitive dysfunction. Over 30% of DBS surgical failures are attributed to inappropriate patient selection [28]. In order to justify the potential surgical risks of DBS, patients must be experiencing significant disability from their disorder, although what defines "significant disability" is subjective and needs to be individualized to each patient [20]. The current goal of DBS in PD is to intervene to maintain motor function and quality of life before disability becomes debilitating [20].

DBS for PD motor symptoms is recommended when pharmacotherapy stops providing adequate symptom relief. In patients with PD, a patient's responsiveness to dopaminergic medication (i.e., levodopa) often is predictive of a patient's motor response to DBS. Signs and symptoms resistant to levodopa are often resistant to DBS [20, 28]. Ideal candidates for DBS targeting motor symptoms have dopa-responsive motor symptoms, few comorbidities, fluctuating motor symptoms and no or minimal cognitive or behavioral disorders. PD symptoms such as dysarthria, dysphagia, micrographia, severe postural instability, freezing of gait, cognitive dysfunction and dysautonomia are less responsive to DBS targeting the STN, GPi, or Vim [20, 31].

A detailed understanding of a patient's cognitive status is essential. Typically, patients with dementia or significant cognitive impairment are excluded from surgery. Patients with diminished cognitive abilities may have the following challenges: a diminished motor response post-surgery; difficulty cooperating with the awake surgical procedure; difficulty accurately describing symptoms, making adjusting the DBS settings and medications post-surgery more challenging; and, most concerning, a worsening of their cognitive status post-surgery [27, 30]. Unfortunately, there is minimal consensus regarding what level of cognitive impairment should exclude patients from this therapy, so the ultimate decision is left to the clinical judgment of the multidisciplinary team [27].

There is concern that mood disorders (depression and anxiety) can worsen following surgery. In addition, untreated mental health conditions may result in poor compliance following surgery [27]. Patients with severe, unresolved psychotic symptoms should be excluded from consideration for this procedure, at least until the psychotic episode resolves [20, 28]. Patients are often awake during the electrode lead placement, which can be quite stressful. Any neurologically compromised patient may show exacerbation of symptoms under stress. For those with cognitive deficits, severe autonomic dysfunction or severe ataxia, DBS surgery may provide an unacceptable risk of significant complications. This appears to be more concerning in patients undergoing bilateral STN DBS than GPi DBS [30, 32].

5. Surgical outcomes

In one of the most comprehensive randomized, controlled trials comparing DBS to best medical therapy, DBS was found to be more effective than best medical therapy in improving motor function and quality of life. Weaver et al. [31] found that DBS patients gained an average of 4.6 h of "on" time per day (the amount of time when patients experience relief from Parkinson's symptoms) with reductions in the amount of "on" time with dyskinesia and "off" time (the time when PD patients are not experiencing relief from their symptoms). Self-reported improvements in motor functioning showed a 29% gain. On the contrary, most patients undergoing best medical therapy did not show any improvement in motor functioning after 6 months of treatment. Understandably, these improved motor functioning scores were associated with a significant improvement in quality-of-life measurements.

Those motor and non-motor symptoms which show a strong dopaminergic response typically respond the best to DBS therapy [33]. Outcomes often depend on a variety of factors including target selection, programming settings, electrode placement, medical management and patient expectations [33]. More severe apathy, depression and axial symptoms prior to DBS surgery are predictors of negative subjective perception of outcome following surgery [33]. While desires for improvements in gait, non-motor symptoms, interpersonal relationships, and professional life often influence a patient's decision to pursue DBS surgery, these expectations are not often met post-surgically [33]. Patients may struggle with a new body image and changes in their relationships with others due to changes in caregiving needs [27]. In addition, while DBS has been shown to positively impact a patient's quality of life, several studies have shown no improvement in caregiver burden following surgery [33]. Where DBS does result in less caregiving needs, spouse caregivers may find themselves struggling to redefine their role in their relationship now that they are no longer needed in the same capacity [27].

Several studies have found slight reductions in cognitive function test results in patients who underwent DBS therapy, compared to the best medical therapy group, relating to reductions in executive functioning, verbal associative fluency, working memory and visuomotor speed [27, 31, 34]. Studies show varied results but there is suggestion that STN-DBS, more than the GPi-DBS, may result in slightly higher risk of cognitive decline after surgery [34, 35]. A meta-analysis of 41 studies looking at the effect of DBS in PD on cognition, found STN DBS correlating with slight declines in psychomotor speed, memory, attention, executive functioning and moderate declines in phonemic and semantic fluency [36]. Higher DBS pulse widths have been associated with declines in cognitive functioning in patients with ET [27]. This cognitive impact seems unresponsive to changes in DBS settings or on/off motor states suggesting it is related to lead position [33]. A variety of reasons for this response have been considered including: cortical or subcortical microtrauma following implantation of the electrode, changes in frontostriatal neuronal activation secondary to DBS, changes in neuronal activation secondary to reduced dopaminergic therapy following surgery, advancing age and lower cognitive reserve [35].

While GPi STN is thought to result in less worsening of impulse control disorders and psychiatric conditions, studies suggest that STN DBS may result in greater reduction in medication when targeting PD motor symptoms [27]. Caution should be taken with too rapid reduction in dopaminergic therapy as this could worsen apathy [33]. While there is evidence that candidates for DBS surgery have a higher-than-expected suicide rate after STN-DBS, correlating with an increase in post-operative depression and impulse control disorders [33], a systematic review by the Congress of Neurological Surgeons did not find an increased association with suicidal behaviors with STN v GPi targets [4]. Further supporting STN DBS for medication reduction, a retrospective study found reduced risk of psychosis in patients with DBS for at least 8 years compared with medically managed patients with no significant risk differences with respect to dementia, institutionalization or death [37]. This study found that the rate of persistent psychosis reduced 74% in DBS treated patients compared with medically managed patients, presumably related to the reduction in dopaminergic therapy following STN-DBS.

6. Neuromodulation as a treatment for cognitive impairment in PD

As has been discussed above, abnormalities of various functional networks underlie the cognitive impairment of PD patients. Accordingly, approaches that modulate these abnormal networks could be potential treatment options. Efforts have been made exploring the safety and efficacy of neuromodulation in patients with cognitive problems in the past decade. However, robust evidence is lacking.

In 2009, a case report described an individual with Parkinson-dementia syndrome who was implanted with two electrodes in the STN and two in the NBM [38]. Stimulation of the bilateral STNs alleviated motor symptoms and stimulation of the bilateral NBMs resulted in better cognitive function. At a later report, the authors noted that the improvement in ADLs and activities of interest was due to improvement in apraxia, which only occurred with the activation of the NBM leads, not the STN leads [10].

Gratwicke et al. [3] conducted a randomized, double-blind, crossover study of 6 patients with PDD who were treated with NBM-DBS. They were appropriate DBS surgical candidates except for their diagnosis of PDD. They were still cognitively well enough to provide informed consent and meet pre-set criteria on the Mini-Mental State Examination as well as having minimal atrophy on brain MRI. All patients safely tolerated DBS surgery and low-frequency stimulation but did not show any improvement in their cognitive outcomes; yet there was an improvement noted in their neuropsychiatric scores (in particular, visual hallucinations, a parietal lobe function) on NBM-DBS. This team conducted a similar study on 6 patients with dementia with Lewy bodies (DLB) [39]. These results, combined with their previous study on PDD, showed no significant improvement in cognitive outcomes but did note possible improvement in neuropsychiatric symptoms. These studies offer further suggestions that NBM stimulation may modulate cholinergic transmission.

The DEMPARK-DBS study [40] is embarking on a sham-controlled trial of combined STN and NMB DBS for PD with dementia to evaluate the safety of bilateral STN-DBS in PDD patients and to study if NBM-DBS impacts cognitive decline. Patients with dementia are typically excluded from DBS therapy due to concerns about potential further deterioration of their cognitive status; however, many could benefit from the reduction in dopaminergic therapy that often occurs following STN-DBS implantation as this can reduce the risk of delirium or hyperdopaminergic behaviors which can exacerbate PDD symptoms. Implantation into the NBM target alone would not address motor or non-motor symptoms associated with advanced PD. This will be the first controlled study to compare STN-NBM-DBS in patients with PDD as well as to evaluate the safety of STN-DBS in patients with PDD.

Typically, frequencies in the high gamma range (100–180 Hz) are used to target motor symptoms; however, theta stimulation (which the authors define as 5–12 Hz) has been associated with various cognitive functions [35, 41]. Hippocampal theta oscillations are involved with episodic and spatial memory encoding and retrieval [41]. STN theta oscillations have been found to be involved with executive functions such as verbal fluency, working memory, sensorimotor conflict and response inhibition [35]. In 2018, a pilot study looked at the effect of theta and gamma stimulation on cognitive function [35]. Theta frequency stimulation was found to improve cognitive performance whereas gamma frequency stimulation worsened cognitive performance. In 2020, another study further investigated the effect of theta versus gamma frequencies on verbal fluency and executive function in PD patients [41]. Results found improvements in episodic category verbal fluency during theta versus gamma frequency STN stimulation, confirming the role of theta oscillations in hippocampal-dependent memory processes [41]. Since theta frequencies do not improve motor functions, the authors propose further investigation into the possibility of interleaving theta and gamma stimulation to address both the motor and cognitive symptoms of PD.

7. The future of DBS technology

As we have discussed, the benefits of DBS are often limited by side effects and rapid battery drain. Recent and future DBS technologies are focusing on reducing side effects, maximizing benefit, and prolonging battery life. The presence of multiple DBS manufacturers has resulted in a rapid advancement in this technology due to global competition. Newer technologies include segmented leads, directional stimulation, increased battery longevity, increased programming flexibility, remote programming, expanded MRi compatibility and neural recording capabilities [42].

Previously, the FDA approved implanted leads were omnidirectional, putting stimulation out in all directions, in a sphere-like shape. The challenge with these omnidirectional leads is that in creating a stimulation field strong enough to address the symptoms of concern, non-desired side effects often occurred as a result of stimulating adjacent structures. "Field shaping," where programmers can focus the stimulation on desired targets and move away from targets of concern has been a recent focus. Recently, several "directional" leads have received FDA approval. These directional leads allow the programmers to steer the stimulation away from structures that may be contributing to side effects and towards structures of clinical interest. DBS systems that offer multiple independent current control, where each individual lead contact has its own current source, provide additional precision in programming, compared with single-source current source systems, where all electrodes share a single current source [42, 43].

Conventional DBS (cDBS) technology uses an open-loop platform that, oftentimes, makes balancing stimulation to maximize benefits but minimize side effects challenging. In addition, limited battery capacity makes cDBS cumbersome due to the need for numerous battery replacement surgeries over an individual's lifespan. As noted earlier, cDBS settings result in a in a continuous stimulation field. These settings are created by the clinician and adjustments are made as needed based on a patient's response at a future clinical visit. This continuous stimulation does not match the fluctuating clinical state of the patient, often making patients more prone to side effects and using more energy than may be required [43].

Newer technologies are exploring a closed-loop or adaptive DBS (aDBS) system that can make real-time adjustments in stimulation based on continuous feedback. The ability to adjust stimulation parameters to better match the fluctuating state of the patient may result in fewer side effects and less energy drain on the implanted battery. By recording local field potentials (LFPs), new DBS IPGs provide an opportunity to correlate clinical symptoms with this input signal. Studies are underway to help standardize interpretation of these signals. The ultimate goal is to create a standardized interpretation of these signals and to optimize artificial intelligence-based programming, reducing the time burden on clinicians fr0m the current "trial and error" approach and improving differentiation of stimulation needs for various PD phenotypes [42, 43].

8. Conclusion

While there is growing evidence that neuromodulation of the cholinergic network may have a role in addressing neuropsychiatric symptoms in patients with PD, exacerbation of cognitive impairment, in particular a reduction in verbal fluency, following DBS is a concern. Lower pulse widths and the use of theta frequency stimulation appear to dampen the impact of DBS on cognitive performance. Newer and emerging technologies including closed-loop adaptive DBS, multiple-source stimulation, and directional current steering may help reduce negative outcomes and improve DBS efficacy although there is still limited data on the impacts of these on cognition [33].

Conflict of interest

Kia Shahlaie – Consultant for Abbott.
Laura Sperry – Consultant for Abbott, DBS Advisory Panel for Medtronic.

Author details

Kiarash Shahlaie[1], Laura Sperry[1], Luhua Wei[2] and Lin Zhang[1*]

1 University of California, Davis Health, Sacramento, CA, USA

2 Peking University First Hospital, Beijing, China

*Address all correspondence to: mdzhang@ucdavis.edu

References

[1] Buter TC, van den Hout A, Matthews FE, Larsen JP, Brayne C, Aarsland D. Dementia and survival in Parkinson disease: A 12-year population study. Neurology. 2008;**70**(13):1017-1022

[2] Aarsland D, Kurz MW. The epidemiology of dementia associated with Parkinson disease. Journal of the Neurological Sciences. 2010;**289**(1-2):18-22

[3] Gratwicke J, Zrinzo L, Kahan J, Peters A, Beigi M, Akram H, et al. Bilateral deep brain stimulation of the nucleus basalis of meynert for parkinson disease dementia: A randomized clinical trial. JAMA Neurology. 2018;**75**(2):169-178

[4] Rughani A, Schwalb JM, Sidiropoulos C, Pilitsis J, Ramirez-Zamora A, Sweet JA, et al. Congress of neurological surgeons systematic review and evidence-based guideline on subthalamic nucleus and globus pallidus internus deep brain stimulation for the treatment of patients with Parkinson's disease: Executive summary. Neurosurgery. 2018;**82**(6):753-756

[5] Aarsland D, Creese B, Politis M, Chaudhuri KR, Ffytche DH, Weintraub D, et al. Cognitive decline in Parkinson disease. Nature Reviews Neurology. 2017;**13**(4):217-231

[6] Halliday GM, Leverenz JB, Schneider JS, Adler CH. The neurobiological basis of cognitive impairment in Parkinson's disease. Movement Disorders. 2014;**29**(5):634-650

[7] Dubois B, Tolosa E, Katzenschlager R, Emre M, Lees AJ, Schumann G, et al. Donepezil in Parkinson's disease dementia: A randomized, double-blind efficacy and safety study. Movement Disorders. 2012;**27**(10):1230-1238

[8] Emre M, Aarsland D, Albanese A, Byrne EJ, Deuschl G, Deyn PP d, et al. Rivastigmine for dementia associated with Parkinson's disease. The New England Journal of Medicine. 2004;**351**(24):2509-2518

[9] Gratwicke J, Kahan J, Zrinzo L, Hariz M, Limousin P, Foltynie T, et al. The nucleus basalis of Meynert: A new target for deep brain stimulation in dementia? Neuroscience and Biobehavioral Reviews. 2013;**37**:2676-2688

[10] Kumbhare D, Palys V, Toms J, Wickramasinghe CS, Amarasinghe K, Manic M, et al. Nucleus basalis of Meynert stimulation for dementia: Theoretical and technical considerations. Frontiers in Neuroscience. 2018;**12**:614

[11] Ray NJ, Bradburn S, Murgatroyd C, Toseeb U, Mir P, Kountouriotis GK, et al. In vivo cholinergic basal forebrain atrophy predicts cognitive decline in de novo Parkinson's disease. Brain. 2018;**141**(1):165-176

[12] Schulz J, Pagano G, Fernández Bonfante JA, Wilson H, Politis M. Nucleus basalis of Meynert degeneration precedes and predicts cognitive impairment in Parkinson's disease. Brain. 2018;**141**(5):1501-1516

[13] Barrett MJ, Sperling SA, Blair JC, Freeman CS, Flanigan JL, Smolkin ME, et al. Lower volume, more impairment: Reduced cholinergic basal forebrain grey matter density is associated with impaired cognition in Parkinson disease. Journal of Neurology, Neurosurgery, and Psychiatry. 2019;**90**(11):1251-1256

[14] Gang M, Baba T, Hosokai Y, Nishio Y, Kikuchi A, Hirayama K, et al.

Clinical and cerebral metabolic changes in Parkinson's disease with basal forebrain atrophy. Movement Disorders. 2020;**35**(5):825-832

[15] Schumacher J, Thomas AJ, Peraza LR, Firbank M, Cromarty R, Hamilton CA, et al. EEG alpha reactivity and cholinergic system integrity in lewy body dementia and Alzheimer's disease. Alzheimer's Research & Therapy. 2020;**12**(1):46

[16] Díez-Cirarda M, Strafella AP, Kim J, Peña J, Ojeda N, Cabrera-Zubizarreta A, et al. Dynamic functional connectivity in Parkinson's disease patients with mild cognitive impairment and normal cognition. Neuroimage: Clinical. 2018;**17**:847-855

[17] Zhang C, Wu C, Zhang H, Dou W, Li W, Sami MU, et al. Disrupted resting-state functional connectivity of the nucleus basalis of meynert in Parkinson's disease with mild cognitive impairment. Neuroscience. 2020;**442**:228-236

[18] Maiti B, Koller JM, Snyder AZ, Tanenbaum AB, Norris SA, Campbell MC, et al. Cognitive correlates of cerebellar resting-state functional connectivity in Parkinson disease. Neurology. 2020;**94**(4):e384-e396

[19] Pandey S, Sarma N. Deep brain stimulation: Current status. Neurology India. 2015;**63**(1):9-18

[20] Marks WJ. Deep Brain Stimulation Management. Cambridge, New York: Cambridge University Press; 2011

[21] Doshi PK. Expanding indications for deep brain stimulation. Neurology India. 2018;**66**(Supplement):S102-S112

[22] Rodriguez-Oroz MC, Obeso JA, Lang AE, Houeto J-L, Pollak P, Rehncrona S, et al. Bilateral deep brain stimulation in Parkinson's disease: A multicentre study with 4 years follow-up. Brain. 2005;**128**(10):2240-2249

[23] Lee DJ, Lozano AM. The future of surgical treatments for Parkinson's disease. Journal of Parkinson's Disease. 2018;**8**(s1):S79-S83

[24] Benabid AL, Pollak P, Gervason C, Hoffmann D, Gao DM, Hommel M, et al. Long-term suppression of tremor by chronic stimulation of the ventral intermediate thalamic nucleus. Lancet. 1991;**337**(8738):403-406

[25] FitzGerald J. Neuromodulation: Deep Brain Stimulation Targets. Available from: https://www.neuromodulation.com/fact_sheet_brain_targets. [Accessed: November 5, 2021]

[26] Okun MS, Rodriguez RL, Mikos A, Miller K, Kellison I, Kirsch-Darrow L, et al. Deep brain stimulation and the role of the neuropsychologist. The Clinical Neuropsychologist. 2007;**21**(1):162-189

[27] Mole JA, Prangnell SJ. Role of clinical neuropsychology in deep brain stimulation: Review of the literature and considerations for clinicians. Applied Neuropsychology Adult. 2019;**26**(3):283-296

[28] Bronstein JM, Tagliati M, Alterman RL, Lozano AM, Volkmann J, Stefani A, et al. Deep brain stimulation for Parkinson disease: An expert consensus and review of key issues. Archives of Neurology. 2011;**68**(2):165

[29] Dayal V, Limousin P, Foltynie T. Subthalamic nucleus deep brain stimulation in Parkinson's disease: The effect of varying stimulation parameters. Journal of Parkinson's Disease. 2017;**7**(2):235-245

[30] Hariz MI. Complications of deep brain stimulation surgery. Movement Disorders. 2002;**17**(Suppl 3):S162-S166

[31] Weaver FM, Follett K, Stern M, Hur K, Harris C, Marks WJ, et al. Bilateral deep brain stimulation vs best medical therapy for patients with advanced Parkinson disease: A randomized controlled trial. JAMA. 2009;**301**(1):63-73

[32] Hariz MI, Rehncrona S, Quinn NP, Speelman JD, Wensing C. Multicenter study on deep brain stimulation in Parkinson's disease: An independent assessment of reported adverse events at 4 years. Movement Disorders. 2008;**23**(3):416-421

[33] Rossi M, Bruno V, Arena J, Cammarota Á, Merello M. Challenges in PD patient management after DBS: A pragmatic review. Movement Disorders Clinical Practice. 2018;**5**(3):246-254

[34] Rothlind JC, Cockshott RW, Starr PA, Marks WJ. Neuropsychological performance following staged bilateral pallidal or subthalamic nucleus deep brain stimulation for Parkinson's disease. Journal of the International Neuropsychological Society. 2007;**13**(1):68-79

[35] Scangos KW, Carter CS, Gurkoff G, Zhang L, Shahlaie K. A pilot study of subthalamic theta frequency deep brain stimulation for cognitive dysfunction in Parkinson's disease. Brain Stimulation. 2018;**11**(2):456-458

[36] Combs HL, Folley BS, Berry DTR, Segerstrom SC, Han DY, Anderson-Mooney AJ, et al. Cognition and depression following deep brain stimulation of the subthalamic nucleus and globus pallidus pars internus in Parkinson's disease: A meta-analysis. Neuropsychology Review. 2015;**25**(4):439-454

[37] Mahlknecht P, Peball M, Mair K, Werkmann M, Nocker M, Wolf E, et al. Has deep brain stimulation changed the very long-term outcome of Parkinson's disease? A controlled longitudinal study. Movement Disorders Clinical Practice. 2020;**7**(7):782-787

[38] Freund H-J, Kuhn J, Lenartz D, Mai JK, Schnell T, Klosterkoetter J, et al. Cognitive functions in a patient with Parkinson-dementia syndrome undergoing deep brain stimulation. Archives of Neurology. 2009;**66**(6):781-785

[39] Gratwicke J, Zrinzo L, Kahan J, Peters A, Brechany U, McNichol A, et al. Bilateral nucleus basalis of Meynert deep brain stimulation for dementia with Lewy bodies: A randomised clinical trial. Brain Stimulation. 2020;**13**(4):1031-1039

[40] Daniels C, Steigerwald F, Capetian P, Matthies C, Malzahn U, Heuschmann PU, et al. Combined subthalamic and nucleus basalis of Meynert deep brain stimulation for Parkinson's disease with dementia (DEMPARK-DBS): Protocol of a randomized, sham-controlled trial. Neurological Research and Practice. 2020;**2**:41

[41] Lam J, Lee J, Williams M, Cohn M, Wilson M, Mark C, et al. Cognitive effects of theta frequency bilateral subthalamic nucleus stimulation in Parkinson's disease: A pilot study. Brain Stimulation. 2021;**14**(2):230-240

[42] Krauss JK, Lipsman N, Aziz T, Boutet A, Brown P, Chang JW, et al. Technology of deep brain stimulation: Current status and future directions. Nature Reviews Neurology. 2021 Feb;**17**(2):75-87

[43] Habets JGV, Heijmans M, Kuijf ML, Janssen MLF, Temel Y, Kubben PL. An update on adaptive deep brain stimulation in Parkinson's disease. Movement Disorders. 2018;**33**(12):1834-1843

Chapter 11

Parkinson's Disease, Headache and Pain

Marc E. Lenaerts

Abstract

Parkinson's disease (PD) is a vast and complex syndrome. Far more than a mere disorder of motor function, it encompasses autonomic, cognitive, emotional and systemic symptoms. Moreover, pain has increasingly been recognized as an associated feature. Within pain and headache, migraine can bear a unique relation with PD. We hereby review the scientific literature on the relation between PD, pain and migraine and analyze the pathophysiological underpinnings and suggest adjustments in the management to tentatively improve clinical outcomes in this setting.

Keywords: Parkinson's disease (PD), cervical dystonia, migraine, headache, pain, comorbidity, comprehensive management

1. Introduction

Parkinson's disease (PD) is a very complex condition, and increasing emphasis is given on the non-motor symptoms. Mindful of the extent of its pathology in the CNS (central nervous system) and of the complexity of its symptomatology approaching PD comprehensively including pain has vast clinical benefits. As such, the study of comorbidities in PD as well as its clinical ramifications with various pathophysiologic processes brings much benefit for the comprehensive care of this disease.

Here, we concentrate on the relations between PD on one hand, and pain and headaches on the other. At the core of PD symptomatology is hypertonia that causes abnormal musculoskeletal dynamics including among others, painful muscle contractions, acceleration of joint degeneration and encroachment of neural structures in the spine. Abnormal central pain mechanisms might also be involved. The relation with migraine is more elusive but likely relates to pathologic central pain processing and neurotransmitter shifts, particularly dopamine.

2. Epidemiology

Pain was already mentioned by James Parkinson himself is his 1817 seminal article "An essay on the shaking palsy" [1].

Pain is highly prevalent in PD, and several epidemiological studies have highlighted this issue [2–6]. It affects women disproportionately [7].

Few studies have investigated the comorbidity of migraine and PD. This merits several considerations. Both conditions are diagnosed with clinical criteria, even PD that could otherwise be diagnosed with certainly with pathology. Some of the basic aspects that we know of some of pathogenesis of the two conditions, one with degenerating neurons in the substantia nigra and one with dysregulation on the trigemino-cervical complex, do not raise a high suspicion of comorbidity. The age of onset as well as the gender predominance is likewise pointing away from comorbidity. Thus, it seems at first glance that comorbidity would be unlikely, or even that the two conditions would partly mutually exclusive, or protective of one another.

One-year prevalence of migraine is high, about 12% population (chronic migraine about 2%); and that of PD moderate, about 0.5% population, making statistical evaluations more cumbersome by requiring relatively high numbers of observations [8–10].

In an in-depth analysis of 237 patients suffering from PD, 66 had a history of migraine, a lifetime prevalence of 28% [11]. The prevalence of current migraine was 13%. These are similar to those in the general population [12]. More interestingly, among these 66 comorbid patients, the prevalence of current migraine was significantly lower than in 66 matched non-PD controls (47% vs. 68%), suggesting a possible surprising benefit from chronic dopamine therapy or, interestingly, an ongoing protective effect of PD on migraine [11].

In a large Taiwanese, 2.5-year cohort of one group of over 40,000 of 40–90-year-old migraine sufferers and an equal same-age group of controls, the prevalence of PD in the first group was at 1.64 odds above that in the second, and the incidence rate was increased as well [13].

A survey of 223 patients with PD reported a migraine prevalence of 19% and another of 71 patients one of 11% [14, 15].

A case–control study of 109 patients with PD demonstrated no significant effect of the emergence of PD motor symptoms on the course of migraine [16].

A cross-sectional analysis of 43 patients with PD with headache (12 with migraine and 31 with tension-type headache) demonstrated no correlation between PD stages and the presence or characteristics of headache including migraine [17].

In a recent survey, the largest-to-date, of 436 patients with PD and 401 controls, PD was associated with a significantly lower rate of migraine (one-year and lifetime prevalence) by almost half, and this was not the case for headaches in general. Moreover, the onset of PD was associated with a substantial reduction in migraine symptom burden when compared with prior to onset. This was not because of age which we know reduces migraine frequency, for the decrease was far more pronounced than in migraine controls without PD [18].

In summary, there is limited literature on the comorbidity between PD, on one hand, and pain and migraine, on the other. Results of studies vary, in part due to methodology, and so far no definite conclusion can be drawn, more investigations being warranted.

3. Pathophysiology

Dopamine modulates pain and levodopa increases pain thresholds [19, 20].

Pain can relate to the motor function in PD and should always be analyzed within that mind frame. Rigidity causes pain *via* muscle hyperactivity, contractures, tendon pain and joint wear [21]. Nonetheless, there is no clear time correlation between pain levels and motor scores [3, 5].

Several anatomical targets of PD pathology (Lewy bodies, degeneration) are involved in pain, emotion and autonomic control: basal ganglia; medial spino-reticulo-thalamic pathway, including locus coeruleus, periaqueductal gray and thalamus; lateral spino-thalamic pathway (modulated by DBS) [22–24].

The role of dopamine is most interesting. Dopamine-blocking agents help the symptoms of migraine (and not only the nausea but the pain itself), dopamine-enhancing or mimicking agents help PD and dopamine is key in placebo response.

Dopamine seems involved in behavioral and autonomic modifications during migraine attacks: appetite, vigilance, energy and blood pressure [25, 26]. Some mutations in dopamine D2 receptor (DRD2) and some in catechol-oxy-methyl-transferase link to migraine [27–29]. Central catecholamines including dopamine modulate pain, pain sensitization and other symptoms [30, 31].

Dopamine receptors are found in the nucleus tractus solitarius, dorsal vagus and area postrema, all involved in the gastro-intestinal symptoms of migraine [32]. Also, D1 receptors found in renal arteries might influence the diuresis of migraine postdromes and D2 receptors in the sympathetic ganglia contribute to migraine hypotension and syncope by reducing norepinephrine release [33, 34].

Migraine prodromes (yawning hunger, hypervigilence), accompanying symptoms (anorexia, nausea, vomiting, hypotension), are partly under dopamine control. Dopamine agonists such as apomorphine cause similar symptoms as side effects and these side effects occur. In migraine sufferers, these effects can occur at lower than average doses [35–37], and apomorphine can trigger migraine [38].

The clinical severity and responsivity to dopamine was investigated in patients with PD with or without migraine. In a trial of 18 patients with PD among whom 10 with migraine, UPDRS (Unified Parkinson's Disease Rating Scale) showed longer on-times, shorter off-times and lower levodopa requirements but no difference in hallucinations [39].

The dopamine-dependent late phase of CNV (contingent negative variation) electrophysiology test is abnormal but normalizes with migraine episode resolution and is modulated by the dopaminergic apomorphine [40, 41]. Hallucinations can be observed in both PD and migraine. In migraine, CSD (cortical spreading depression, mechanism of the aura) can cause hallucinations and seems under serotonergic and cholinergic control, themselves relevant to PD [42, 43].

Valproate and flunarizine, used in migraine prophylaxis, can induce parkinsonism [44, 45].

Dopamine-blocking agents such as promethazine and prochlorperazine are well known to help the gastro-intestinal symptoms of migraine symptoms but also reduce pain independently. Domperidone had equal effect to acetylsalicylic acid or metoclopramide or prochlorperazine alone [35, 46–49].

However, increasingly the gastro-intestinal symptoms of migraine are treated with serotonin 5 HT-3 receptor antagonists ondansetron or granisetron for tolerability reasons, and thorazine infusions for refractory status migrainosus should be avoided in PD.

The substantia nigra possesses a high concentration of serotonin 1—B, D and F—receptors that are the target of sumatriptan [50] and this could alter tolerability of sumatriptan in PD. The substantia nigra is activated after occipital aura on functional MRI (magnetic resonance imaging) [51]; therefore, PD could influence the expression of migraine auras.

Hormonal fluctuations can influence several neurologic conditions [52]. Estrogens specifically influence involves the striatum. PD tremor probably, and migraine certainly, is menstrually exacerbated [52–54]. The incidence of PD might be reduced with the implementation of hormone replacement therapy [55, 56].

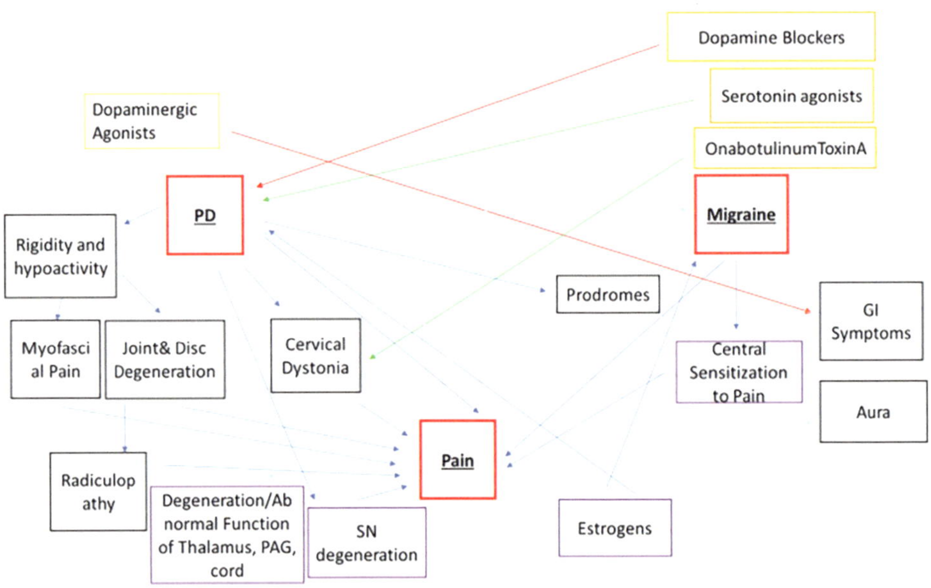

Figure 1.
The multiple interrelations between PD, migraine and pain. This illustrates the complex relations between PD, pain and migraine. Abbreviations: SN: Substantia Nigra; PAG: Periaqueductal gray matter. Boxes: Red: Key conditions; black: Syndromes; purple: Pathophysiology and pathology. Orange: Treatments. Arrows: Represent influence. Blue: Clinical and physiological; dark: Strong evidence; light: Hypothetical. Red and green: Pharmacologic; red: Negative synergy; green: Positive synergy.

Post-menopausal hormone replacement therapy shows a modest benefit in PD and a more definite one in migraine [57, 58].

PD can present with cervical dystonia, which contributes to cervicogenic headaches, but also aggravates migraine. This becomes very pertinent when patients are treated with botulinum toxin for both dystonia and migraine.

The relation between microbiome and nervous system is under increasing scrutiny: The former can contribute to autoimmune conditions and alter biochemical processes affecting PD and migraine; autonomic dysfunction in these two conditions can alter the microbiome, maybe with synergy when comorbid [57].

Beta-blockers presumably affect migraine not *via* blood pressure but *via* central catecholamines (as per CNV studies) [59]. Cortical hyperexcitability in migraine depends on central catecholamine activity. Dopamine has once been coined the "migraine accelerator." Postural stability is often affected in migraine overall, not just its vestibular form [60]. PD causes more profound postural instability.

The prevalence of depression is increased in migraine as well as in PD (**Figure 1**).

PD can, *via* abnormal tone and posture, cause myofascial pain and degenerative disk and joint disease, leading to pain directly and by neural compression, and cervicogenic headache. The possible degeneration and dysfunction of structures involved in pain such as thalamus, PAG, cord, contributes to pain, and that of the substantia nigra might influence migraine auras. Central sensitization in migraine can amplify systemic pains. The dopamine deficit in migraine could have a partial protective effect on migraine. PD treatment enhancing dopaminergic activity might aggravate the nausea of migraine; mirroring this, dopamine blockers, used to control migraine nausea, aggravate PD symptoms. Serotonergic agents might benefit PD. BotulinumToxinA for chronic migraine benefits cervical dystonia encountered in PD.

4. Syndromic presentations

4.1 General clinical principles

Pain syndromes in PD are attributable to either unrelated etiologies or features of the condition itself or often to a combination thereof. It is beneficial to approach pain in PD with a somewhat unifying concept [61]. It can in turn be classified within the following useful clinical frames: movement-related dystonic or akathitic, musculoskeletal, radicular or central [62] (**Table 1**). Note that choreic and athetotic movements are typically not significantly painful. Additional pain syndromes seen in PD more than the general populations but not specific to it are pain linked to constipation and the discomfort associated with orthostatic hypotension and metaphorically referred to as "coat-hanger" syndrome [63]. Aiding to classify the patient's syndrome in the aforementioned scheme (and adding a visceral pain category), the KPPS (King's PD Pain Scale) is a useful questionnaire [64].

4.2 Dystonia

Dystonia, primary or pharmacologically induced, can generate impacting painful syndromes including, if scapular, a frozen shoulder and, if cervical, cervicogenic headache [65, 66]. Dystonia is painful compared with the non-statically sustained chorea or athetosis. Akathisia is an unpleasant symptom rather than painful.

Dystonia can be present with levodopa end-of-dose fluctuation. This can be managed with extended-release levodopa or the addition of dopa metabolism to prolong the therapeutic effect, and in rare instances, even apomorphine can afford fast relief [67, 68]. A similar reasoning applies to the early AM dystonia where apomorphine might be even more necessary [62]. LCIG (levodopa/carbidopa intestinal gel) therapy can also be beneficial [69].

Dopamine agonists also show benefit in dystonia-related pain [70].

Botulinum toxin is an excellent approach for focal, such as cervical or scapular, dystonia [71].

Deep brain stimulation has shown to be effective against cervical dystonia [72].

4.3 Musculoskeletal pain

Although as stated above time correlation between motor fluctuations and pain levels is not firmly established, the chronic abnormal muscle contractions, tendinous strain, abnormal posture with uneven joint wear and pressure point distribution, and most importantly limited amount and range of motion, all contribute to musculoskeletal pain. The frequency, duration, intensity and anatomical distribution are highly variable. The clinician ought to assess these multiple aspects of the syndrome to better diagnose and manage these pains, all the while addressing the specific and commonly observed contribution of the abnormal motor function. For instance, upper truncal dystonia can contribute to frozen shoulder, cervicalgia, cervicogenic headache and camptocormia, which can induce spine pain at any level. NSAIDs, muscle relaxants, physical therapy and, at times, surgery, are all part of the therapeutic armamentarium. Cannabinoids are increasingly considered but there is no consensus recommendation yet [73]. Additional beneficial aspects of therapy at large encompass the elements of social and artistic activity, such as painting, music and dancing [74]. Treating associated depression and anxiety is inherently beneficial. Choosing a pharmacologic agent that enhances dopaminergic activity is worthwhile, such as citalopram, nortriptyline or venlafaxine [75–77].

Pain syndrome	Dystonia	Akathisia	Musculoskeleletal	Radiculopathic	Central
Pathophysiology	Dopaminergic deficit Excessive contractions from early AM akinesia or mid-day off phenomenon	Dopaminergic deficit	Abnormal postures Muscle and tendon contractures Abnormal joint wear	Spine degenerative disease, precipitated by abnormal posture	Unclear, possible dopaminergic deficit
Symptomatology	Posture-related nociceptive pain Any area of body Common in cervico-scapular area Can lead to cervicogenic headache and frozen shoulder syndrome	More discomfort than severe pain Restlessness Include restless legs syndrome	Pain in muscle, tendons, fascias and joint Nociceptive mechanical pain exacerbated by excessive (in) activity	Lancinating pain radiating in radicular territory	Highly variable locations and types and intensity Can be holosomatic, truncular, prosopalgic Often complex and atypical in description

Five main pain syndromes in PD with their pathophysiologic and clinical characteristics.

Table 1.
Classification of pain syndromes in PD (modified from Ford) [18].

4.4 Radiculalgia

Nerve root pain is not uncommon in PD with a survey estimating the prevalence between 10 and 29% [78]. Camptocormia can undoubtedly contribute to spine degeneration and foraminal stenoses. Tricyclic antidepressants, SNRI (serotonin-norepinephrine-reuptake inhibitors) and anticonvulsant neuromodulating drugs are part of a wide choice of pharmacologic agents to choose from in helping neuropathic pain. Gabapentin has shown to potentially have additional motor benefit in PD pain [79].

4.5 Central pain

Central pain syndromes are highly variable, protean, at times outright atypical. Pain can be diffuse, more focused on truncal or perineal areas. Prosopalgia can be observed. Often it is accompanied by numbness, paresthesia and/or allodynia. These are typically unrelated to the level of motor function. They are typically dismissed for long by providers and generate understandable accrued frustration in patients. Their etiology remains elusive and abnormal central catecholaminergic activity, including dopamine, remains likely. Cautious history and *ad hoc* ancillary investigations are warranted to ensure the more common and/or concerning nociceptive etiologies are ruled out. Cautious assessment of psychotherapeutic support is advised. Management includes neuromodulatory drugs such as gabapentin, pregabalin, duloxetine [79, 80]. Biofeedback and cognitive-behavioral therapy and supportive psychotherapy should be discussed [62, 81]. NSAIDs (Non-Steroid Anti-Inflammatory Drugs) and regular or opioid analgesics are neither typically helpful nor recommended.

4.6 Akathisia

Albeit not typically painful *per se*, akathisia is uncomfortable and merits attention and care. Related to ventral tegmental dopaminergic insufficiency, it can be diffused and occur anytime, and it can also be more focal in time and distribution such as in the case of restless leg syndrome. Management options include dopaminergic drugs such ropinirole, levodopa especially extended-release or other avenues increasing dopaminergic activity in the brain stem [82].

5. Practice guidelines

Like cognitive, affective and autonomic symptoms, pain is an additional non-motor sphere of symptoms that can also fluctuate. It significantly impacts quality of life in PD too. Screening for depression in patients with migraine, PD and even more so both is paramount.

Patients with PD will consult for their pain either to their movement disorder specialist or to general neurologist or other providers. It is important for the former to be involved in case the specific management of the parkinsonian syndrome needs to be managed in depth, as discussed below. Indeed, often, dopaminergic adjustment is beneficial to pain in PD. This is particularly relevant given the propensity for pain to be at times the presenting symptom of PD [5, 83, 84].

Pain in PD is complex, often multifactorial, and the relationship with PD itself is far more complex that might initially appear and requires a thorough and cautious approach. After a comprehensive history and physical exam, judicious use of ancillary investigation might be warranted. Multifaceted therapy is typically necessary and pharmacotherapy, and physical and occupational therapies, psychotherapeutic measures, social interventions, procedures and surgery might be indicated. Moreover, physical therapy can be considered in the broader sense and encompass, if supported by evidence, thermotherapy, osteopathic and chiropractic measures, water exercise, (electro-)acupuncture, etc. As an example, acupuncture shows benefit in PD pain [85]. Patient education is not least crucial, for patient's emotional comfort as well as active participation to treatment. Special attention is recommended for the most at-risk and vulnerable patients. Ensuring patients remain engaged in family, social and, if applied, work activities is paramount. Additional attention to balance is advised in patients with PD suffering from migraine. Dysautonomia being common in PD and migraine, great caution is required using medications affecting blood pressure in comorbid patients. Orthostatic blood pressure assessments are essential.

A summary of management of pain syndromes in PD is outlined in **Table 2**.

The care of migraine rests on four pillars (**Figure 2**):

1. Lifestyle modification: proper sleep hygiene, quality diet with regular meals and limited artificial and fermented foods and drinks, regular exercise and stress management;

2. Abortive treatment: acute relief of the migraine attack symptoms: pain, gastrointestinal symptoms such as nausea and vomiting, sensoriphobia (photophobia, phonophobia, kinesiophobia, etc.) and others; insurance patient can return to a functional and productive state;

3. Rescue therapy: measures to help patient who remains severely symptomatic of the attack after abortive treatment;

4. Prophylactic treatment: applies if attacks are weekly or more frequent, if the abortive treatment is insufficient (along with rescue measures) or contraindicated; this part of therapy aims at reducing the burden of migraine overall: attack frequency, duration, intensity, impact; and doing so in respect of patient's ability to function and be productive.

Lifestyle modification has substantial overlap with PD, including stress management and relaxation therapy, regular sleep, regular physical activity.

Abortive treatments include the following:

Non-specific agents such as acetaminophen, non-steroid anti-inflammatory drugs and combination medications (e.g., acetaminophen and caffeine) as well as, albeit rarely advised, opioids. These have no specific impact on, nor are to be modified in, PD.

Specific agents include ergot-derivatives, which activate the 5 HT receptor as well as the dopamine receptor, thus often requiring a dopamine blocker toward off gastrointestinal symptoms, which can negatively impact PD; triptans (5 HT 1 B/D agonists); gepants (CGRP receptor blockers) and a ditan (like triptans, a 5 HT agonists but on a separate receptor subtype (F) without vasoconstrictive effect). Thus, mainly the dihydroergotamine must be the subject of particular caution in PD.

Prophylactic treatments include the following:

Antidepressants: tricyclic such as SNRI (serotonin-norepinephrine reuptake inhibitors); some with enhancing effect on dopamine (see section on pain).

DOI: http://dx.doi.org/10.5772/intechopen.103051

Pain Syndrome	Dystonia	Akathisia	Musculoskeleletal	Radiculopathic	Central
	Levodopa (extended release) Dopaminergic agents MAO-i, COMT-i DBS (seep brain stimulation) Apomorphine	Amantadine Beta-blockers Benzodiazepines, Mirtazapine Vit B6	NSAIDs Muscle relaxants Physical therapy Pain management procedures Surgery	Neuropathic pain medication such as amitriptyline, gabapentin or pregabalin Physical therapy Pain management procedures Surgery	Neuromodulating agents such as gabapentin, pregabalin, duloxetine or amitriptyline Biofeedback and CBT (cognitive-behavioral therapy)

Table 2.
Management of pain syndromes in PD (modified from Ford) [18].

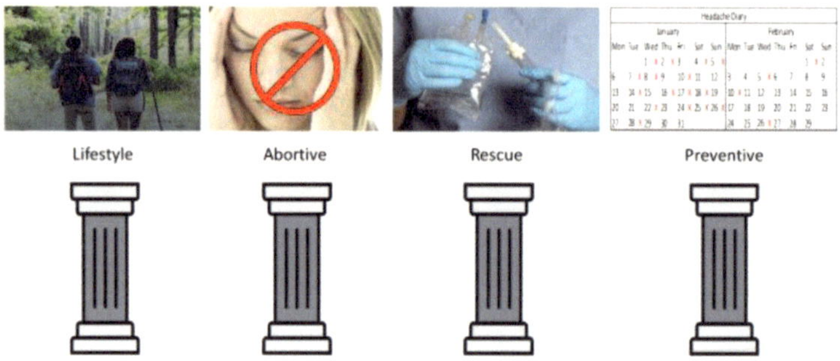

Figure 2.
The four pillars of migraine treatment. Migraine is best managed comprehensively with a plan for healthy lifestyle adjustment, abortive treatment to stop the ongoing symptoms, rescue treatment if the latter fails, and preventive (prophylactic) care to reduce burden over time and decrease the need for abortive and rescue interventions.

Anticonvulsants: Topiramate is neutral on PD but can add its cognitive side effects to the potential existing PD-related dysfunction; valproate has been shown to cause tremor and maybe secondary parkinsonism, while gabapentin, albeit a weak agent, seems to be beneficial on PD motor symptoms (see section on pain).

Antihypertensives: Beta-blockers can be beneficial in akathisia; angiotensin conversion enzyme inhibitors and angiotensin receptor blockers are neutral in PD and so are calcium channel blockers; hypotension can in any case, however, have more likely side effect in patients with PD who have orthostatic hypotension.

Botulinum Toxin A injections can most definitely benefit PD-related cervical dystonia (see section on pain).

Other medications such as Memantine can also be considered.

An increasing number of FDA-approved options are at the disposal of the clinician for the non-pharmacologic management of headache, which is attractive in the pharmaco-therapeutically loaded regimen of PD management. These include the following:

Trigeminal nerve stimulator.
Peripheral remote neuromodulating stimulator.
Transcranial magnetic simulator.

A number of procedures are also now available, often, however, off-label, and include the following:

Anesthetic blocks:

Occipital nerve injections (greater, lesser, third or all occipital nerves) with local anesthetic.
Supra-orbital nerve anesthetic blocks.
Spheno-palatine ganglion anesthetic block.

Other:

Trigger point injections.
Lidocaine IV infusion.
Ketamine IV infusion.
Thorazine infusion (not recommended in PD).

As much as the role of physical therapy is known to benefit pain, relative immobility has the inverse effect.

Table 3 relates the main pharmacotherapies for migraine to their potential impact, positive and negative, on PD symptoms and treatment.

CATEGORY	Name(s)	Indication	Side effects relevant to PD	Positive synergy	Negative synergy	Caveats/ other
Beta-blockers	Propranolol, metoprolol	Prophylaxis	Orthostatic hypotension Fatigue Impotence	Can help if associated essential tremor	—	—
Angiotensin conversion enzyme inhibitors	Lisinopril	Prophylaxis	Hypotension	—	—	—
Angiotensin receptor blockers	Candesartan	Prophylaxis	Hypotension	—	—	—
Calcium channel blocker	Verapamil	Prophylaxis	Hypotension, arrhythmia	—	—	Avoid with clozapine
Calcium channel blocker	Flunarizine	Prophylaxis	Sedation; depression; hyperphagia; tremor	—	Can aggravate parkinsonism	Avoid in PD; QT prolongation
Tricyclic antidepressants	Amitriptyline, nortriptyline	Prophylaxis	Anticholinergic Alpha-adrenergic (tachyarrhythmias)	Mood improvement Xerostomia might help sialorrhea	Constipation Confusion	Avoid in elderly especially if cognitive concerns
SNRIs (serotonin-norepinephrine reuptake inhibitors)	Venlafaxine	Prophylaxis	Abnormal dreams; sexual dysfunction	Mood improvement	Affected dreams if already having RBD (REM-sleep behavior disorder)	—
Anticonvulsant	Topiramate	Prophylaxis	Cognitive (language) slowing; paresthesia; dysgeusia; anorexia; cramps	Can help if associated essential tremor	Cognitive slowing; muscle cramps	Avoid if cognitive concerns
Anticonvulsant	Divalproex	Prophylaxis	Tremor (even at rest); hyperphagia;	Mood stabilization	Added tremor	Possible liver toxicity
Anti-CGRP monoclonal antibodies	Eptinezumab, erenumab, fremanezumab, galcanezumab	Prophylaxis	Local injection site reaction	—	—	—

CATEGORY	Name(s)	Indication	Side effects relevant to PD	Positive synergy	Negative synergy	Caveats/ other
NMDA-receptor antagonist	Memantine	Prophylaxis	Nausea, dizziness, paradoxical confusion	Cognitive improvement	—	—
Chemodenervation	OnabotulinumToxinA	Prophylaxis	Weakness facial and neck muscles	Benefit for dystonia and sialorrhea	Can aggravate camptocormia	—
Natural supplements	Riboflavin; Coenzyme Q 10; magnesium	Prophylaxis	—	Might benefit when nutrition is challenged; decreased muscle contractions	—	No concern re: interaction
Neurostimulators	Electric: trigeminal, armband; vagal; magnetic: transcranial	Prophylactic and abortive	Discomfort	—	—	No concern re: interaction
Analgesic	Acetaminophen	Abortive	—	Helps other PD-related pains	—	Liver malfunction
NSAIDs	Ibuprofen, naproxen	Abortive	Gastralgia, GI bleed	Helps other PD-related pains	—	Avoid in GI disease and in coronary artery disease
Triptans	Sumatriptan and six other triptans	Abortive	Chest pressure; palpitations; sedation	—	—	Avoid in active atherosclerosis
Ergot derivative	Dihydroergotamine	Abortive or rescue	Chest pressure; palpitations; sedation			Avoid in active atherosclerosis Requires anti-emetic and thus prefers serotonin-3 receptor antagonist
Ditan	Lasmiditan	Abortive	Nausea; sedation	—	—	—

DOI: http://dx.doi.org/10.5772/intechopen.103051

CATEGORY	Name(s)	Indication	Side effects relevant to PD	Positive synergy	Negative synergy	Caveats/ other
Gepants	Ubrogepant; rimegepant; atogepant	Abortive (ubrogepant and rimegepant) and prophylactic (rimegepant and atogepant)	Nausea	—	—	—
Anti-emetics: antidopaminergic	Oral: domperidone Oral or injectable: promethazine, prochlorperazine	Adjuvant	Sedation oculogyric crisis	Help nausea associated with PD meds	Can aggravate PD symptoms	Avoid in PD
Neuroleptic	Injectable thorazine	Thorazine	Sedation, oculogyric crisis	—	Can aggravate PD symptoms	Avoid in PD; QT prolongation
Anti-emetics: anti-serotonergic type 3	Ondansetron, granisetron	Adjuvant	Confusion	Help nausea associated with PD meds	—	No aggravation of PD symptoms
Peripheral nerve blocks	Lidocaine, bupivacaine	Rescue	Procedure-related	Can help other PD-related pains including musculoskeletal	—	—

Pharmacotherapy for migraine by category, indication (prophylactic, abortive, rescue), with emphasis on side effects relevant to PD, and positive and negative synergies for PD and other caveats re: PD.

Table 3.
Medications for migraine and potential impact on PD.

6. Discussion

As we universally understand diseases better, we humbly reminded of their complexities and ramifications. Initially and for a long time considered a condition of primarily motor dysfunction, which it does remain, PD is now considered a multifaceted condition and pain and headaches are integral to the syndrome. Much remains to be studied to understand the complex epidemiology linking PD to the painful conditions. In PD as well as migraine, the natural evolution over the decades calls for a cautious interpretation of data and further refined studies, to understand the potential influencing role of one onto the other. Migraine manifests most of its symptoms in the early and middle part of life but singular presentations occur later, including silent auras and white matter hyperintensities that could have more impact on PD, a condition affecting mostly middle and later life. Chronic migraine has profound influence on the brain ability to process pain, likely beyond head pain, and even structural changes in the pain matrix are observed [86]. This could in turn be relevant to the other pain syndromes associated with PD.

From a clinical practice standpoint, the multitude of available treatments for PD, pain and headaches makes co-management complex and one can anticipate future discoveries on interactions, contraindications and synergies, leading to additional guidelines.

7. Conclusions

Scientific literature calls for increased awareness of the relation between PD, headache and pain syndromes. Comorbidity is subtle, clinical presentations varied and co-management delicate. More epidemiologic studies with wider population and sharp diagnostic accuracy, more understanding of the pathophysiology of each conditions, are warranted. Genetic investigations including areas relevant dopamine regulation might shed additional light on comorbidity. Increasing awareness includes better education and clinical guidelines.

It is suggested to integrate the assessment of pain and headaches in every patient suffering from PD.

From the standpoint of what physicians stand for, we can use these data to improve the quality of the care we deliver to patients with these comorbidities but also apply similar reasoning and principles to all comorbidities. It is about just doing best state-of-the art healthcare. At the core is the principle of holistic medicine to its true acceptation.

DOI: http://dx.doi.org/10.5772/intechopen.103051

Author details

Marc E. Lenaerts
Neurology and Headache Medicine, Departments of Neurology and Anesthesiology/Pain Management, University of California, Davis, CA, USA

*Address all correspondence to: mlenaerts@ucdavis.edu

References

[1] Parkinson J. An Essay on the Shaking Palsy. London: Sherwood, Neely, Jones; 1817

[2] Ford B. Pain in PD. Clinical Neuroscience. 1998;**5**:63-72

[3] Tinazzi M, Del Vesco C, Fincati E, et al. Pain and motor complications in PD. Journal of Neurology, Neurosurgery, and Psychiatry. 2006;**77**:822-825

[4] Beiske AG, Loge GH, Ronningen A, et al. Pain in PD: Prevalence and characteristics. Pain. 2009;**141**:173-177

[5] Buhnam C, Wrobel N, Grashorn W, et al. Pain in PD: A cross-sectional survey of its prevalence, specifics and therapy. Journal of Neurology. 2017;**264**:758-769

[6] Broen MP, Braaksma MM, Patijn J, et al. Prevalence of pain in PD: A systematic review using the QUADAS tool. Movement Disorders. 2012;**27**: 480-484

[7] Zella MAS, May C, Muller T, et al. Landscape of pain in PD: Impact of gender differences. Neurological Research. 2019;**41**:87-97

[8] Merikangas K. Contributions of epidemiology to our understanding of migraine. Headache. 2013;**53**:230-246

[9] Natoli JL, Manack A, Dean B, et al. Global prevalence of chronic migraine: A systematic review. Cephalalgia. 2010;**30**:599-609

[10] Marttila RJ. Epidemiology. In: Koeller WC, editor. Handbook of PD. New York: Marcel Dekker; 1992. pp. 35-57

[11] Brabanti P, Fabbrini G, Vanacore N, et al. Dopamine and migraine: Does PD modify migraine course? Cephalalgia. 2000;**20**:720-723

[12] Lipton RB, Stewart WF, Diamond S, et al. Prevalence and burden of migraine in the United States; data from the American Migraine Study II. Headache. 2001;**41**:646-657

[13] Wang HI, Ho YC, Huang YP, et al. Migraine is related to an increased risk of PD: A population-based, propensity score-matched, longitudinal follow-up study. Cephalalgia. 2016;**36**:1316-1323

[14] Lorenz I. A survey of migraine in PD. Cephalalgia. 1989;**9**:83-86

[15] Indo T, Naito A, Sobue I. Clinical characteristics of headache in PD. Headache. 1983;**23**:211-212

[16] de Olivera VC, Araujo Leite MA, de Souza JA, et al. The behavior of migraine in patients with PD. Neurology International. 2015;**7**:6133

[17] Sampaio Rocha-Filho PA, Leite Souza-Lima CF. PD and headaches: A cross-sectional study. Headache. 2020;**60**:967-973

[18] Suzuki K, Okuma Y, Uchiyama T, et al. The prevalence, course and clinical correlates of migraine in PD: A multicenter case-controlled study. Cephalalgia. 2018;**38**:1535-1544

[19] Gerderlat-Mas A, Simonetta-Moreau M, Thalamas C, et al. Levodopa raises objective pain thresholds in PD: A R III reflex study. Journal of Neurology, Neurosurgery, and Psychiatry. 2007; **78**:1140-1142

[20] Brefel-Courbon C, Payoux P, Thalamas C, et al. Effect of levodopa on pain threshold in PD: A clinical and PET study. Movement Disorders. 2005; **12**:1557-1563

[21] Broetz D, Eichner M, Gasser T, et al. Radicular and non-radicular back pain in PD: A controlled study. Movement Disorders. 2007;**22**:853-856

[22] Saadé NE, Atweh SF, Bahuth NB, et al. Augmentation of nociceptive reflexes and chronic deafferentation pain by chemical lesions of either dopaminergic terminals or midbrain dopaminergic neurons. Brain Research. 1997;**751**:1-12

[23] Blanchet PJ, Brefel-Courbon C. Chronic pain and pain processing in PD. Progress in Neuro-Psychopharmacology and Biological Psychiatry. 2018; **87**:200-206

[24] Zhang L, Wang XH, Sperry L, et al. Target selection recommendations based on impact of deep brain stimulation surgeries on non-motor symptoms of PD. Chinese Medical Journal. 2015;**128**:3371-3380

[25] Akerman S, Goadsby PJ. Dopamine and migraine: Biology and clinical implications. Cephalalgia. 2007;**27**:1308-1314

[26] Mascia A, Áfra J, Schoenen J. Dopamine in migraine: A review of pharmacological, biochemical, neurophysiological and therapeutic data. Cephalalgia. 1988;**18**:174-182

[27] Peroutka SJ, Wilhoit T, Jones K. Clinical susceptibility to migraine with aura is modified by dopamine D2 receptor Nco I alleles. Neurology. 1997;**49**:201-206

[28] Del Zompo M, Cherchi A, Ponti M, et al. Association between dopamine receptors D 2, D3 and D4 receptor genes and migraine without aura in a Sardinian sample. Cephalalgia. 1997;**17**:329

[29] Erdal ME, Herken H, Yilmaz M, et al. Significance of the COMT gene polymorphism in migraine. Molecular Brain Research. 2001;**94**:193-196

[30] Noseda R, Burstein R. Migraine pathophysiology: Anatomy of the trigemino-vascular pathway and associated neurological symptoms, CSD, sensitization and modulation of pain. Pain. 2013;**154**(Suppl 1):S44-S53

[31] Charbit AR, Akerman S, Goadsby PJ. Dopamine: What's new in migraine? Current Opinion in Neurology. 2010;**23**:275-281

[32] Hyde TM, Knable MB, Murray AM. Distribution of dopamine D1-D4 receptors in human dorsal vagal complex. Synapse. 1996;**24**:224-232

[33] Kohli JD, Glock D, Goldberg LI. Selective DA1 versus DA1 antagonist activity of domperidone in the periphery. European Journal of Pharmacology. 1983;**89**:137-141

[34] Sicuteri F, Bonucci M, Cangi F, et al. Syncope and dopamine-receptor hyperactivity: Myths and facts about basilar artery migraine. In: Carroll JD, Pfaffenrath V, Sjaastad O, editors. Migraine and Betablockade. Molndal: Hassle AB; 1985. pp. 147-160

[35] Peroutka SJ. Dopamine and migraine. Neurology. 1997;**49**:650-656

[36] Del Zompo M, Lai M, Loi V, et al. Dopamine hypersensitivity in migraine: Role of apomorphine syncope. Headache. 1995;**35**:222-224

[37] Fanciullacci M, Michelacci S, Curradi C, et al. Hyperresponsiveness of migraine patients to the hypotensive action of bromocriptine. Headache. 1980;**20**:99-102

[38] Sabatini U, Rascol O, Rascol A, et al. Migraine attacks induced by subcutaneous apomoprhine in two migrainous Parkinsonian patients.

Clinical Neuropharmacology. 1990; **13**:264-267

[39] Cubo E, Kompoliti K, Leurgans SE, et al. Dopaminergic sensitivity in patients with migraine and PD. Clinical Neuropharmacology. 2004;**27**:30-32

[40] Kropp P, Gerber WD. Contingent negative variation during migraine attack and interval: Evidence for normalization of slow cortical potentials during the attack. Cephalalgia. 1995;**15**:123-128

[41] Timsit-Berthier M, Mantanus H, Marissiaux P, et al. CNV and dopamine receptor reactivity: Correlation with the apomorphine test. Electroenc ephalography and Clinical Neurophysiology. 1986;**38**:403-405

[42] Manford M, Andermann F. Complex visual hallucinations: Clinical and biological insights. Brain. 1998;**121**:1819-1840

[43] Baizabal-Carvallo JF, Alonzo-Juarez M. Valproate-induced rest tremor and parkinsonism. Acta Neurologica Belgica. 2021;**121**:515-519

[44] Muralidharan Q, Rahman J, Banerjee D, et al. Parkinsonism: A rare adverse effect of valproic acid. Cureus. 2020;**23**:12

[45] Lin W, Lin CL, Hsu C, et al. Flunarizine induced parkinsonism in migraine group: A nationwide population-based study. Frontiers in Pharmacology. 2019;**10**:1495

[46] McGregor A, Wilkinson M, Bancroff K. Domperidone plus paracetamol in the treatment of migraine. Cephalalgia. 1993;**13**:124-127

[47] Tek DS, McClellan DS, Olshaker JS, et al. A prospective, double-blind study of metoclopramide hydrochloride for the control of migraine in the emergency department. Annals of Emergency Medicine. 1990;**19**: 1083-1087

[48] Amery WY, Waelkens J. Prevention of the last chance: An alternative pharmacological treatment of migraine. Headache. 1983;**23**:37-38

[49] Ellis DL, Delaney J, DeHart A, et al. Metoclopramide in the treatment of migraine headache. Annals of Emergency Medicine. 1993;**22**:191-195

[50] Castro ME, Pascual J, Romón T, et al. Differential distribution of ^{3}H-Sumatriptan binding sites in human brain: Focus on brainstem and spinal cord. Neuropharmacology. 1997; **36**:535-542

[51] Welch KMA, Cao Y, Aurora S, et al. MRI of the occipital cortex, red nucleus and substantia nigra during visual aura of migraine. Neurology. 1998;**51**:1 465-1469

[52] Roeder H, Leira E. Effects of the menstrual cycle on neurological disorders. Current Neurology and Neuroscience Reports. 2021;**21**:34

[53] Barth C, Villringer A, Sacher J. Sex hormones affect neurotransmitters and shape the adult female brain during hormonal transition periods. Frontiers in Neuroscience. 2015;**9**:37

[54] McGregor A. Menstrual migraine: Therapeutic approaches. Therapeutic Advances in Neurological Disorders. 2009;**2**:327-336

[55] Song YJ, Li SR, Li XW, et al. The effect of estrogen replacement therapy on Alzheimer's disease and PD in post-menopausal women: A meta-analysis. Frontiers in Neuroscience. 2020;**14**:157

[56] Wang P, Li J, Qiu S, et al. Hormone replacement therapy and PD risk in women: A meta-analysis of 14 studies. Neuropsychiatric Disease and Treatment. 2015;**11**:59

[57] The Parkinson Study Group POETRY Investigators. A randomized pilot trial of estrogen replacement therapy in post-menopausal women with PD. Parkinsonism & Related Disorders. 2011;**17**:757-760

[58] McGregor A. Menstrual and peri-menopausal migraine: A narrative review. Maturitas. 2002;**142**:24-30

[59] Linssen AM, Vuurman EF, Sambeth A, et al. Contingent negative variation as a dopamine biomarker: Evidence from dose-related effects of methylphenidate. Psychopharmacology. 2011;**218**:533-542

[60] Akdal G, Balci BD, Angin S, et al. A longitudinal study of balance in migraineurs. Acta Oto-Laryngologica. 2012;**132**:27-32

[61] Wasner G, Deuschl G. Pains in PD; many syndromes under one umbrella. Nature Reviews. Neurology. 2012;**8**:284-294

[62] Ford B. Pain in PD. Movement Disorders. 2010;**25**:S98-S103

[63] Beasdale-Barr KM, Mathias CJ. Neck and other muscle pains in autonomic failure: Their association with orthostatic hypotension. Journal of the Royal Society of Medicine. 1998;**91**:355-359

[64] Chaudhuri KR, Riz Perez-Lloret S, Rey MV, Dellapina E, et al. Emerging analgesic drugs for PD. Expert Opinion on Emerging Drugs. 2012;**17**:157-171

[65] Cattaneo C, Kulisevsky J, Tubazio V, et al. Long-term efficacy of safinamide on PD chronic pain. Advances in Therapy. 2018;**35**:515-552

[66] Chaudhuri KR, Rizos A, Trenkwalder C, Rascol O, Pal S, Martino D, et al. King's PD pain scale, the first scale for pain in PD: An international validation. Movement Disorders. 2015;**30**:1623-1631

[67] Riley D, Lang AE, Blair RDG, et al. Frozen shoulder and other shoulder disturbances in PD. Journal of Neurology, Neurosurgery, and Psychiatry. 1989;**52**:63-66

[68] Barbanti P, Fabbrini G, Pauletti C, et al. Headache in cranial and cervical dystonia. Neurology. 2005;**64**:1308-1309

[69] Zibetti M, Merola A, Artusi CA, et al. Levodopa/carbidopa intestinal gel infusion in advanced PD: A seven-year experience. European Journal of Neurology. 2014;**21**:312-318

[70] Rascol O, Zesiewicz T, Chaudhuri KR, et al. A randomized, controlled, exploratory pilot study to evaluate the effects of Rotigotine transdermal patch in PD-associated chronic pain. Journal of Clinical Pharmacology. 2016;**56**:852-861

[71] Rodrigues FB, Duarte GS, Marques RE, et al. Botulinum toxin type A for cervical dystonia. Cochrane Database of Systematic Reviews. 2020;**11**:CD 003633

[72] Kaelin-Lang A, Hana Y, Burgunder JM, et al. Bilateral pallidal stimulation improves cervical dystonia for more than a decade. Parkinsonism & Related Disorders. 2020;**81**:78-81

[73] Shohet A, Khlebtovsky A, Roizen N, et al. Effect of medical cannabis on thermal quantitative measurements of pain in patients with PD. European Journal of Pain. 2017;**21**:486-493

[74] Zhang S, Liu D, Ye D, et al. Can music-based movement therapy improve motor dysfunction in patients with PD? Systematic review and meta-analysis. Neurological Sciences. 2017;**38**:1629-1636

[75] Devos D, Dujardin K, Poirot I, et al. Comparison of desipramine and citalopram treatments for depression in PD: A double-blind, randomized,

placebo-controlled study. Movement Disorders. 2008;**23**:850-857

[76] Menza M, Dobkin RD, Marin H, et al. A controlled trial of antidepressants in patients with PD and depression. Neurology. 2009;**72**:886-892

[77] Richard IH, Mcdermott MP, Kurlan R, et al. A randomized, double-blind, placebo-controlled trial of antidepressants in PD. Neurology. 2012;**78**:1229-1236

[78] Goetz CG, Tanner CM, Levy M, et al. Pain in PD. Movement Disorders. 1986;**1**:45-49

[79] Olson WL, Gruenthal M, Mueller ME, et al. Gabapentin for PD: A double-blind, placebo-controlled, cross-over trial. The American Journal of Medicine. 1997;**102**:60-66

[80] Djaldeti R, Yust-Katz S, Kolianov V, et al. The effect of duloxetine on primary pain symptoms in PD. Clinical Neuropharmacology. 2007;**30**:201-205

[81] Quinn NP, Lang AE, Koller WC, et al. Painful PD. Lancet. 1986; **1**:1366-1369

[82] Comella CL, Goetz CG. Akathisia in PD. Movement Disorders. 1994;**5**: 545-549

[83] Farnikova K, Krobot A, Kanovsky P. Musculoskeletal problems as an initial manifestation of PD: A retrospective study. Journal of the Neurological Sciences. 2012;**319**:102-104

[84] Lin CH, Wu RM, Chang H, et al. Preceding pain symptoms and PD: A nationwide population-based cohort study. European Journal of Neurology. 2013;**20**:1398-1404

[85] Yu SW, Lin SH, Tsai CC, et al. Acupuncture effect and mechanism for treating pain in patients with PD. Frontiers in Neurology. 2019;**10**:114

[86] Naguib LE, Abdel Azim GS, Abdellatif MA. A volumetric magnetic resonance imaging study in migraine. The Egyptian Journal of Neurology, Psychiatry and Neurosurgery. 2021; **57**:116

Chapter 12

A Potential Innovative Therapy for Parkinson's Disease: Selective Destruction of the Pathological Assemblies of Alpha-Synuclein

Judit Oláh, Attila Lehotzky, Tibor Szénási and Judit Ovádi

Abstract

With the aging of the population, Parkinson's disease poses a serious socio-economic problem; there is no effective therapy that can arrest/revert the progression of the disease. The hallmarks of Parkinson's disease and other synucleinopathies are the disordered alpha-synuclein and TPPP/p25. These proteins have neomorphic moonlighting characteristics by displaying both physiological and pathological functions. Physiologically TPPP/p25 regulates the dynamics/stability of the microtubules and is crucial for oligodendrocyte differentiation; while alpha-synuclein is involved in neuronal plasticity modulation and synaptic vesicle pool maintenance. In healthy brain, alpha-synuclein and TPPP/p25 occur predominantly in neurons and oligodendrocytes, respectively; however, they are co-enriched and co-localized in both cell types in brain inclusions in the cases of Parkinson's disease and multiple system atrophy, respectively. The pathomechanisms of these diseases are largely unknown; the fatal species are the small, soluble homo- and hetero-associations of alpha-synuclein. These proteins with their high conformational plasticity and chameleon feature are challenging drug targets. Nevertheless, the contact surface of TPPP/p25-alpha-synuclein assemblies has been validated as a specific drug target. This new strategy with innovative impact, namely targeting the interface of the TPPP/p25-alpha-synuclein complex, could contribute to the development of anti-Parkinson drugs with unique specificity.

Keywords: alpha-synuclein, TPPP/p25, pathological assemblies, drug target, innovative therapy

1. Introduction

With the aging of society, neurological disorders have become more and more widespread resulting in serious social and economic problems. Parkinson's disease (PD) is the second most common neurodegenerative disease [1]. The etiology of this disease is initiated by unfolded/misfolded proteins, which form homologous and/or heterologous oligomers leading to the formation of aggregates and inclusions such as Lewy bodies predominantly comprised of alpha-synuclein (SYN) as histopathological hallmarks [1, 2].

At the present time, there is no proven therapy that can counteract the progression of the disease. The symptomatic therapies may reverse or slow down the progression of the symptoms, but cannot arrest/revert the neurodegenerative process [3]. The motor impairments of PD are attributed to the loss of dopaminergic neurons in the substantia nigra pars compacta; the phenotype is characterized by rigidity, resting tremor and bradykinesia [1]. The gold standard drug in the clinical practice is the L-dopa (or levodopa), precursor of dopamine, which relieves these motor symptoms by the replacement of the lost dopamine; however, large variability in drug response in terms of efficacy and adverse reactions have been observed [3, 4]. These side effects of conventional anti-parkinsonian drugs have compelled the researchers to seek novel alternatives such as gene therapy, stem cells transplants and neuroprotective agents [3]. The latest progression for the therapy suggests further opportunities (applications of antibodies, antisense-oligonucleotides and small molecules) that decrease the SYN level and its aggregation in the brain, some of them are now under clinical trials [3, 5].

One of the important factors in the PD research is related to the finding that SYN displays both physiological and pathological functions [5]; consequently, besides the specific and effective destruction of the accumulated SYN leading to the formation of its toxic assemblies/aggregations, the optimal SYN level has to be maintained/ensured for its physiological functions. In this chapter, the structural and functional potentials of SYN and Tubulin Polymerization Promoting Protein (TPPP/p25), hallmarks of PD [6], are reviewed leading to their molecular mechanism/pathomechanism in the initiation of PD and other synucleinopathies.

2. SYN and its physiological associations

SYN is an unstructured protein, prototype of the *chameleon* proteins [7]. Although the intrinsically disordered SYN is predominantly unfolded under physiological conditions, helically folded tetrameric structure or the combination of the two also have been suggested as its native structure [8]. In response to environmental changes, the disordered SYN is able to adopt significant conformational changes with different amount of secondary structures determined by pH, temperature, presence of organic solvents, membranes or specific metal ions [7, 9]. The structure of SYN have been studied in details under a plethora of distinct circumstances [10–12]. Structurally SYN comprises three regions: the N-terminal region involved in lipid binding; the highly hydrophobic central NAC region; and the acidic unfolded C-terminus, which exhibits chaperone activity and may counteract the aggregative potency of SYN [5, 13, 14] (**Figure 1**). The disordered C-terminal segment of SYN (45 aa) was found to modulate its aggregation, however, a terminal peptide (30 aa) was ineffective as a competitor in the aggregation process, which is characteristic for chameleon proteins [7].

The central hydrophobic region of SYN corresponding to residues 71–82 was found to be essential for its misfolding and aggregation, while a second critical region (residues 45–57) is of great importance in mediating β-strand to β-strand interactions in the fibril conformation [8]. Mutations are localized (18–53 aa) within the N-terminal region of SYN involved in lipid-binding. Based on comparative analysis of SYN structure, the 32–58 aa region was assigned as a crucial one to ensure the stability and secondary structure of SYN [15]. This issue is in agreement with another study which revealed the prominent role of a similar segment (39–45 aa) of the protein in membrane penetration [16]. SYN mutants with increased oligomerization efficacy are more inclined to penetrate the membrane [17].

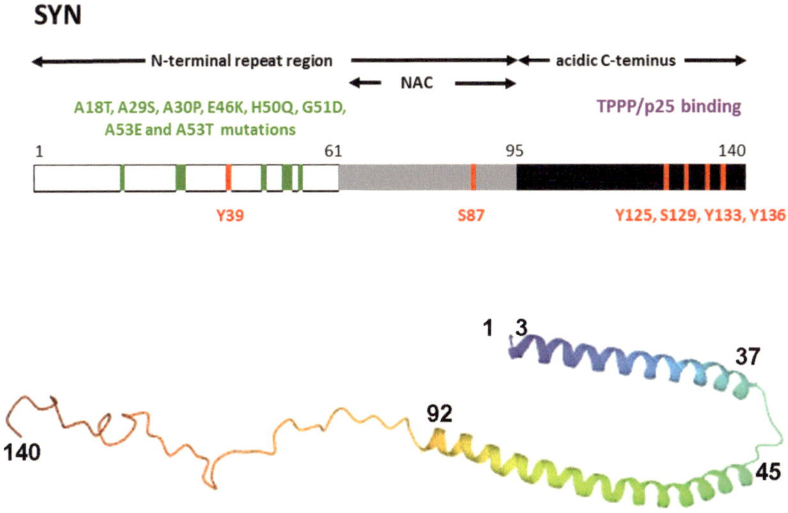

Figure 1.
Schematic representation of SYN. Familial mutations related to PD (green), and phosphorylation sites (red) are indicated. 3D structure of the human micelle-bound alpha-synuclein determined by NMR (DOI: 10.2210/pdb1XQ8/pdb) [14].

In normal brain, SYN binds to the surface of synaptic vesicles [5, 18]. Although it is highly disordered when isolated in solution; however, its micelle-bound form displays a partial helical structure that could be formed into curved α-helices [14, 19] (**Figure 1**). In spite of the data accumulated so far, the physiological function of SYN is still unclear in details. Membrane bound conformations of SYN are likely mediate its physiological function including the modulation of neuronal plasticity, synaptic vesicle pool maintenance, and dopamine metabolism [5, 13]. Moreover, it has been proposed that it can function as a microtubule regulatory protein (dynamase) [20–22]; as a disordered hub protein it also interacts with at least 50 ligands and other proteins [23].

The role of molecular chaperones in the regulation of the physiological function of SYN has been recently reviewed [24]. These interactions reduce the amount of free SYN in the cells and thus prevent its structural transition towards pathological states. Heat shock proteins (Hsp) are molecular chaperones that assist in proper conformational binding of proteins; they display protective effect against their toxicity and counteracts aggregation [25, 26]. SYN interacts with Hsp90 and Hsp70 as shown by co-immunoprecipitation [27]. The modulation of the proteolytic degradation of SYN by inhibiting Hsp90 function or by promoting Hsp70 function resulted in enhanced degradation of the aggregated protein. In fact, this issue has been suggested for treatment of PD against SYN toxicity [25]. Small molecules, which either directly interact with SYN or modulate molecular chaperones, were found to decrease SYN aggregation in vitro or in some animal models of PD; however, there is no clinical proof for their efficacy yet [25].

3. SYN mutations and pathological assemblies

SYN was the first identified causative gene of familial PD, all identified mutations can be found in the N-terminal region that affect the oligomerization, fibrillation and/or aggregation of SYN leading to the formation of the toxic species, see [1, 5, 6] and references therein. Until now, the following mutants have been identified to be involved in PD: A18T, A29S, A30P, E46K, H50Q, G51D, A53E and A53T [28] (**Figure 1**). There are mutants (A18T, A29S, E46K, H50Q and A53T) that increase SYN aggregation, others (G51D and A53E) slow down its aggregation; while the A30P mutation increases the oligomerization, yet hinders the fibrillation [29, 30]. G51D mutation, although the slowest to aggregate, is the most potent of the known early onset mutations supporting the hypothesis that increased lifetime of smaller oligomers can impart toxic effects [8]. The post-translational modifications, such as Ser129, Ser87 and Tyr125 phosphorylation, could also display various effects on the SYN assembly. The phosphorylation of SYN on Ser129 is negligible in normal brain, but it is the dominant form in Lewy bodies [31]. However, the effects of these modifications on the drug/ligand binding of SYN have not been clarified yet.

Two cellular pathways are involved in SYN clearance trying to maintain its physiological protein level: the ubiquitin-proteasome system (UPS) [32] and the autophagy-lysosomal pathway [33–35]. UPS is involved in proteolytic degradation of short-lived, damaged and misfolded protein; while the degradation of the long-lived and aggregated protein as well as that of the damaged organelles are achieved by macroautophagy (autophagy) and the selective chaperone-mediated autophagy (CMA) [36–38]. Macroautophagy degrades cellular waste through the fusion of the autophagosomes, carrying the material, with the lysosomes containing hydrolyses. Whereas CMA degrades soluble cytosolic proteins containing a specific CMA motif related to the pentapeptide KFERQ. The cytosolic chaperone heat-shock cognate 70 kDa protein (Hsc70) recognizes this motif, then it delivers the targeted protein to the lysosomes, and after binding to the lysosomal-associated membrane protein 2A (LAMP-2A), the targeted protein is translocated into the lysosomal lumen.

Genetic and post-mortem studies have suggested that modifications occur in both macroautophagy and CMA in the case of PD [39]. Mutations or post-translational modifications of SYN can also affect its turnover by CMA, such as the A30P and A53T mutants, related to familial cases of PD, which are not efficiently degraded through CMA, they can bind LAMP-2A, but are not internalized inside the lysosomes [40]. The protein level of the LAMP-2A, a key CMA marker, can be decreased in the substantia nigra of PD brains as compared to controls [41], while its protein level correlates with increased SYN accumulation in the affected PD brain regions.

The inhibition of the chaperone-SYN interaction facilitates the binding of SYN forming amphipathic helix into the lipid bilayer of the mitochondria membrane leading to membrane disruption [24]. SYN interaction with mitochondria occurs at higher protein expression or impaired chaperone-SYN ratio; therefore, the pathological conditions result in the failing of its CMA-derived proteolytic degradations [24]. Therapeutic strategies aiming to increase the SYN degradation through activation of these clearance pathways have thus been deeply explored in order to re-establish physiological levels of the protein and prevent its accumulation in PD [25, 42, 43]. The most interactions of SYN with mitochondria occur in cells in the case of oxidative stress [44] that can promote SYN aggregation associated with mitochondrial dysfunction [45, 46]. The localization of the enriched SYN on the mitochondrial membrane can produce destructive effect. Cellular oxidative stress is known to be a common factor driving synucleinopathy progression [44, 47].

Under oxidative stress conditions DJ-1, a cellular protease, is translocated from the cytoplasm to the mitochondria [48, 49]. DJ-1 is able to interact with both monomeric and oligomeric SYN counteracting its oligomerization propensity [50]. The crucial role of DJ-1 to control the aggregated SYN in proximity of mitochondria is also reflected by the fact that DJ-1 has been found in the proximity of Lewy bodies [51, 52]. Mutations within DJ-1 associated with PD reduce the capacity of DJ-1 to prevent toxic SYN assemblies [53–55]. The ability of DJ-1 to inhibit SYN aggregation appears to be dependent on the oxidation of its Cys106 residue (Cys_{106}-SO_2^- form) [50, 56, 57]. SYN overexpression activates CMA by elevating the levels of LAMP-2A; however, DJ-1 deficiency suppressed this effect. Experiments with DJ-1 knockout (KO) mice and DJ-1 siRNA knockdown SH-SY5Y cells confirmed that DJ-1 deficiency increased the accumulation and aggregation of SYN in both models, by accelerating the degradation of LAMP-2A, a lysosome-associated membrane protein. DJ-1 deficiency also downregulated the level of lysosomal Hsc70 [52]. These findings provide evidence for the molecular interaction between PD-related proteins via the CMA pathway.

In recent years, emerging evidence points out that microglial and astrocytic dysfunction may also play an important role in the pathogenesis of PD [40]. Several genes associated with PD are also expressed in glial cells, displaying comparable or even higher levels than in neurons, which are also involved in inflammatory response, oxidative stress, lysosomal and mitochondrial function, and autophagy. Perturbations in DJ-1 may alter different glial processes that can impact neuronal survival, DJ-1-deficient microglia displayed elevated intracellular reactive oxygen species and nitric oxide leading to increased dopaminergic neurotoxicity [58]. Recently it has been suggested that primary cortical astrocytes form DJ-1 KO mice may provide decreased neuroprotection to surrounding neurons due to alterations in pro-inflammatory mediator expression [52].

The cytoskeletal microtubule system plays a crucial role in several physiological and pathological processes which is achieved by the decoration of this filamentous network with proteins/enzymes as well as post-translational modifications [59]. The microtubule associated proteins/enzymes regulate these intracellular processes such as cell division, differentiation, autophagy, intracellular trafficking and aggresome formation by modulating microtubule dynamics and stability. Destabilization of the microtubule network, low tubulin acetylation levels and axonal transport deficits have been observed in PD [60, 61]. SYN has been described as a microtubule dynamase [21] and it also interacts with microtubule stabilizing proteins such as tau and TPPP/p25 [22, 59]. SYN binds within the microtubule-binding domain of tau and may promote its hyperphosphorylation resulting in impaired axonal transport [62]. The microtubule associated tau and TPPP/p25 stabilize the microtubule network [22, 59].

4. TPPP/p25, a multifunctional microtubule associated protein

Physiologically, TPPP/p25 modulates the dynamics and stability of the microtubule network by bundling the microtubules and enhancing the tubulin acetylation due to the inhibition of tubulin deacetylases [59, 63]. In normal brain, TPPP/p25 is expressed in oligodendrocytes (OLGs) and a key factor in the growth of projections in the course of differentiation requested for the axon ensheathment [64]. Therefore, the optimal endogenous TPPP/p25 level plays key physiological functions in the formation of differentiated OLGs, which are key players in myelin sheath formation.

TPPP/p25 is an intrinsically disordered protein without a well-defined 3D structure, whose middle, highly flexible CORE region is straddled by the unstructured N- and C-termini [65] (**Figure 2**). Two human gene sequences have been identified, which encode homologous proteins displaying approximately 60% identity with TPPP/p25. These proteins are N-terminal-free forms denoted as TPPP/p18 and TPPP/p20 [66]. The similarity of TPPP/p25 to TPPP/p20 is manifested in their intrinsically disordered characteristics and association to microtubules [66]. 3D

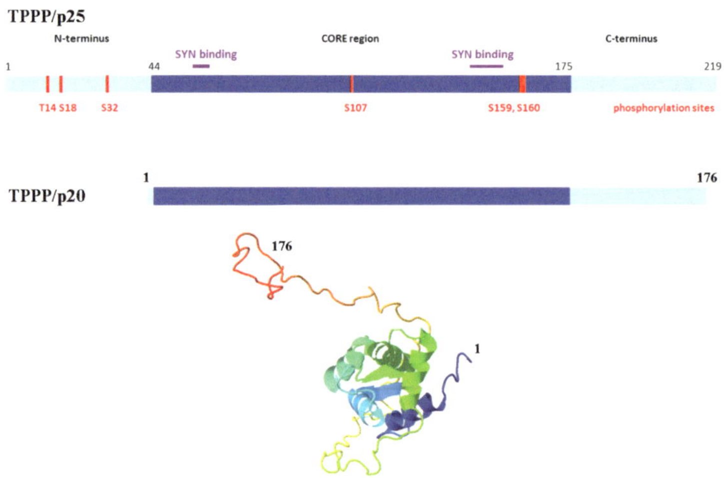

Figure 2.
Schematic representation of TPPP/p25. Phosphorylation sites (red) are indicated. 3D structure of the homologous TPPP/p20 determined by NMR (DOI: 10.2210/pdb2JRF/pdb) [67].

structure of TPPP/p20, but not TPPP/p25, has been determined by NMR (from TPPP/p20 the unfolded N-terminal tail of TPPP/p25 is missing) [67]. TPPP/p20 is involved in developmental processes of the musculoskeletal system [68], and surprisingly, not in neurodegenerative, rather in cancerous processes due to its modulation of the cell proliferation, see [59] and references therein.

TPPP/p25 occurs in monomeric and dimeric forms, the dimeric form displays enhanced tubulin polymerization promoting activity [69]. The UPS is the major system responsible for the elimination of the disordered TPPP/p25 suggested by the finding that MG132, a well-established inhibitor of proteasome, enhanced the intracellular TPPP/p25 level [70, 71]. The stabilization of TPPP/p25 against the proteolytic degradation is resulted from the structural changes of the protein coupled with its dimerization which is essential for the maintenance of the stability of the myelin sheath.

The forms of plasticity of synapsis within the OLG lineage as well as the connection of the OLG and myelin dysfunction in neurodevelopmental disorders with cognitive symptoms have recently been described [72]. The OLG precursor cells proliferate and some of them differentiate. A subset of these new OLGs integrates into sheaths on unmyelinated axon segments. In this process, TPPP/p25 could be a key player since its endogenous expression is involved in the differentiation of the dividing progenitor cells under post-transcriptional control [64]. In the course of this process, the plasticity of the myelin sheath might be modified.

Recently in has been shown that TPPP/p25 KO mice have shorter lamellar microtubules, and consequently shorter and thinner myelin sheaths [73]. Cultured TPPP/p25 KO OLGs also displayed additional aberrant features, including more proximal branches, mixed microtubule polarity and accumulation of myelin basic protein mRNA. In the brain of these mice, decreased myelination have been observed, although no gross differences were found in neurofilament staining, indicating that axonal tracts and neuronal morphology is largely intact [73]. Concerning the behavior of TPPP/25 KO mice, their anxiety behavior has been similar as in the case of wild type mice, however, they lack fear responses. Deficits in fear-conditioning, which is a memory dependent task, as well as in spatial memory tests support possible short-term memory defects [74]. Experiments with TPPP/p25 KO mice that exhibit hypomyelination with aberrant myelin sheaths and motor coordination deficits have suggested that microtubule nucleation outside the cell body at Golgi outposts by TPPP/p25 is critical for the elongation of the myelin sheath [73]. In fact, elevation of the TPPP/p25 level was detected in rat brain in the course of aging [75], however, it is unclear whether it is due to increased demand or aberrant accumulation. The latter issue may be related to the development of different neurological disorders such as Alzheimer's disease (AD), PD, multiple system atrophy (MSA) and diffuse Lewy body disease (DLBD); however, increased TPPP/p25 level was detected with remyelinating lesions in the case of multiple sclerosis [76].

5. From TPPP/p25-SYN interaction to their co-localization in Lewy body

TPPP/p25, as a *moonlighting* protein, performs distinct functions under physiological and pathological conditions without alterations at gene level [77]. This feature of TPPP/p25 manifested primarily itself in its association with SYN, the hallmark of PD. Pathologically, TPPP/p25 interacts with SYN resulting in its oligomerization/aggregation [78]. Studies with various truncated and deletion mutants of the human TPPP/p25 produced by recombinant techniques revealed significantly reduced, but not abolished interaction with SYN [79, 80]. These findings indicated that the lack of identified binding segments of the wild type TPPP/p25 could be replaced by other segments [81]. Although it has been well-established that SYN is also a disordered protein; notwithstanding, the *neomorphic chameleon* characteristic was introduced for TPPP/p25 to indicate the distinction of the two disordered proteins. Namely, the modifications of TPPP/p25 at gene level is able to maintain its associative potency [81]; in contrast to this, the deletion of the last 20 amino acid residues of SYN abolished its interaction with TPPP/p25 [80].

The unfolded SYN and TPPP/p25 are expressed distinctly in neurons [82, 83] and OLGs [64, 75], respectively, in healthy brain; however, they are co-enriched and co-localized in pathological inclusions in the cases of PD and MSA [84]. The interaction of SYN and TPPP/p25 has been proven at atomic, molecular and cellular levels as well as in post-mortem brain tissues [6, 59]. Short peptide fragments have been produced by proteolytic degradation of the interacting proteins as well as by chemical synthesis based upon the interface segments identified experimentally using the wild type proteins [79, 80]. The interactive and aggregative potencies of the wild type and truncated forms of SYN and/or TPPP/p25 were visualized by immunofluorescence microscopy (**Figure 3**). Massive co-aggregation of the two hallmark proteins were achieved by the contact surface-containing fragments instead of the full proteins.

The interaction of TPPP/p25 with SYN has been extensively characterized at atomic, molecular, cellular and tissue levels using wild type and mutant human recombinant proteins and living human cell models [6, 59, 85]. The interaction of SYN and TPPP/p25 in living cells was visualized by immunofluorescent confocal microscopy coupled with Bifunctional Fluorescent Complementation (BiFC) technology using mVenus vectors [81]. The immunofluorescence images presented in **Figure 4** verify the hetero-association of TPPP/p25 and SYN at cellular level; the hetero-association (green fluorescence) is reduced due to the addition of unlabeled TPPP/p25 as a competitor, which provides evidence for the dynamic and specific association of the two disordered proteins [81].

The hetero-association induced by the excess SYN and TPPP/p25 results in the appearance of massive aggregates [79–81]. The co-enrichment and co-localization of TPPP/p25 and SYN specific for synucleinopathies were established in post-mortem human brain tissues of patients with PD and other neurological disorders (**Figure 5**). TPPP/p25 is enriched in filamentous SYN bearing Lewy bodies of PD

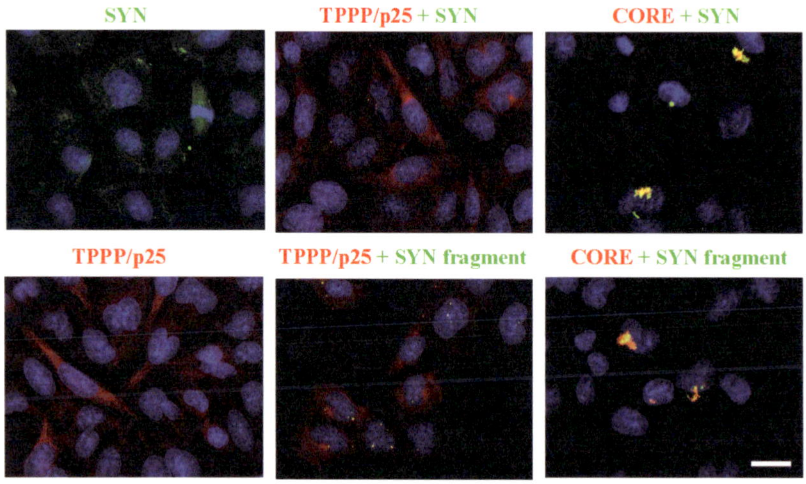

Figure 3.
Intracellular co-enrichment and co-localization of wild type SYN and TPPP/p25 as well as their fragments in CHO10 cells [80]. Uptake of SYN and/or TPPP/p25 by CHO10 cells from the medium following their premixing as detected by immunofluorescence microscopy. Nuclei were counterstained with 4,6-diamidino-2-phenylindole (blue). Scale bar: 5 μm.

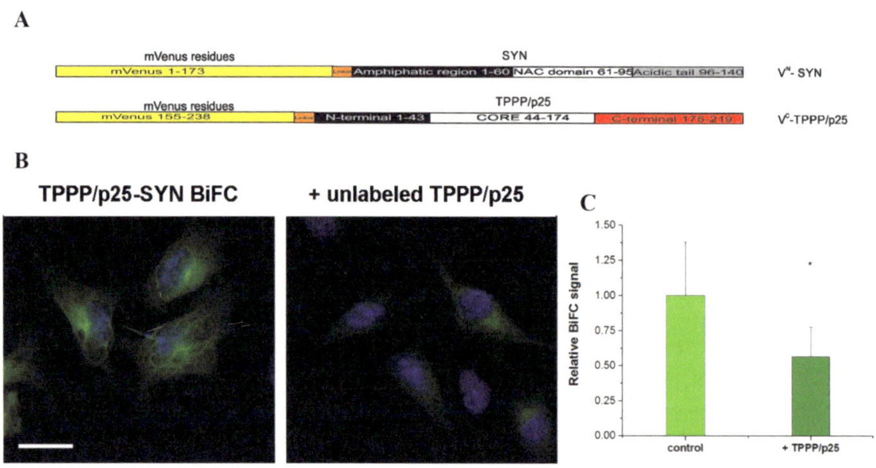

Figure 4.
Dynamic association of TPPP/p25 with SYN in living HeLa cells as visualized by BiFC technology [81]. (A) Scheme of BiFC constructs for co-transfection of TPPP/p25 and SYN. (B): Visualization of the association of mV^{N}-SYN and V^{C}-TPPP/p25 (green). Effect of the unlabeled TPPP/p25 on the association of TPPP/p25 with SYN (BiFC) signal. Bar: 10 μm. (C) Quantification of the relative BiFC signal.

and DLBD, as well as in glial inclusions of MSA [84]. In contrast to synucleinopathies, no co-localization was found between TPPP/p25 and phosphorylated tau in inclusions of Pick's disease (PiD), progressive supranuclear palsy (PSP), and corticobasal degeneration (CBD). It is worth noting that clustered immunoreactivity of TPPP/p25 was found along filaments of unstructured but not compact neurofibrillary tangles in the case of AD. Based on these findings TPPP/p25 was suggested to be a novel marker of alpha-synucleinopathies [84].

Co-immunoprecipitation analysis carried out on HEK293T and oligodendroglial KG1C cell lines with ectopically expressed SYN and TPPP/p25 corroborated the specific interaction of the two proteins; moreover, TPPP/p25 is able to induce SYN oligomerization [86, 87]. Recently an oligodendroglial cell model of MSA has been studied, in which after the overexpression of TPPP/p25 and uptake of human

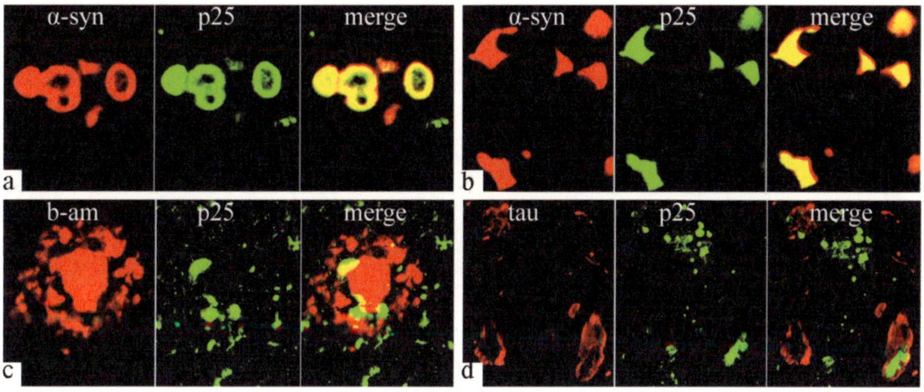

Figure 5.
SYN and TPPP/p25 in post-mortem brain samples in the cases of PD (a), MSA (b), DLBD and AD (c) and AD (d), respectively [84].

pre-formed SYN fibrils, the cells formed insoluble, highly aggregated, pathological assemblies [86]. Mavroeidi and his co-workers have also revealed that these assemblies resulted in the disruption of the microtubule and myelin networks [86] indicating the toxic potential of the pathological TPPP/p25-SYN assembly. In addition, the formation of the glial cytoplasmic inclusion was suggested due to the endogenously expressed hallmark proteins. In the case of MSA, early relocation of TPPP/p25 (from the myelin sheath and the nucleus to the cytoplasm) has been observed [88, 89].

In normal brain SYN and TPPP/p25 are expressed predominantly in neurons and in OLGs, respectively [64, 75, 82, 83]. However, these two hallmark proteins are co-enriched and co-localized in Lewy bodies and glial cytoplasmic inclusions characteristic for PD and MSA, respectively [84, 87, 90]. The intra- and extracellular transmission of SYN forms between neurons as well as between neurons and OLGs in the case of PD and MSA has been established [91, 92]. In addition, the presence of both proteins in the extracellular space has been reported inasmuch as their occurrence in the cerebrospinal fluid (CSF) [93–95], their cellular uptake from the medium were also detected [79, 96]. Consequently, the cell-to-cell transmission as a pathological situation can be mimicked in cells models such as HeLa by taking up SYN and/or TPPP/p25 from the medium [79–81].

The mechanism of this process is unclear yet, however, the liberation of the endocytosed materials in the cytoplasm by the mechanism of "endosomal escape" to reach autophagic vacuole has been proposed [97]. This mechanism could take place in the case with the exogenously applied SYN and/or TPPP/p25. Endocytosis has a special relevance in the brain, because of its involvement in neurotransmitter and neurotrophic signaling. Since neuronal cells are highly polarized, they require a highly specialized and complex endocytic machinery. Alterations in this complex system have also been described in PD [40]. Besides conventional endocytosis, exosomal transport, receptor-mediated internalization, passive diffusion, or even direct penetration of the plasma membrane have been suggested as possible pathways for SYN uptake [98].

6. Innovative strategy for PD and MSA therapy

In a recent review Devos and co-workers have reported that "Despite decades of successful preclinical neuroprotective studies, no drug has then shown efficacy in clinical trials." [99]. According to this and other publications, effective neuroprotective therapy is still an unmet need both in PD and MSA. Symptomatic treatments are available, although MSA patients usually show poor l-Dopa responsiveness [100]. Concerning possible disease-modifying therapies, the following strategies are under clinical trials: targeting SYN pathology such as active and passive immunization, anti-aggregative small molecules, RNA interference techniques and an increase in SYN clearance, intervening neuroinflammation or neuronal loss (by stem cells) [25, 92, 100–102]. Remyelinating molecules are also being tested in clinical trials in the case of MSA, since this disease is accompanied by myelin loss as well [100].

A recently reported innovative strategy is based upon the effective and specific inhibition/destruction of the pathological TPPP/p25-SYN complex/assembly by peptide fragments of the partner proteins [81]. The highly flexible foldamers that can recognize oligomers and proteins are among potential therapeutics. These foldamers are endowed with variable pharmacokinetic properties; nonetheless, their constructions with suitable recognition surfaces are still challenging; they have to display contiguous recognition surface or long sequences with broadly distributed recognition contacts, see [103] and references therein. Foldamer-based protein mimetics have been designed by following the principles of multivalent biomolecule-recognizing ligands [103, 104]. In fact, the fragment-based foldamer approach displays unnatural protein mimetics that are capable of specific molecular recognition and inhibition of multifunctional target.

The recognition that the TPPP/p25-derived SYN aggregation is involved in the pathomechanism of the synucleionopathies, but not in that of the tauopathies, underlined that the TPPP/p25-SYN complex is a potential drug target [79–81]. However, the complex as a whole could not be considered as an optimal drug target since both proteins display physiological functions as well, but the interface of their complex occurring only under pathological conditions was proposed to be an excellent target. Thus, the interface of the complex of the two hallmark proteins has been validated at molecular and cellular levels [79–81]. The binding segments of TPPP/p25 involved in its interaction with SYN was identified (147–156 aa) [79–81] (**Figure 6**). The interface has been considered as a potential drug target, which is found to be distinct from the physiological TPPP/p25-tubulin one (178–187 aa). These findings showed the role of the middle, CORE region of TPPP/p25 in the formation of the pathological TPPP/p25-SYN complex; in addition, the stable complex was created by the interaction between the two unstructured proteins with sufficient avidity. Thus, short peptide fragments by targeting the interface of the pathological complex could function as potential anti-Parkinson agents.

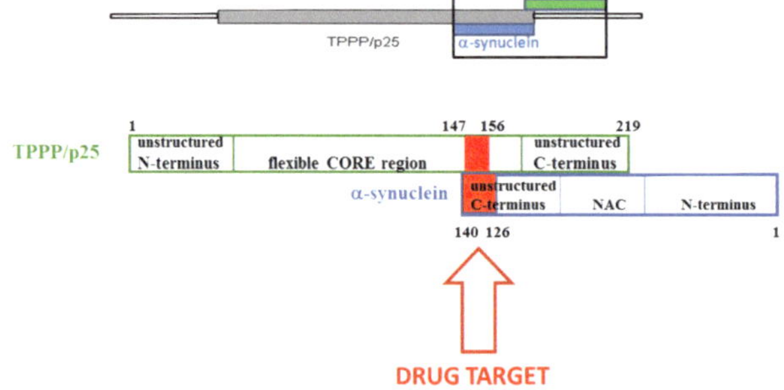

Figure 6.
Distinct segments of TPPP/p25 involved in the physiological (tubulin) and pathological (SYN) interactions. Identified interface segments of the pathological TPPP/p25-SYN complex [6, 79].

The effectiveness of these fragments can be tested by in vitro competition experiments by ELISA using human recombinant proteins and by BiFC approach coupled by fluorescence microscopy [79–81]. The inhibition of the direct association of SYN with TPPP/p25 can be visualized and the inhibitory effect of the fragments can be quantified by the reduction of the fluorescence signal (green). This two-steps-assay seems to be applicable to screen potential drug-like molecules for their anti-Parkinson activity. The innovative interface-targeting methodology allows one to further develop it to disease-related/unrelated interface targeting.

The recognition of the endogenous expression of SYN and TPPP/p25 in neurons and OLGs, respectively, offers opportunity for the selective influence of PD and MSA such as disease-dependent interface targeting of the pathological TPPP/p25-SYN complex. Let us consider the specific interface-targeting fragments that can inhibit and/or destruct the TPPP/p25-SYN assemblies. The nature of the interface fragments for elimination of the pathological complex has to be determined by their origin (TPPP/p25 or SYN fragments).

As illustrated in the scheme (**Figure 7**), in the case of PD the inclusions are formed predominantly in neurons, SYN, and not TPPP/p25, is expressed endogenously in these cells; in this situation a TPPP/p25 fragment can be effective to destruct the pathological complex in neurons without displaying side effects. Conversely, for the treatment of MSA, when the inclusions are formed in OLGs that express endogenously TPPP/p25, it is expected that SYN-based fragments could be effective to diminish the co-assemblies of SYN and TPPP/p25 in OLGs and no unwanted side effect occurs. These issues are based upon the recognition that TPPP/p25 is enriched in Lewy bodies of neurons exclusively in the case of PD, while SYN accumulates in OLGs in cytoplasmic inclusions according to the etiology of MSA.

PD, DLBD and MSA have some common features such as inclusion bodies comprised of SYN and TPPP/p25 as well as decline in motor, cognitive, behavioral and autonomic functions. However, these diseases may be distinguished based on affected cell types and brain structures, the relative onset and prognosis [105, 106]. Cognitive impairment precedes parkinsonism in the case of DLBD, while PD dementia starts 1 year or more after the diagnosis of PD; DLBD patients show more profound cognitive impairments. Approximately ~30% of MSA patients also suffers from cognitive impairment, in particular executive dysfunction. The hippocampus is one of the most vulnerable brain regions affected

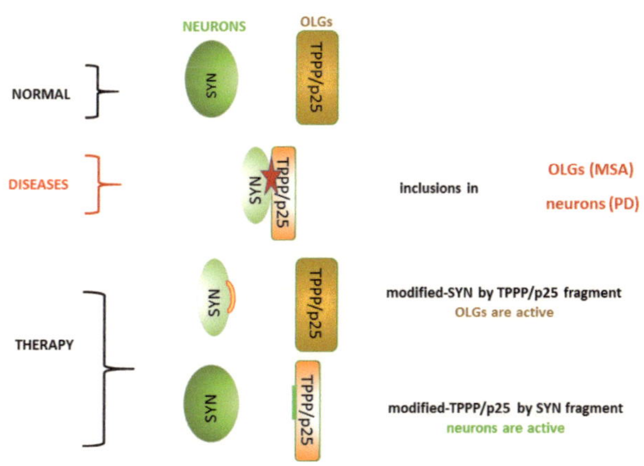

Figure 7.
Disease-dependent interface targeting of the pathological TPPP/p25-SYN complex. Targeting the interface by SYN or TPPP/p25 fragments for MSA and PD therapies.

by synucleinopathies, and its dysfunction may result in cognitive deficits and depression. Oligomerization/aggregation of SYN was found to induce deficits in synaptic transmission and hippocampal neurogenesis, which may contribute to the appearance of cognitive deficits. Short-term memory defects have also been observed in TPPP/p25 KO mice, which exhibit hypomyelination [73, 74]. Recently it has been proposed that OLGs and myelin sheaths play crucial roles in memory and learning [72].

Clinically, the differentiation between PD and MSA is challenging, especially at the early stages of diseases [107]. In contrast to PD, no causal SYN mutations for MSA have been found to date. However, neuropathological hallmarks of both MSA and PD could be observed in the case of the G51D SYN mutant [108]. Two possible scenarios have been proposed to explain the origin of SYN in OLGs and SYN accumulation in glial cytoplasmic inclusions characteristic for MSA brains: either OLGs overexpress SYN under pathological conditions or they take up the neuronal protein from their environment, such as CSF [98]. The latter one, the cell-to-cell transmission has been proven. Recent studies have suggested that the SYN structures/aggregates formed in the cases of different synucleinopathies are distinct that could contribute to the discrimination between PD and MSA [107]. Nevertheless, it is important to notice that the aggregated structures amplified from CSF were similar to those ones amplified from the brain [107]. Biomarkers in CSF, such as phosphorylated/total tau, SYN and β-amyloid$_{1-42}$, can be useful to distinguish PD or MSA patients from healthy controls, and SYN and total-tau could also be used to distinguish between MSA from PD [109]. The analysis of the hallmark TPPP/p25 occurring in the CSF and inclusions of patients might provide more unambiguous information about the nature of synucleinopathies.

Acknowledgements

This work was supported by the Hungarian National Research, Development and Innovation Office Grants OTKA [K-112144 and PD-124061] to J. Ovádi and T. Szénási, the Richter Gedeon Nyrt granted project 6567-19 403 VT (2018-2020) to J. Ovádi, and János Bolyai Research Scholarship of the Hungarian Academy of Sciences to J. Oláh, respectively.

Conflict of interest

The authors declare no conflict of interest.

Abbreviations

SYN	alpha-synuclein
AD	Alzheimer's disease
BiFC	bifunctional fluorescent complementation
CSF	cerebrospinal fluid
CMA	chaperone-mediated autophagy
CBD	corticobasal degeneration
DLBD	diffuse Lewy body disease
Hsc70	heat-shock cognate 70 kDa protein
Hsp	heat shock proteins
LAMP-2A	lysosomal-associated membrane protein 2A

MSA	multiple system atrophy
OLG	oligodendrocyte
PD	Parkinson's disease
PiD	Pick's disease
PSP	progressive supranuclear palsy
TPPP/p25	Tubulin Polymerization Promoting Protein
UPS	ubiquitin-proteasome system

Author details

Judit Oláh, Attila Lehotzky, Tibor Szénási and Judit Ovádi*
Institute of Enzymology, Research Center for Natural Sciences, Eötvös Loránd Research Network, Budapest, Hungary

*Address all correspondence to: ovadi.judit@ttk.hu

References

[1] Kalia LV, Lang AE. Parkinson's disease. Lancet. 2015;386(9996):896-912.

[2] Spillantini MG, Schmidt ML, Lee VM, Trojanowski JQ, Jakes R, Goedert M. Alpha-synuclein in Lewy bodies. Nature. 1997;388(6645):839-840.

[3] Oertel W, Schulz JB. Current and experimental treatments of Parkinson disease: A guide for neuroscientists. Journal of neurochemistry. 2016;139 Suppl 1:325-337.

[4] Politi C, Ciccacci C, Novelli G, Borgiani P. Genetics and Treatment Response in Parkinson's Disease: An Update on Pharmacogenetic Studies. Neuromolecular medicine. 2018;20(1):1-17.

[5] Mochizuki H, Choong CJ, Masliah E. A refined concept: alpha-synuclein dysregulation disease. Neurochemistry international. 2018;119:84-96.

[6] Olah J, Ovadi J. Pharmacological targeting of alpha-synuclein and TPPP/p25 in Parkinson's disease: challenges and opportunities in a Nutshell. FEBS letters. 2019;593(13):1641-1653.

[7] Uversky VN. A protein-chameleon: conformational plasticity of alpha-synuclein, a disordered protein involved in neurodegenerative disorders. J Biomol Struct Dyn. 2003;21(2):211-234.

[8] Meade RM, Fairlie DP, Mason JM. Alpha-synuclein structure and Parkinson's disease - lessons and emerging principles. Molecular neurodegeneration. 2019;14(1):29.

[9] Silva BA, Breydo L, Uversky VN. Targeting the chameleon: a focused look at alpha-synuclein and its roles in neurodegeneration. Molecular neurobiology. 2013;47(2):446-459.

[10] Surguchov A. Synucleins: are they two-edged swords? J Neurosci Res. 2013;91(2):161-166.

[11] Alderson TR, Markley JL. Biophysical characterization of alpha-synuclein and its controversial structure. Intrinsically Disord Proteins. 2013;1(1):18-39.

[12] Fauvet B, Mbefo MK, Fares MB, Desobry C, Michael S, Ardah MT, et al. alpha-Synuclein in central nervous system and from erythrocytes, mammalian cells, and Escherichia coli exists predominantly as disordered monomer. The Journal of biological chemistry. 2012;287(19):15345-15364.

[13] Bellucci A, Mercuri NB, Venneri A, Faustini G, Longhena F, Pizzi M, et al. Review: Parkinson's disease: from synaptic loss to connectome dysfunction. Neuropathology and applied neurobiology. 2016;42(1):77-94.

[14] Ulmer TS, Bax A, Cole NB, Nussbaum RL. Structure and dynamics of micelle-bound human alpha-synuclein. The Journal of biological chemistry. 2005;280(10):9595-9603.

[15] Siddiqui IJ, Pervaiz N, Abbasi AA. The Parkinson Disease gene SNCA: Evolutionary and structural insights with pathological implication. Scientific reports. 2016;6:24475.

[16] Tsigelny IF, Sharikov Y, Kouznetsova VL, Greenberg JP, Wrasidlo W, Overk C, et al. Molecular determinants of alpha-synuclein mutants' oligomerization and membrane interactions. ACS chemical neuroscience. 2015;6(3):403-416.

[17] Afitska K, Fucikova A, Shvadchak VV, Yushchenko DA. Modification of C Terminus Provides New Insights into the Mechanism of alpha-Synuclein Aggregation. Biophysical journal. 2017;113(10):2182-2191.

[18] Bisaglia M, Mammi S, Bubacco L. Structural insights on physiological functions and pathological effects of alpha-synuclein. FASEB journal : official publication of the Federation of American Societies for Experimental Biology. 2009;23(2):329-340.

[19] Borbat P, Ramlall TF, Freed JH, Eliezer D. Inter-helix distances in lysophospholipid micelle-bound alpha-synuclein from pulsed ESR measurements. Journal of the American Chemical Society. 2006;128(31):10004-10005.

[20] Toba S, Jin M, Yamada M, Kumamoto K, Matsumoto S, Yasunaga T, et al. Alpha-synuclein facilitates to form short unconventional microtubules that have a unique function in the axonal transport. Scientific reports. 2017;7(1):16386.

[21] Cartelli D, Aliverti A, Barbiroli A, Santambrogio C, Ragg EM, Casagrande FV, et al. alpha-Synuclein is a Novel Microtubule Dynamase. Scientific reports. 2016;6:33289.

[22] Carnwath T, Mohammed R, Tsiang D. The direct and indirect effects of alpha-synuclein on microtubule stability in the pathogenesis of Parkinson's disease. Neuropsychiatric disease and treatment. 2018;14:1685-1695.

[23] Dev KK, Hofele K, Barbieri S, Buchman VL, van der Putten H. Part II: alpha-synuclein and its molecular pathophysiological role in neurodegenerative disease. Neuropharmacology. 2003;45(1): 14-44.

[24] Aspholm EE, Matecko-Burmann I, Burmann BM. Keeping alpha-Synuclein at Bay: A More Active Role of Molecular Chaperones in Preventing Mitochondrial Interactions and Transition to Pathological States? Life. 2020;10(11).

[25] Teil M, Arotcarena ML, Faggiani E, Laferriere F, Bezard E, Dehay B. Targeting alpha-synuclein for PD Therapeutics: A Pursuit on All Fronts. Biomolecules. 2020;10(3).

[26] Saibil H. Chaperone machines for protein folding, unfolding and disaggregation. Nature reviews Molecular cell biology. 2013;14(10):630-642.

[27] Uryu K, Richter-Landsberg C, Welch W, Sun E, Goldbaum O, Norris EH, et al. Convergence of heat shock protein 90 with ubiquitin in filamentous alpha-synuclein inclusions of alpha-synucleinopathies. The American journal of pathology. 2006;168(3):947-961.

[28] Rosborough K, Patel N, Kalia LV. alpha-Synuclein and Parkinsonism: Updates and Future Perspectives. Current neurology and neuroscience reports. 2017;17(4):31.

[29] Ranjan P, Kumar A. Perturbation in Long-Range Contacts Modulates the Kinetics of Amyloid Formation in alpha-Synuclein Familial Mutants. ACS chemical neuroscience. 2017;8(10):2235-2246.

[30] Lazaro DF, Rodrigues EF, Langohr R, Shahpasandzadeh H, Ribeiro T, Guerreiro P, et al. Systematic comparison of the effects of alpha-synuclein mutations on its oligomerization and aggregation. PLoS genetics. 2014;10(11):e1004741.

[31] Fujiwara H, Hasegawa M, Dohmae N, Kawashima A, Masliah E, Goldberg MS, et al. alpha-Synuclein is phosphorylated in synucleinopathy lesions. Nature cell biology. 2002;4(2):160-164.

[32] Beyer K, Domingo-Sabat M, Ariza A. Molecular pathology of Lewy body diseases. International journal of molecular sciences. 2009;10(3):724-745.

[33] Webb JL, Ravikumar B, Atkins J, Skepper JN, Rubinsztein DC. Alpha-Synuclein is degraded by both autophagy and the proteasome. The Journal of biological chemistry. 2003;278(27):25009-25013.

[34] Cuervo AM, Stefanis L, Fredenburg R, Lansbury PT, Sulzer D. Impaired degradation of mutant alpha-synuclein by chaperone-mediated autophagy. Science. 2004;305(5688):1292-1295.

[35] Lee HJ, Khoshaghideh F, Patel S, Lee SJ. Clearance of alpha-synuclein oligomeric intermediates via the lysosomal degradation pathway. The Journal of neuroscience : the official journal of the Society for Neuroscience. 2004;24(8):1888-1896.

[36] Lamb CA, Yoshimori T, Tooze SA. The autophagosome: origins unknown, biogenesis complex. Nature reviews Molecular cell biology. 2013;14(12):759-774.

[37] Lilienbaum A. Relationship between the proteasomal system and autophagy. International journal of biochemistry and molecular biology. 2013;4(1):1-26.

[38] Nedelsky NB, Todd PK, Taylor JP. Autophagy and the ubiquitin-proteasome system: collaborators in neuroprotection. Biochimica et biophysica acta. 2008;1782(12):691-699.

[39] Arotcarena ML, Teil M, Dehay B. Autophagy in Synucleinopathy: The Overwhelmed and Defective Machinery. Cells. 2019;8(6).

[40] Navarro-Romero A, Montpeyo M, Martinez-Vicente M. The Emerging Role of the Lysosome in Parkinson's Disease. Cells. 2020;9(11).

[41] Alvarez-Erviti L, Rodriguez-Oroz MC, Cooper JM, Caballero C, Ferrer I, Obeso JA, et al. Chaperone-mediated autophagy markers in Parkinson disease brains. Archives of neurology. 2010;67(12):1464-1472.

[42] Parekh P, Sharma N, Gadepalli A, Shahane A, Sharma M, Khairnar A. A Cleaning Crew: The Pursuit of Autophagy in Parkinson's Disease. ACS chemical neuroscience. 2019;10(9):3914-3926.

[43] Mputhia Z, Hone E, Tripathi T, Sargeant T, Martins R, Bharadwaj P. Autophagy Modulation as a Treatment of Amyloid Diseases. Molecules. 2019;24(18).

[44] Barnham KJ, Masters CL, Bush AI. Neurodegenerative diseases and oxidative stress. Nature reviews Drug discovery. 2004;3(3):205-214.

[45] Binolfi A, Limatola A, Verzini S, Kosten J, Theillet FX, Rose HM, et al. Intracellular repair of oxidation-damaged alpha-synuclein fails to target C-terminal modification sites. Nature communications. 2016;7:10251.

[46] Park JH, Burgess JD, Faroqi AH, DeMeo NN, Fiesel FC, Springer W, et al. Alpha-synuclein-induced mitochondrial dysfunction is mediated via a sirtuin 3-dependent pathway. Molecular neurodegeneration. 2020;15(1):5.

[47] Lashuel HA, Overk CR, Oueslati A, Masliah E. The many faces of alpha-synuclein: from structure and toxicity to therapeutic target. Nature reviews Neuroscience. 2013;14(1):38-48.

[48] Bolliger L, Junne T, Schatz G, Lithgow T. Acidic receptor domains on both sides of the outer membrane mediate translocation of precursor proteins into yeast mitochondria. The EMBO journal. 1995;14(24):6318-6326.

[49] Dolgacheva LP, Sirota TV, Teplova VV. [Participation of a Ca^{2+}–binding glycoprotein with a molecular weight of 40 kDa in the electrogenic Ca^{2+} transport

system in mitochondria]. Biofizika. 1994;39(6):1029-1032.

[50] Zondler L, Miller-Fleming L, Repici M, Goncalves S, Tenreiro S, Rosado-Ramos R, et al. DJ-1 interactions with alpha-synuclein attenuate aggregation and cellular toxicity in models of Parkinson's disease. Cell death & disease. 2014;5:e1350.

[51] Jin J, Meredith GE, Chen L, Zhou Y, Xu J, Shie FS, et al. Quantitative proteomic analysis of mitochondrial proteins: relevance to Lewy body formation and Parkinson's disease. Brain research Molecular brain research. 2005;134(1):119-138.

[52] Xu CY, Kang WY, Chen YM, Jiang TF, Zhang J, Zhang LN, et al. DJ-1 Inhibits alpha-Synuclein Aggregation by Regulating Chaperone-Mediated Autophagy. Frontiers in aging neuroscience. 2017;9:308.

[53] Malgieri G, Eliezer D. Structural effects of Parkinson's disease linked DJ-1 mutations. Protein science : a publication of the Protein Society. 2008;17(5):855-868.

[54] Repici M, Straatman KR, Balduccio N, Enguita FJ, Outeiro TF, Giorgini F. Parkinson's disease-associated mutations in DJ-1 modulate its dimerization in living cells. Journal of molecular medicine. 2013;91(5):599-611.

[55] Moore DJ, Zhang L, Troncoso J, Lee MK, Hattori N, Mizuno Y, et al. Association of DJ-1 and parkin mediated by pathogenic DJ-1 mutations and oxidative stress. Human molecular genetics. 2005;14(1):71-84.

[56] Shendelman S, Jonason A, Martinat C, Leete T, Abeliovich A. DJ-1 is a redox-dependent molecular chaperone that inhibits alpha-synuclein aggregate formation. PLoS biology. 2004;2(11):e362.

[57] Kumar R, Kumar S, Hanpude P, Singh AK, Johari T, Majumder S, et al. Partially oxidized DJ-1 inhibits alpha-synuclein nucleation and remodels mature alpha-synuclein fibrils in vitro. Communications biology. 2019;2:395.

[58] Ashley AK, Hinds AI, Hanneman WH, Tjalkens RB, Legare ME. DJ-1 mutation decreases astroglial release of inflammatory mediators. Neurotoxicology. 2016;52:198-203.

[59] Olah J, Lehotzky A, Szunyogh S, Szenasi T, Orosz F, Ovadi J. Microtubule-Associated Proteins with Regulatory Functions by Day and Pathological Potency at Night. Cells. 2020;9(2).

[60] Cartelli D, Cappelletti G. Microtubule Destabilization Paves the Way to Parkinson's Disease. Molecular neurobiology. 2017;54(9):6762-6774.

[61] Pellegrini L, Wetzel A, Granno S, Heaton G, Harvey K. Back to the tubule: microtubule dynamics in Parkinson's disease. Cellular and molecular life sciences : CMLS. 2017;74(3):409-434.

[62] Jensen PH, Hager H, Nielsen MS, Hojrup P, Gliemann J, Jakes R. alpha-synuclein binds to Tau and stimulates the protein kinase A-catalyzed tau phosphorylation of serine residues 262 and 356. The Journal of biological chemistry. 1999;274(36):25481-25489.

[63] Hlavanda E, Kovacs J, Olah J, Orosz F, Medzihradszky KF, Ovadi J. Brain-specific p25 protein binds to tubulin and microtubules and induces aberrant microtubule assemblies at substoichiometric concentrations. Biochemistry. 2002;41(27):8657-8664.

[64] Lehotzky A, Lau P, Tokesi N, Muja N, Hudson LD, Ovadi J. Tubulin polymerization-promoting protein (TPPP/p25) is critical for

oligodendrocyte differentiation. Glia. 2010;58(2):157-168.

[65] Zotter A, Bodor A, Olah J, Hlavanda E, Orosz F, Perczel A, et al. Disordered TPPP/p25 binds GTP and displays Mg2+–dependent GTPase activity. FEBS letters. 2011;585(5):803-808.

[66] Vincze O, Tokesi N, Olah J, Hlavanda E, Zotter A, Horvath I, et al. Tubulin polymerization promoting proteins (TPPPs): members of a new family with distinct structures and functions. Biochemistry. 2006;45(46):13818-13826.

[67] Aramini JM, Rossi P, Shastry R, Nwosu C, Cunningham K, Xiao R, et al. Solution NMR structure of Tubulin polymerization-promoting protein family member 3 from *Homo sapiens*. http://wwwpdborg/pdb/explore/exploredo?structureId=2JRF. 2007.

[68] Staverosky JA, Pryce BA, Watson SS, Schweitzer R. Tubulin polymerization-promoting protein family member 3, Tppp3, is a specific marker of the differentiating tendon sheath and synovial joints. Developmental dynamics : an official publication of the American Association of Anatomists. 2009;238(3):685-692.

[69] Olah J, Zotter A, Hlavanda E, Szunyogh S, Orosz F, Szigeti K, et al. Microtubule assembly-derived by dimerization of TPPP/p25. Evaluation of thermodynamic parameters for multiple equilibrium system from ITC data. Biochimica et biophysica acta. 2012;1820(7):785-794.

[70] Lehotzky A, Tirián L, Tőkési N, Lénárt P, Szabó B, Kovács J, et al. Dynamic targeting of microtubules by TPPP/p25 affects cell survival. Journal of cell science. 2004;117:6249-6259.

[71] Lehotzky A, Olah J, Szunyogh S, Szabo A, Berki T, Ovadi J. Zinc-induced structural changes of the disordered tppp/p25 inhibits its degradation by the proteasome. Biochimica et biophysica acta. 2015;1852(1):83-91.

[72] Xin W, Chan JR. Myelin plasticity: sculpting circuits in learning and memory. Nature reviews Neuroscience. 2020;21(12):682-694.

[73] Fu MM, McAlear TS, Nguyen H, Oses-Prieto JA, Valenzuela A, Shi RD, et al. The Golgi Outpost Protein TPPP Nucleates Microtubules and Is Critical for Myelination. Cell. 2019;179(1):132-146 e14.

[74] Nguyen H, Meservey LM, Ishiko-Silveria N, Zhou M, Huang TT, Fu MM. Fear Deficits in Hypomyelinated Tppp Knock-Out Mice. eNeuro. 2020;7(5).

[75] Takahashi M, Tomizawa K, Fujita SC, Sato K, Uchida T, Imahori K. A brain-specific protein p25 is localized and associated with oligodendrocytes, neuropil, and fiber-like structures of the CA hippocampal region in the rat brain. J Neurochem. 1993;60:228-235.

[76] Hoftberger R, Fink S, Aboul-Enein F, Botond G, Olah J, Berki T, et al. Tubulin polymerization promoting protein (TPPP/p25) as a marker for oligodendroglial changes in multiple sclerosis. Glia. 2010;58(15):1847-1857.

[77] Ovadi J. Moonlighting proteins in neurological disorders. IUBMB life. 2011;63(7):453-456.

[78] Lindersson E, Lundvig D, Petersen C, Madsen P, Nyengaard JR, Hojrup P, et al. p25alpha Stimulates alpha-synuclein aggregation and is co-localized with aggregated alpha-synuclein in alpha-synucleinopathies. The Journal of biological chemistry. 2005;280(7):5703-5715.

[79] Tokesi N, Olah J, Hlavanda E, Szunyogh S, Szabo A, Babos F, et al.

Identification of motives mediating alternative functions of the neomorphic moonlighting TPPP/p25. Biochimica et biophysica acta. 2014;1842(4):547-557.

[80] Szunyogh S, Olah J, Szenasi T, Szabo A, Ovadi J. Targeting the interface of the pathological complex of alpha-synuclein and TPPP/p25. Biochimica et biophysica acta. 2015;1852(12):2653-2661.

[81] Szenasi T, Olah J, Szabo A, Szunyogh S, Lang A, Perczel A, et al. Challenging drug target for Parkinson's disease: Pathological complex of the chameleon TPPP/p25 and alpha-synuclein proteins. Biochimica et biophysica acta Molecular basis of disease. 2017;1863(1):310-323.

[82] Maroteaux L, Campanelli JT, Scheller RH. Synuclein: a neuron-specific protein localized to the nucleus and presynaptic nerve terminal. The Journal of neuroscience : the official journal of the Society for Neuroscience. 1988;8(8):2804-2815.

[83] Bates CA, Zheng W. Brain disposition of alpha-Synuclein: roles of brain barrier systems and implications for Parkinson's disease. Fluids Barriers CNS. 2014;11:17.

[84] Kovacs GG, Laszlo L, Kovacs J, Jensen PH, Lindersson E, Botond G, et al. Natively unfolded tubulin polymerization promoting protein TPPP/p25 is a common marker of alpha-synucleinopathies. Neurobiology of disease. 2004;17(2):155-162.

[85] Olah J, Bertrand P, Ovadi J. Role of the microtubule-associated TPPP/p25 in Parkinson's and related diseases and its therapeutic potential. Expert review of proteomics. 2017;14(4):301-309.

[86] Mavroeidi P, Arvanitaki F, Karakitsou AK, Vetsi M, Kloukina I, Zweckstetter M, et al. Endogenous oligodendroglial alpha-synuclein and TPPP/p25alpha orchestrate alpha-synuclein pathology in experimental multiple system atrophy models. Acta neuropathologica. 2019;138(3):415-441.

[87] Hasegawa T, Baba T, Kobayashi M, Konno M, Sugeno N, Kikuchi A, et al. Role of TPPP/p25 on alpha-synuclein-mediated oligodendroglial degeneration and the protective effect of SIRT2 inhibition in a cellular model of multiple system atrophy. Neurochemistry international. 2010;57(8):857-866.

[88] Ota K, Obayashi M, Ozaki K, Ichinose S, Kakita A, Tada M, et al. Relocation of p25alpha/tubulin polymerization promoting protein from the nucleus to the perinuclear cytoplasm in the oligodendroglia of sporadic and COQ2 mutant multiple system atrophy. Acta neuropathologica communications. 2014;2:136.

[89] Song YJ, Lundvig DM, Huang Y, Gai WP, Blumbergs PC, Hojrup P, et al. p25alpha relocalizes in oligodendroglia from myelin to cytoplasmic inclusions in multiple system atrophy. The American journal of pathology. 2007;171(4):1291-1303.

[90] Jellinger KA, Wenning GK. Multiple system atrophy: pathogenic mechanisms and biomarkers. J Neural Transm (Vienna). 2016;123(6):555-572.

[91] Menendez-Gonzalez M, Padilla-Zambrano HS, Tomas-Zapico C, Garcia BF. Clearing Extracellular Alpha-Synuclein from Cerebrospinal Fluid: A New Therapeutic Strategy in Parkinson's Disease. Brain sciences. 2018;8(4).

[92] Valdinocci D, Radford RAW, Goulding M, Hayashi J, Chung RS, Pountney DL. Extracellular Interactions of Alpha-Synuclein in Multiple System Atrophy. International journal of molecular sciences. 2018;19(12).

[93] Marques O, Outeiro TF. Alpha-synuclein: from secretion to dysfunction and death. Cell death & disease. 2012;3:e350.

[94] Andersen AD, Binzer M, Stenager E, Gramsbergen JB. Cerebrospinal fluid biomarkers for Parkinson's disease - a systematic review. Acta neurologica Scandinavica. 2017;135(1):34-56.

[95] Vincze O, Olah J, Zadori D, Klivenyi P, Vecsei L, Ovadi J. A new myelin protein, TPPP/p25, reduced in demyelinated lesions is enriched in cerebrospinal fluid of multiple sclerosis. Biochemical and biophysical research communications. 2011;409(1):137-141.

[96] Danzer KM, Kranich LR, Ruf WP, Cagsal-Getkin O, Winslow AR, Zhu L, et al. Exosomal cell-to-cell transmission of alpha synuclein oligomers. Molecular neurodegeneration. 2012;7:42.

[97] Lee HJ, Suk JE, Bae EJ, Lee JH, Paik SR, Lee SJ. Assembly-dependent endocytosis and clearance of extracellular alpha-synuclein. The international journal of biochemistry & cell biology. 2008;40(9):1835-1849.

[98] Fouka M, Mavroeidi P, Tsaka G, Xilouri M. In Search of Effective Treatments Targeting alpha-Synuclein Toxicity in Synucleinopathies: Pros and Cons. Frontiers in cell and developmental biology. 2020;8:559791.

[99] Devos D, Hirsch E, Wyse R. Seven Solutions for Neuroprotection in Parkinson's Disease. Movement disorders : official journal of the Movement Disorder Society. 2020.

[100] Meszaros L, Hoffmann A, Wihan J, Winkler J. Current Symptomatic and Disease-Modifying Treatments in Multiple System Atrophy. International journal of molecular sciences. 2020;21(8).

[101] Stoker TB, Barker RA. Recent developments in the treatment of Parkinson's Disease. F1000Research. 2020;9.

[102] Zhang CL, Han QW, Chen NH, Yuan YH. Research on developing drugs for Parkinson's disease. Brain research bulletin. 2020.

[103] Fulop L, Mandity IM, Juhasz G, Szegedi V, Hetenyi A, Weber E, et al. A foldamer-dendrimer conjugate neutralizes synaptotoxic beta-amyloid oligomers. PloS one. 2012;7(7):e39485.

[104] Rinaldi S. The Diverse World of Foldamers: Endless Possibilities of Self-Assembly. Molecules. 2020;25(14).

[105] Yang W, Yu S. Synucleinopathies: common features and hippocampal manifestations. Cellular and molecular life sciences: CMLS. 2017;74(8):1485-1501.

[106] Hansen D, Ling H, Lashley T, Holton JL, Warner TT. Review: Clinical, neuropathological and genetic features of Lewy body dementias. Neuropathology and applied neurobiology. 2019;45(7):635-654.

[107] Shahnawaz M, Mukherjee A, Pritzkow S, Mendez N, Rabadia P, Liu X, et al. Discriminating alpha-synuclein strains in Parkinson's disease and multiple system atrophy. Nature. 2020;578(7794):273-277.

[108] Katzeff JS, Phan K, Purushothuman S, Halliday GM, Kim WS. Cross-examining candidate genes implicated in multiple system atrophy. Acta neuropathologica communications. 2019;7(1):117.

[109] Cong S, Xiang C, Wang H, Cong S. Diagnostic utility of fluid biomarkers in multiple system atrophy: a systematic review and meta-analysis. Journal of neurology. 2020.